The Hadassah Jewish Family BOOK OF HEALTH AND WELLNESS

The Hadassah Jewish Family BOOK OF HEALTH AND WELLNESS

Robin E. Berman, M.D.

Arthur Kurzweil

Dale L. Mintz, MPA, CHES

An Arthur Kurzweil Book

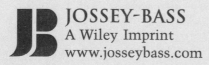

JOSSEY-BASS
A Wiley Imprint
www.josseybass.com

Published by Jossey-Bass
A Wiley Imprint
989 Market Street, San Francisco, CA94103–1741   www.josseybass.com

The contents of this work are intended to further general scientific research, understanding, and discussion only and are not intended and should not be relied upon as recommending or promoting a specific method, diagnosis, or treatment by physicians for any particular patient. The publisher and the author make no representations or warranties with respect to the accuracy or completeness of the contents of this work and specifically disclaim all warranties, including without limitation any implied warranties of fitness for a particular purpose. In view of ongoing research, equipment modifications, changes in governmental regulations, and the constant flow of information relating to the use of medicines, equipment, and devices, the reader is urged to review and evaluate the information provided in the package insert or instructions for each medicine, equipment, or device for, among other things, any changes in the instructions or indication of usage and for added warnings and precautions. Readers should consult with a specialist where appropriate.

The fact that an organization or Web site is referred to in this work as a citation and/or a potential source of further information does not mean that the author or the publisher endorses the information the organization or Web site may provide or recommendations it may make. Further, readers should be aware that Internet Web sites listed in this work may have changed or disappeared between when this work was written and when it is read. No warranty may be created or extended by any promotional statements for this work. Neither the publisher nor the author shall be liable for any damages arising herefrom. Readers should be aware that Internet Web sites offered as citations and/or sources for further information may have changed or disappeared between the time this was written and when it is read.

Jossey-Bass books and products are available through most bookstores. To contact Jossey-Bass directly call our Customer Care Department within the U.S. at 800-956-7739, outside the U.S. at 317-572-3986, or fax 317-572-4002.

Jossey-Bass also publishes its books in a variety of electronic formats. Some content that appears in print may not be available in electronic books.

Library of Congress Cataloging-in-Publication Data
Berman, Robin E., date
    The Hadassah Jewish Family Book of Health and Wellness / Robin E. Berman, Arthur Kurzweil, and Dale L. Mintz. — 1st ed.
        p. cm.
    "An Arthur Kurzweil Book"
    Includes bibliographical references and index.
    ISBN-13: 978-0-7879-8071-9 (alk. paper)
    ISBN-10: 0-7879-8071-4 (alk. paper)
        1. Health—Religious aspects—Judaism. 2. Medicine—Religious aspects—Judaism.
3. Healing—Religious aspects—Judaism. 4. Medical laws and legislation (Jewish law)
5. Medical ethics. 6. Jewish ethics.
    I. Kurzweil, Arthur. II. Mintz, Dale L. III. Title.
    BM538.H43B47 2006
    613.2088'296—dc22   2005028781

Printed in the United States of America
FIRST EDITION
HB Printing   10 9 8 7 6 5 4 3 2 1

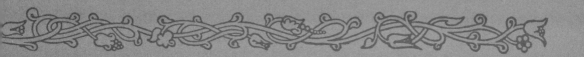

Contents

∽ PART THREE ∽
Nutrition

∽ PART FOUR ∽
Jewish Genetic Diseases

*This book is dedicated to
the extraordinary women who,
every day,
make a positive difference
in people's lives.*

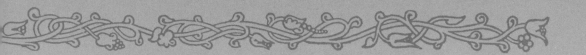

Acknowledgments

While my two coeditors and I are offering our own individual words of acknowledgments here, I want to begin on behalf of all three of us by expressing our thanks to the contributors to this volume. As you look through the list of contributors, you will see individuals from all parts of the Jewish world, as well as clergy and laypeople, professionals and nonprofessionals. Each brings a particular expertise and wisdom, and all come together to promote good health and wellness. Thank you for joining together to make this book.

At Jossey-Bass, many people also came together, as part of its professional staff, to bring out this volume. The publishing of a book requires the skills and talents of many people. In particular, I'd like to thank Joanne Clapp Fullagar, who guided the book through its various stages of production and brought her vast experience and ceaseless dedication, as she always does, to this project.

Seth Schwartz, on the editorial staff of Jossey-Bass, once again went beyond the call of duty for the sake of this book. I have seen Seth and his passion for books enhance every book project in which we have been involved. Thank you for your warmth and professionalism.

Catherine Craddock's skills and experience were of significant help at one stage of this book in particular.

Alan Rinzler, executive editor at Jossey-Bass, brought the germ of the idea of this book ("germ" might not be the right metaphor for a book on health and wellness) to me and joined me in developing it every step of the way. Alan, your creativity, your gifts as an editor, and your heartfelt love of Jewish heritage and tradition are what made this book happen. Thank you for your friendship and for so many other things—including the inspiration to search for two partners who could join forces to make this book an important one.

Those two partners, my coeditors, Dale Mintz and Robin Berman, brought vital nourishment to this ambitious project.

Thank you, Robin, for your medical experience, expertise, and enlightened perspectives. Thank you for your wisdom and unique spirit. Your friendship means so much to me. Your achievements move me deeply. Until history ends and beyond, may our souls continue to mingle.

Thank you, Dale. As National Director of Hadassah's Department of Women's Health and Advocacy, you brought not only your own professionalism, knowledge, and commitment but also the light that shines from Hadassah, the Women's Zionist Organization of America, and its sterling reputation in so many areas and especially in regard to health care.

My daughter, Malya Kurzweil, helped me, as always, whenever I needed her assistance. I am one of many who especially know her for her breadth of knowledge, her quick mind, her sense of humor, and her impressive record of achievements. Thanks, Malya. And thank you to my other children, Miriam and Moshe. Miriam, our conversations about this book will remain in my memory. I'm sure they helped me. I see that with each passing day we come to each other with more things to discuss and explore. How lucky I am. And Moshe, while you did not have any direct impact on this book, I have no doubt that our philosophical and spiritual discussions, our shared observations about life, and our ongoing chess tournament keep me at my best.

Special thanks go to my parents, Saul and Evelyn Kurzweil. Our daily conversations and discussions keep me on my toes and continue the way you have always encouraged my curiosity, scholarship, and spiritual life.

My sincere gratitude and love go to Dr. Helen Hecht. You are a remarkable human being, an extraordinary physician, and a treasured friend. And may our memory of Dr. Harold Wise always be for a blessing.

It is important for the reader to know that without the editorial skills and talents of Rebecca Allen, this book would never have happened. It would not be accurate to say that Rebecca assists me with some of my editorial work, because in addition to her assistance, Rebecca teaches me, offers wonderful suggestions and new approaches and ideas, and is ultimately exactly what a busy writer and editor wants in a colleague. She is quick, creative, dedicated, enthusiastic, and professional. Her devotion to Jewish tradition and to the Jewish people is constant and is an inspiration. Thank you, Rebecca, for your many contributions to this book and for your words of Torah.

Heal us, *Hashem*, then we will be healed; save us, then we will be saved, for you are our praise. Bring complete recovery for all our ailments; for you are God, king, the faithful and compassionate healer. Blessed are you, *Hashem*, who heals the sick of his people Israel.

Arthur Kurzweil

My thanks go first and foremost to my parents, Nathaniel and Sylvia Ely, both of blessed memory, who nurtured and sustained me in every possible way, my mother in particular, who encouraged me to think in a creative independent manner.

I thank all of my teachers, too numerous to mention, who were there as mentors and guides in my never-ending quest of alternative approaches to healing.

Thanks to Arthur Kurzweil, my colleague on this project, who has always expressed respect in our friendship.

The authors of the various essays that appear in this publication should be acknowledged for their attention and care to the issues that are addressed. Final thanks to everyone at Hadassah who took part in the completion of the project.

Robin E. Berman

There are many people to thank who were instrumental in the development and production of this book: Hadassah's president, June Walker, and the Executive Committee for their commitment to educating our membership and Marlene Post for her foresight in making women's health a priority during her presidency.

To the Hadassah volunteers, past and present, who have given their time, expertise, and passion: Patricia Levinson, Janice Greenwald, Estie Lipsit, Miki Schulman, Karen Venezky, Sue Mizrahi, Doris Greenberg, Nancy Shuman, Laura Schiff, Lynn Klein, and Ruth Zimbler, for their unending belief that Hadassah's commitment to educating members about their health was and will continue to be their priority.

My gratitude also goes to Hadassah's Legal and Creative Services departments, for their support, commitment, and hard work associated with a project of this magnitude. For the support from Bonnie Dimun and Deborah Nagler my special thanks.

My family, Steve, Eric, Jaclyn, Paige, Adam, and Jordan, who remind me always of the importance of love and caring.

And finally, I've saved the best for last, to Ellen Marks and Diana Crown, my right and left hands, I am more than grateful.

Dale L. Mintz

Introduction

∽ Why a Hadassah Jewish Family Health Book?

Some teachers teach that human beings are merely physical bodies. We are born. We live. We die.

Biology textbooks sometimes break the average body down into its chemical makeup and tell us how much a body is worth. For example, decades ago, the U.S. Bureau of Chemistry (now called the Food and Drug Administration) reportedly calculated that the chemical and mineral composition of the human body breaks down as follows:

- 65 percent oxygen
- 18 percent carbon
- 10 percent hydrogen
- 3 percent nitrogen
- 1.5 percent calcium
- 1 percent phosphorous
- 0.35 percent potassium
- 0.25 percent sulfur
- 0.15 percent sodium
- 0.15 percent chlorine
- 0.05 percent magnesium
- 0.0004 percent iron
- 0.00004 percent iodine

In addition, it was discovered that our bodies contain trace quantities of fluorine, silicon, manganese, zinc, copper, aluminum, and arsenic. The value was about a dollar.

However, the Web site of the Indiana University School of Medicine reports a study indicating that, when broken down into "fluids, tissues and germ fighting," our bodies are worth more than $45 million. The figure was based on a survey published in *Wired* magazine, which said:

> Vital organs are no longer the most valuable body parts. Rather, bone marrow heads the list . . . priced at $23 million, based on 1,000 grams at $23,000 per gram. DNA can fetch $9.7 million, while extracting antibodies can bring $7.3 million. A lung is worth $116,400, a kidney $91,400 and a heart $57,000. Women's eggs are costlier than men's sperm. The survey found that a fertile woman could sell 32 egg cells over eight years for $224,000; however, for a man to earn the same amount, he would have to make 12 sperm donations a month for 20 years.

The Web site adds: "Although this break down is illegal, unethical and also impossible, you should not feel like a million dollars anymore. You can feel like $45 million, instead!"

Some teachers do not teach us that we are just bodies. They teach that we are bodies with souls.

But the great Jewish sages throughout the centuries teach neither of these perspectives. They do not teach us that we are just *bodies.* They do not teach us that we are bodies with *souls.* Rather, Jewish tradition teaches that each of one of us is a *soul—that has a body.*

Given the assumption that we are all souls who have been offered a body to use for a certain, very limited, time period, one can begin to understand the reason for a Jewish book on health. For good health is not just a desirable condition; it is a profound responsibility. *Our bodies are on loan to us, and we have an obligation to take care of them.*

ABOUT THIS BOOK

A quick glance at the table of contents of this book reflects well the reason for a book on health for Jewish families. In Jewish life, we are asked to find the right path for living, and we call the ways of that path the *mitzvot* (plural). The Jewish people, led by our great teachers, continue to look carefully at life and to work out the correct paths for ourselves.

To offer just one modern example, it is clear from all the traditional sources in Jewish history—from the Bible to the Talmud to the codes of Jewish law and beyond—that we must not knowingly do damage to our bodies. When we put that principle—that negative *mitzvah*—together with the fact that we now know the dangers of cigarette smoking, suddenly the question of whether to smoke becomes not only a health concern but a spiritual question and a question of Jewish law.

This book, then, is a book about the *mitzvah* of taking care of the body that is on loan to each of us.

Some of the many topics explored in this book are as follows:

* Judaism on healing
* *Brit milah* (ritual circumcision)
* Infertility issues from a Jewish perspective
* Caring for the elderly
* Is smoking kosher?
* Jewish medical ethics
* Jewish meditation
* Abortion in Jewish law
* Stem cell research and Jewish law
* Jewish genetic diseases
* Jewish approaches to AIDS

Jews, of course, do not have bodies that function any differently from those of others in the human family. However, we urge you to examine the chapters in Part Four, especially those in the "Special Focus: Specific Genetic Conditions." These chapters focus on Jewish genetic diseases, that is, diseases of genetic origins that tend, statistically, to appear more frequently within Jewish families. Many of us who attended colleges and universities in the late 1960s and 1970s can recall the concerted effort to encourage Jewish students to get tested to see if they were carriers of the gene that can result in Tay-Sachs disease. Today, just a few decades later and as a result of that testing and heightened awareness, Tay-Sachs has essentially been eradicated from the Jewish community. Great progress has been made regarding the battles against Jewish genetic diseases.

There are other compelling reasons for a book on health for Jews and Jewish families. For example, although Jews surely do not have a monopoly on attentive child care, there is little question but that Jewish families have always treated its children with the utmost care and attention, to the point of ancient Jewish sources describing all Jewish children as little messiahs. Sections in this book on child care in general, as well as specific issues like circumcision and breast-feeding, are sure to inform and inspire readers.

Many medical issues that are in the headlines today are also clearly Jewish issues. For example, the ethical and moral questions surrounding the issue of stem cell research is one that many Jewish ethicists have examined in detail. The same is true for the subject of abortion, as well as various aspects of infertility.

JEWS AND HEALING

It has often been noted that Jewish tradition has always been greatly concerned for all the details of life and its many issues. To offer one example, Jewish tradition is not satisfied with a big, bold statement like "love thy neighbor as thyself," as found in the book of Leviticus of the Torah. Our sages have asked: What is love? What is a "neighbor"? What does it mean to love oneself? These questions prompt more questions. And those lead to still more.

In the same way, Jewish tradition is not satisfied, for example, with a simple recommendation that we visit people who are sick. Rather, visiting the sick is a special category of *mitzvah* and even has a special Hebrew name (*bikkur cholim*), as well as a vast literature, developed throughout the centuries, with the fine details of the art and imperative of visiting someone who is ill. In addition, Jewish tradition teaches that visiting the sick is not just a nice thing to do. It has important healing properties in itself. This book explores the many sides of visiting the sick and ways to do it with grace and effectiveness.

Other health issues have also been closely examined, discussed, and developed by the great Jewish sages. For example, the guiding principles recommended and required of caregivers over the ages, including family members, physicians, and other health care professionals, could fill volumes. Caregiving is not just a human activity; it is a spiritual act, an art, and a sacred responsibility. This book explores many aspects of caregiving and visiting the sick, as well as honoring the elderly and other related issues, from a Jewish perspective.

Similarly, although prayer in Jewish life is a daily activity, prayer becomes especially emphasized in Judaism in response to illness and suffering. Across the Jewish spectrum of observance and belief, from the most liberal to the most traditional, all of the various so-called "movements" among American Jewry in recent years have been making special efforts to teach about the relationship between prayer and illness and the importance and necessity of prayer in our lives, especially in response to sickness. We know that the section of this book on prayer will provide wise counsel and guidance for family caregivers and for those who are ill.

An unfortunate modern quip states that most Jewish holidays can be summarized as "They tried to kill us; we survived; let's eat." Although we know that the beautiful range of Jewish holy days on the Jewish calendar hardly reflects this joke, we also know that the two most popular Jewish holidays in American life are Hanukkah and Passover, both of which celebrate victories from oppression and both of which use food as part of the celebration. And Jews understand that eating is an important and emphasized part of every weekly Sabbath, as well as the other major festivals. But as Part Three, "Nutrition," explores, food in Jewish life is not just things like gefilte fish, potato latkes, and hamantashen.

Proper diet and eating habits are surely topics of interest. We would like to note that although we are not advocating that everyone become a vegetarian, we have included a long section on Jewish vegetarianism because it is, for many, a healthy option, and it also holds a special place among many Jews, from the most traditional to the most liberal.

ABOUT THE EDITORS

This book has been compiled and edited by three members of the Jewish community who have much in common and also have their differences. We are a family, as Rabbi Adin Steinsaltz so aptly points out in *We Jews: Who Are We and What Should We Do?* (Jossey-Bass, 2005). We are not a religion, we are not a race, and we are not a nation. We are a family. And as with all families, the Jewish family tree has many branches.

- Robin E. Berman is not only the president and medical director of the National Gaucher Foundation but also a physician with a practice of integrative medicine, which utilizes both conventional and alternative, or nonstandard, approaches to healing. In addition, with her husband and family, she leads a traditional Jewish life.
- Arthur Kurzweil, a writer, editor, publisher, and Jewish educator, has lectured and taught widely in synagogues and to Jewish groups all across the spectrum of Jewish affiliations and denominations.
- Dale L. Mintz, a certified health educator formerly with the American Heart Association and now National Director of Hadassah's Department of Women's Health and Advocacy, finds her religious affiliation in the world of liberal Judaism.

The diversity of the editors of this book, like the diversity within the Jewish world itself, is reflected within these pages. We have looked for excellent teachings about a wide variety of health issues from a similarly wide variety of experts. Just as the Jewish world consists of many viewpoints and approaches, so does this book. We do not claim that the book represents every subject and issue or every point of view, but we are committed to presenting a healthy cross-section of views and concerns from many precincts within the Jewish family.

Hadassah's Commitment to Health Care

In 1912, Henrietta Szold, returning from her first visit to Palestine impelled by the need for access to medicines and health care, founded Hadassah. Her vision initiated the creation of a health care system first in Palestine and subsequently in the state of Israel. Over the years, Hadassah has built and continues to maintain two world-class hospitals in Jerusalem, ninety clinics, and the state-of-the-art Center for Emergency Medicine, along with a college, a career counseling center, and youth rescue schools and centers. As a result of Szold's foresight, there is Hadassah, the Women's Zionist Organization of America, Inc., whose volunteers and professionals have worked with passion and devotion for nearly a century to improve health care for all of Israel's citizens. In addition, its mission now includes American educational programs on health, advocacy, Jewish education, and public policy.

In 1995, the Department of Women's Health and Advocacy (WHA) was established. It is dedicated to educating women about healthy life choices and promoting wellness and disease prevention for a more informed Jewish woman. WHA programs encourage screenings and self-examinations to foster awareness of the changes in our bodies and to enable us to communicate better with our health care providers.

It is no accident that this book contains Jewish text and materials along with articles on health and wellness that expand the knowledge of the reader. It is dedicated to a purposeful expression of Hadassah's commitment to the traditions of Judaism and maintaining good health.

And we want to make clear to the reader what this book is and what it is not:

• If you are ill or feel that you need medical attention, seek the help of a professional health care provider in whom you have confidence. This book can be supportive, inspiring, and informative as a supplement to sound medical care.

• Many questions generated by health care issues have important ramifications in Jewish law. Because, as a matter of principle, every case is different and unique according to Jewish law, this book does not provide *any* halakhic (Jewish legal) opinions that you can necessarily apply to a particular situation. Our best advice is that for Jewish legal opinions, you must consult a qualified rabbi with an understanding heart.

• All the authors represented in this volume speak for themselves and do not necessarily reflect the personal views of the editors, the publisher, or Hadassah. The editors have included pieces that they feel can be informative, stimulating, provocative, and nourishing to readers. The editors are well aware that, like themselves, the Jewish community is diverse and that members of the community often hold diverse views on important matters. This is not only true between "movements" (for example, where a Reform rabbi might disagree with an Orthodox rabbi) but also within the same movement (for example, when two Orthodox rabbis disagree with each other). The important thing is that we increase our concern for healthy living, learn how best to take care of ourselves and our loved ones, and encourage research and education to advance the cause of good health for all.

The good news is that there are so many places to go to find important information on every topic related to health. Most of us, for example, have already discovered firsthand how effective the Internet can be for research. The bad news, however, is that there is so much information, some of it with conflicting facts and advice, that it is difficult for a layperson to evaluate it. Our advice is to read this book and gain a better understanding of the ways in which creative and informed Jews—in many cases the leading visionaries of their generation—have looked at and are still looking at the many issues related to health, the care of the body, medical ethics issues, diseases, issues of health care, and more.

Speak to local Jewish community leaders and your local rabbi for help in finding additional resources in the Jewish world.

- Don't forget your local public library reference librarian as a source for information, answers to questions, and recommendations for further reading. If your local synagogue has a library, its librarian can also be helpful.
- Most important, keep in mind the teaching of the great Jewish teachers of wisdom throughout the centuries: *as the Temple of the Soul, the human body must be honored.*

Robin E. Berman, M.D.
Arthur Kurzweil
Dale L. Mintz, M.P.A., C.H.E.S.
Editors

Health in the Jewish Tradition

Chapter 1

Hadassah's Commitment

✍ *Jewish Perspective on Health*

Why is Hadassah involved with health education? Hadassah's commitment to health care is certainly in keeping with its primary mission, and that alone could justify our involvement. But are the principles of outreach, prevention, early detection, and treatment of disease Jewish issues? Are we, as Jews, to work for these ends? The answer is a resounding *yes!*

Medicine and religion have a unique relationship. Because God is the ultimate source of all healing, the first question, from a religious standpoint, is this: Does human healing interfere with divine providence? Adherents of certain faiths believe that it does. Judaism, however, enjoins us to seek and provide medical assistance.

Leviticus 19:16 states, "Do not stand by the blood of your fellow." Maimonides explains this in *Mishneh Torah, Hilkhot Rotzei'ah:* "Whoever is able to save another, and does not, transgresses the commandment." The Torah, therefore, obligates us to heal the sick as a religious precept included in the category of saving a life.

From the Sources

For each one person who dies a natural death, there are ninety-nine others who die through their own negligence.

Yurushalmi, Shabbat 14:14.

From the Sources

The *Jewish Encyclopedia* says:

- The Rabbis regarded the laws of health as of greater importance than those of a mere ritualistic character. "You have to be more careful in cases where danger is involved than in those which involve a mere matter of ritual" (*Chulin* 10a).
- In time of plague the Rabbis recommended staying at home and avoiding the society of men.
- Perspiration was considered especially dangerous, and it was therefore forbidden to touch, during meals, any part of the body that is usually covered or to hold bread under the arm, where the perspiration is usually profuse.
- Coins should not be placed in the mouth, as there is the apprehension that they have been touched by persons suffering from contagious diseases.
- Articles of food should not be placed under a bed, because something impure might fall on them.
- It was also forbidden to eat from unclean vessels or from vessels that had been used for unseemly purposes, or to eat with dirty hands. These and many other laws are derived by the Rabbis from the expression, "And ye shall not make your souls abominable."

Hadassah's involvement in health education also fulfills a Jewish moral imperative. Deuteronomy 4:9 says, "Take utmost care and watch yourselves scrupulously." Expanding on this, numerous passages of Talmud require an individual to obtain medical attention when sick. *Baba Kama* 46b states, "The person who is in pain visits a healer." Jewish medical ethics, though, goes beyond caring for ourselves when sick. We are required to take preventive action. Rabbi Joseph Caro, in the *Shulchan Aruch, Orah Hayyim*, obligates us to take all possible measures to ensure health. Maimonides requires us, in *Mishneh Torah, Hilkhot Dei'ot*, to "set your heart that your body should be healthy and strong in order that your soul be upright to know the Lord." Furthermore, Maimonides asserts that each individual is obligated "to avoid whatever is injurious to the body, and to cultivate habits conducive to health and vigor." Hadassah champions all of these Jewish precepts in order to educate its members to be healthy in body, mind, and spirit.

℘ *Edith Diament Gurewitsch, M.D.*

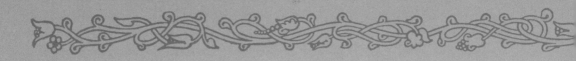

Chapter 2

The Jewish Way of Healing

In times of sickness, many Jews seek spiritual comfort and healing through non-Jewish means. For some people, however, there comes a point when they turn back to the Jewish tradition and community to see what it has to offer. Such seekers can find abundant resources in Judaism, which has addressed questions of health and recovery for millennia. Here's a personal story:

> Shoshanna had never been religious or affiliated with any synagogue. But when she was diagnosed with metastatic breast cancer, she called the Jewish Healing Center. "I rebelled against Judaism all my life," she said. "But now I'm sick and I'm not sure how to cope, and I wonder what I've been rejecting all these years. Maybe Judaism has something to offer me."

To cure the body means to wipe out the tumor, clear up the infection, or regain mobility. To heal the spirit involves creating a pathway to sensing wholeness, depth, mystery, purpose, and peace. Cure of the body may occur without healing of the spirit, and healing without cure. Pastoral caregivers and family members of seriously ill people know that sometimes lives and relationships are healed, even when there is no possibility of physical cure; in fact, serious illness often motivates people to seek healing of the spirit.

Recent research in the mind-body field suggests that the disease process itself may be affected by psychosocial healing; mind and spirit may not be as separate from the biochemistry of physical illness as we once thought. For instance, in *Healing and the Mind*, David Spiegel, M.D., of Stanford University, reports that women

DID YOU KNOW?

Jewish tradition has long recognized that, at times of illness, the body and spirit together need healing. The *Mi Sheberach* prayer, traditionally recited for someone who is ill, asks God for *refuah sh'leima* (a complete healing), and then specifies two aspects: *refuat haguf* (cure of the body) and *refuat hanefesh* (healing of the soul or spirit or whole person).

with metastatic breast cancer who participated in a one-year support group lived significantly longer than women who received similar medical treatment without a support group. Being part of a meaningful community that encourages self-expression can affect the course of an illness.

> Faced with terminal illness, Shoshanna turned toward the Jewish community. Though she was not expecting to find a physical cure, she desperately hoped for healing of the spirit. At fifty years of age, she began her own journey of Jewish learning and spiritual development.

SPIRITUAL HEALING: *BIKKUR CHOLIM*

A fundamental feature of Jewish spiritual healing is *bikkur cholim* (visiting the sick)—a practice that is particularly important in contemporary life, when isolation and lack of community are two of the

From the Sources

Rabbi Abba, son of Rabbi Hanina, said, "One who visits the sick takes away one sixtieth of his pain."

Talmud, *Nedarim* 39b.

greatest burdens people face. At a time of illness, *bikkur cholim* offers the comfort of human connection and interdependence—a sense of desperately needed community.

The *mitzvah*, or obligation, of *bikkur cholim* helps fulfill the obligation to love our neighbors as ourselves and is required of every Jew. Like comforting mourners and performing other acts of kindness, *bikkur cholim* brings goodness to the world.

> In response to his AIDS diagnosis, David tried to meet his emotional needs by working with a therapist and staying in contact with close friends. Then one day he saw an advertisement for a "Spiritual Support Group for HIV-Positive Jews."
>
> Through the group, David had his first positive adult experience of Jewish community. When the group came to a close, David and two other participants joined a local Reform synagogue. His fellow synagogue members provided *bikkur cholim* visits, bolstering David tremendously during his difficult days of illness.

SPIRITUAL HEALING: PRAYER

In addition to *bikkur cholim*, Jewish tradition teaches that we should pray for ourselves and for others during a time of illness. Many modern Jews are resistant to praying in general and especially skeptical about praying for something specific, such as good health.

Yet prayer offers a quiet time for reflection, providing release from anxious thoughts that exacerbate both physical and psychic pain. The mental relaxation of prayer can bring comfort when we take the perspective that our lives are ultimately in God's hands. In addition, when we pray in community and use Jewish liturgy, we not only benefit from the company of other Jews, but we find comfort in knowing that the words of the Psalms and blessings have been spoken by millions of Jews past and present who, like us, yearn for healing.

Here is Eve's story:

> When Eve was diagnosed with lymphoma, she sought the finest medical treatment available. Deeply committed to her Judaism, Eve was

nonetheless unaware of Jewish practices for strengthening the body and spirit at times of illness.

A spiritual counselor introduced Eve to the *Mi Sheberach* prayer. Before going into surgery, she decided to send copies of that prayer to her doctors, both of whom were Jewish. Immediately following the surgery, Eve's doctors prayed on her behalf, and when her husband described this final ritual of the operating room to Eve after she woke from surgery, she was deeply moved and grateful.

OTHER TOOLS FOR HEALING

The Torah—the first five books of the Hebrew scriptures—can be a source of healing for the spirit and psyche. Some rabbis "prescribe" sacred verses for use in meditation. Rabbi Richard Levy of Los Angeles teaches the wisdom of writing the verse and affixing it where one will see it throughout the day: above the desk, on the telephone keypad, on the dashboard.

Some Jews have used the *niggun* (the wordless tune), which has become part of many Jewish worship services. By repeating a wordless tune over and over again, or one with nonsense syllables, one can begin to still the mind and open the heart.

Jewish tradition also offers active modes of spiritual healing. When the experience of illness compromises our sense of power, we need to feel that we are contributing to the good of the world because, for Jews, *tikkun olam* (repair of the world) and *tikkun hanefesh* (repair of the soul) are inseparable.

 DID YOU KNOW?

The Psalms have been Jews' primary devotional literature of healing. These sacred verses invite the person reading them to identify with the psalmist in his pain and longing. Psalms of healing take the reader through a cycle of bewilderment, anguish, complaint, and renewed hope and faith.

> ### *From the Sources*
>
> O Lord my God, I cried out to You, and You did heal me.
>
> Psalms 30:2.

Finally, any amount of personal observance that contributes to feeling that one lives in a meaningful universe is beneficial. Immersion in Jewish ritual can help heal the spirit, highlighting community, connection, meaning, and God.

     Rabbi Nancy Flam

Chapter 3

Ten Jewish Psychological Insights

1. *It is not easy to notice the miracle contained in just being alive. Still, most of us would feel better if we could keep this in mind.*

Being alive and aware are, of course, all we have ever known. Appreciating life is kind of like noticing the vivid light and the white screen that make a movie appear before us. Naturally, if the film starts to sputter and flicker, we notice immediately.

We can all use help with this. Sothe Talmud (*Menachot* 42b) designs a solution, with our saying about one hundred specific blessings a day in thanks for events in our experience, including some for just being awake and aware.

2. *The very first act to perform each morning is also the most important step you will take each day: you bless your life and trust that nothing will be thrown at you that is beyond your reach.*

We sit up in bed, bleary-eyed and dazed, waiting to get our bearings. Before our thoughts fall into order, we already hear the first words in our minds—the *Modeh Ani* prayer. We have programmed these words to appear, welcoming us to the day. They are our reward for past mornings of such repetition.

Accordingly, these are also the first words in the prayer book; they are the very first words we are urged to say at the moment of awakening. It makes gratitude the first feeling of the day, and it places us on the ready: we are about to have the day's series of events placed in our paths. Some will feel pleasant and some otherwise. Several will come to teach us, others to test our learning; all will present us with the chance to find the sparks of truth and love hiding in each moment.

3. *Every life has a unique purpose, and looking for it is part of the mission.*

I am just a tiny, single person, with a life that speeds by. My entire people make up only a small fragment of the world, and my whole world itself quickly disappears in the expanse of space. Yet the Talmud asks me to consider that "for my sake was the world created" (*Sanhedrin* 37a)! Lest I take this as a suggestion of arrogance (rather than an urging to find my mission), the Talmud (*Niddah* 30b) balances out the first statement with a second teaching to consider ourselves potentially wicked at each moment.

As the mystical manual, the *Tanya*, explains this, we carry a continual urge to selfishness (the *yetzer harah*) that skips back and forth on our paths and through our thoughts, looking to fool us and to derail our life's charge into emptiness. Our task becomes that of using the wisdom gained by study and practice, in order to keep this internal adversary at bay. Then we search for the groove in which the music of our lives will be played.

The aim of each life is that of finding the hints that will reveal each of our particular quests. The general prompts come from Jewish tradition. Our own specific clues show themselves in the strange turns of fortune, even in the troubles that tend to trip us, and especially in the set of talents provided each of us.

4. *You already are who you want to be. We each come equipped with the innate talents we seek.*

This does not mean that you have done all that you want to do. Since you are alive, you have yet to discover and fulfill a role. Still, you are already the person that you need to be in order to achieve this. The essence of each person is a pure and indestructible power (*Berachot* 10a) that is forever whispering wise and loving instructions, whenever we want to listen.

This guiding voice is original equipment, and so are the personal talents we will need. Tradition teaches (*Avos* 4:2) that our own efforts are echoed in the innate capacity to fulfill our higher aims. It is as if the path to which we are committed is also cleared before us. This makes sense. People seldom have an intrinsic desire to develop an ability they do not possess. (This does not apply to extrinsic motivation, such as the wish for applause.) There is even a healthy form of guilt that we feel, totally unrelated to social shame, when we do not express our potential. People who cannot draw a picture do not lose sleep over their inability, but those who can create such beauty will feel an itch to do so. Talents unexpressed are usefully burdensome. They push us to polish them into a form that we can then contribute to others.

5. *Feeling more than one way (ambivalence) is a good sign. It means that our loving side and our selfish side are having the right argument.*

If you read the beginning of the Torah, you can notice that nothing but "people" is described as having an allegorical recipe in the Essential Plan of Everything. All the other entities, no matter how tiny or how huge, even the infinite heavens, are called forth without effort and without any constituents whatsoever. Divine "speech" intends it, and it instantly is. The wording is mild and effortless, translated as "let there be . . ." The philosophers call this kind of creation *ex nihilo,* or "out of nothing."

People, on the other hand, are made up of raw materials, and an astonishing combination it is. We are made, first, out of earth—in other words, dirt. Our first ingredient is from the lowest possible level of all. This is how Adam, after he names all the other creatures, names himself. Call me "Adam," he says, "from *adamah,*" which means the ground at one's feet.

Great! So the other creatures get to be an expression of divine speech, and we get to be made of clay! This is an inauspicious start. Of course, you have never seen a piece of clay walk around, so there needs to be a second constituent. Now it gets much better.

The other ingredient is none other than "the breath of God." Not just speech, but breath—this rich symbol of an intimate projection from the cosmic core expresses our second ingredient. In this way, humans comprise the most extraordinary contradiction imaginable: the highest and lowest elements, totally both spiritual and physical, combined fully in every person's nature.

If we are supposed to combine the darkest physicality with the loftiest spiritual light, then what does it mean to be human? It means that, by composition, we stand exactly between heaven and earth, having each as a part of us. In the same way, it also means being unlike either an angel or an animal. It is also the only way our inconsistencies and contradictions really make any sense.

Animals are completely physical in the Jewish view. They can develop, according to their design, and they can vary within the range of that design. Yet they cannot change into anything much different from what they are, nor can they even have the concept of doing so. Their natures are too uniform for transformation, so their acts are all perfect in reflecting their destiny to be whatever they were born to be. Similarly, the higher incorporeal energies that we call angels cannot change any more than animals can change. They are also, according to their designs, performing their function with similar perfection.

As a result, we can become lower than the animals; they have an excuse for brutality, as it is their nature. We have no such excuse, as the breath of God whispers continually (see item 4), making certain that we know better, even when we do worse. Yet we can also be higher than the angels, as they cannot but obey. (We will revisit this in item 10.) When we sanctify our lives and, with that, our world, we are choosing to do so.

The ethical mandate to make such choices leads to our internal argument, which is a good sign. The complacent opposite is not such a good sign. It usually means that our selfish side is pretending to be our conscience but is really offering rationalizations instead. So the rabbinic sages urge us to watch out for any voice inside that seeks to relieve us of obligations. This warning begins in the Torah with the humanoid-snake in the Garden, who convinces Eve to follow her inner sense and ignore the brief life-instructions she has been given. For more on this, refer to Rabbi David Fohrman at http://www.jewishexplorations.com.) It is no coincidence that there is a voice inside us continually suggesting that we have done enough, that we know better than anyone before us, and that we are doing very nicely and can stop growing.

Instead, if you are wrestling, you are on-task. That is where the name Israel (*yisro'el*) comes from. Jacob receives this new name because he wrestles and will not let go without a blessing.

6. *At each difficult moment, the cruelest possible statement to make to someone else is the kindest possible statement you can make to yourself: "Good will also come from this."*

The Hebrew for this statement is *gam zu letovah*, which is literally "also this is for the best" (*Taanit* 20b). Many people see this as a result of two spiritual truths: first, there are no coincidences; second, the Intelligence behind the universe is benevolent. This is consistent in Jewish teaching, without exception. Others believe that there are *only* coincidences and that the belief in providence is wishful thinking. These two positions are obviously opposites. Not so obviously, their difference is oddly irrelevant. Psychologically, certain truths are so powerful that they might as well be true, because implementing them is nothing short of transforming to one's destiny.

In other words, when one insists (like Jacob) on extracting the blessing from every adversity, by the time one is done with fortune it looks just like destiny. So whether we arrive at this strategy psychologically or theologically, it becomes a sail that can harness any wind and propel us forward. As such a gift, it is a kind statement indeed to make to oneself: "Good will also come from this."

As a result, we can say it to ourselves frequently, and it will both guide and comfort us. In contrast, it is one of the worst possible things we can say to other people when they are suffering. In that case, we would, in effect, be blocking the face of their pain, so that we do not have to see it. Anything that makes the anguish of others more opaque to us only magnifies that anguish. So we learn that Abraham, despite his reverence, pushed back at God, point by point, in his efforts to save the people of Sodom. Yet when it came to himself, when he heard that he must destroy his son by his own hand—his only son, whom he loved—he said not a word and rose early to rush ahead. We are not asked to *be* Abraham but to learn this contrast from him.

7. *Mourning has to happen, is not supposed to be a solitary activity, and gradually softens, step by step.*

I remember, as a child, watching a police drama on television and being perplexed after the officers knocked on the door of a new widow, only to have her answer the door herself and, all alone, to answer their questions. I began to wonder if Jews might have perfected the psychological management of bereavement. We have certainly had a lot of opportunities to practice.

The first essential fact of Jewish mourning is that one cannot avoid it. Grief means that one has sustained an unthinkable loss. Immediately, we are supported into the space of seeing what we cannot yet think about. All distraction ends, even the performance of Jewish rituals (*mitvot*). We watch the beloved body and have it watched without interruption, until we place it into the ground, and we protect it under the cover of the earth from which we come, filling the emptiness in that ground ourselves. Then we sit in our home, removing even the distracting concern over the appearance of our faces, unseen behind the cloth-covered mirrors. We sit in our discomfort, not on chairs, helpless like a child who does not even gather his own food. Others serve us, since they are there. We do not mourn alone.

Instead, we seek to reverse the cause of our collective problems; we unify in the love that Israel always has the potential to achieve. Our opinions and judgments disappear. There is only this time for pain in whatever form it takes. We accept the pain of those who weep openly and of those who sink into grief as if a temporary grave. Our first comfort is always from each other. It is the same plan, whether during our collective mourning as a people (*Tisha B'av*) or during personal mourning: joining together, taking care of each other, and all for a prescribed period only.

Throughout the next year, we move through each stage of the path of healing, guided every step by those who have taught others, until they themselves became mourned in this same way.

8. *Slaves of all types work every day. Freedom means having one day a week for peace, reflection, and gratitude.*

After listening to a taped presentation by Jewish educator Dennis Prager, I checked out something that I hope you will also now notice. The blessing that introduces the Sabbath on Friday nights does not itself talk about the seventh-day account. It is customary to read that biblical paragraph first, but this does not form the toast over wine that brings the Sabbath to the family table. What does this long blessing talk about? It talks about being taken and freed from bondage in Egypt.

A slave never gets a day off, which is also to say that anyone who does not get a day off may be enslaved. What can enslave those who live in political freedom? It is not that hard to tell: it is probably whatever they are serving for all seven days each week.

In contrast, the Torah demands, to the point of putting this in the Ten Commandments, that we are not slaves, and we do get a day off. In fact, this is an essential element in the Jewish plan for stress management, as the chapter on that subject describes.

9. *Love means saying it when you're sorry.*

Not all readers may be old enough to remember the promotional tagline for the movie *Love Story:* "Love means never having to say you're sorry." The point was actually that one does not need to require an apology from others. Love does indeed mean, however, needing to apologize to others.

The Jewish official forgiveness day is Yom Kippur, the day of suspending the argument between the two aspects of our natures (see item 5). On this day, an impossible psychological metamorphosis occurs. We get a fresh start with a new record, our failings all erased. We are deep-cleansed, our souls polished bright and new, in pristine readiness to begin again. Yet there is a big exception to all this—one single area where none of this avails us. Our hurts toward others must be wiped clean by virtue of our own efforts.

The process for this is explicit in the Talmud (for example, *Yoma* 87a). I approach the person I have injured or offended and apologize, asking for forgiveness. I offer any appropriate amends, such as making the apology in front of others who may have either witnessed or heard of the original insult. If the other person does not accept my apology, I still owe it. So I return and make the same offer and the same request. I do so a third time, as needed. After that, the apology is complete and so am I, even if the other person is not.

10. *Nothing can destroy your worth. Anyone can turn around, and changing direction has ever more meaning the further you had strayed.*

We have noted (see item 4) that the essential core of each individual is immaculate, adamantine, and holy. This is not just a hidden worth. On the contrary, the Talmud (*Berachot* 10a) teaches that the soul fills the entire body. Further, we have just summarized (item 9) the transformational process of turning our lives around, which occurs most powerfully on Yom Kippur. The word often called "repentance," which is *t'shuvah*, more literally and accurately means "to return." The sages (*Mo'ed Katan* 9b) extend this option, literally, to the worst of us.

What we have not yet noted is the full depth of this transmutation from addictive errors back into resonance with our missions (see item 3). How deep is it? It goes as far as harnessing our errors into virtues (*Yoma* 86b). This would be like a bank saying, "Not only is your loan balance forgiven, but we now owe you the entire amount

Healthy Habits for Mind and Body

- Compose affirmations and create opportunities.
- Positive words and deeds generate positive returns from others.
- When you perceive that there is a problem with someone, speak your mind . . . but just as quickly apologize if you are wrong.
- Give yourself time to meditate each day. Calm your mind and ask for guidance, remaining confident that you will receive answers.
- Engage in long conversations and loving interactions with family and friends, looking for the divine in everything.
- Avoid being influenced by extreme beliefs and values.
- Try to engage in work that you believe in.
- Be patient and understanding with others.
- Be honest with others and especially with yourself.
- Take care of your body by exercising daily, eating a varied diet containing at least five servings of fruits and vegetables, avoiding caffeine, drinking minimal alcohol, and *not smoking.*

Hadassah Health Memo, Spring 2001.

of your debt." If the arithmetic of this is elusive, the psychology of it is sensible and elegant.

Remember, every event is also for good (item 6), even the inevitable trips and falls of life. For instance, social psychology has learned that people who at first dislike each other usually develop stronger bonds than those who liked each other initially. As another example, recovering alcoholics usually make better alcoholism counselors than those who have not struggled with addiction.

There is a resolute psychological power to the process of descending previous to an ascent (see item 5). Jewish mysticism describes the meaning and purpose of the entire physical world in just that way (*derah b'tachtonim*). The prerogative to convert a mistake into a merit motivates change ingeniously. It also brings together the thrust of several of the other Jewish psychological insights described earlier, weaving them into a golden rope that can rescue those most discouraged by the inevitable follies within our lives.

Rick Blum, Ph.D.

Chapter 4

Why Are So Many Hospitals Named After Mount Sinai?

Mount Sinai was the place in the desert where the Jewish people received the Torah. But as we all know, that's not the only Mount Sinai. There is also a Mount Sinai in New York City, and there are Mount Sinais in Los Angeles, Miami, and Toronto—hospitals named, presumably, after the original Mount Sinai.

We understand why a hospital would be named after certain individuals, such as a philanthropist or a famous doctor. But why should Mount Sinai—the site where the Torah was given—be the name of a hospital?

I began asking around, but nobody seemed to know, including friends in the medical profession. So I wrote to the hospitals and received this from the public affairs office of Mount Sinai Hospital of Toronto: as the "site where the Ten Commandments were handed down to Moses, the name 'Mount Sinai' signifies the wellspring of moral law and the source of all compassion."

They weren't giving away too much, but I got the message. Although "Thou shalt heal the sick" is not inscribed in the Ten Commandments (just as "Thou shalt make house calls" was also never written in stone), there was much more to the revelatory goings-on at Sinai than just the Ten Commandments.

It's no mystery why Maimonides has medical centers named after him. Besides being one of the greatest Torah scholars of all time, he was also physician to the royal court of Alexandria in the twelfth century. And after making the long commute home every day by donkey, with hardly a moment to rest, he would receive his fellow Jews at home, providing answers to all their questions—medical, religious, and communal. In his own lifetime, Maimonides was so revered for his wisdom and compassion that the Jews of Yemen included his name in the kaddish prayer.[1]

What about Moses? Although he was not a doctor, he was a compassionate caregiver. The *Midrash* relates that, as a shepherd, Moses once chased after a lost lamb and found the animal bent over and drinking. Realizing that it must have been thirsty and tired, he picked it up and carried it back to the flock. God said that "a person who pities even a helpless beast will surely show compassion for an entire nation." At that moment, Moses merited the prophetic vision of the Burning Bush, in which he was chosen to be the shepherd of his people, to lead the Jews out of Egypt.[2]

Moses is noted for one particularly spectacular foray into practical healing: when poisonous snakes attacked the Jews in the desert, God instructed Moses to fashion a special healing instrument—a pole topped with the form of a copper snake. When the pole was held aloft, those who had been afflicted by a snakebite would gaze on the serpentine image and be cured (Numbers 21:6–10). This was the forerunner of the caduceus—the snake-entwined rod that is today the emblem of the medical profession.

The Talmud (*Rosh Hashana* 29) asks rhetorically: "But is the snake capable of determining life and death?! Rather, when Israel would gaze upward and bind their hearts to their Father in Heaven, they would be healed; and if not, they would perish."

 DID YOU KNOW?

The *Midrash* relates that for those who stood at Sinai, all their afflictions were healed: the crippled could walk, and the blind could see. With the revelation, the world reached a level of moral and spiritual perfection that manifested itself as the disappearance of all physical blemish. The symbiosis of a healthy mind and body is fundamental to Jewish thought.

Fixing their eyes on the snake alone would not yield any cure; nor was it sufficient to just ask God to save them, without the snake-on-a-pole therapy. No, the people had to gaze upon the snake and focus on the fact that only God, who created the snake in the first place, could transform that same venomous creature into a medium of healing.

Remarkably, snakebites today are cured with antivenin manufactured from small quantities of snake venom that stimulate the production of antibodies in the blood. It's the same idea taught by Moses: the source of affliction itself becomes the remedy.

PRAYER AND HEALING TODAY

The connection between prayer and healing is an old one but is being rediscovered in our own time. Various studies have been conducted to determine the efficacy of prayer in healing. Although the scope of the studies has been relatively small (and therefore inconclusive), the results so far indicate that prayer has a decidedly positive effect on recovery rates from serious illnesses.

The topic has been written about in the *New England Journal of Medicine* and other scholarly journals.

Studies at Duke University, Ohio State University, and San Francisco General Hospital have shown a positive correlation between faith and healing. But studies such as these can only measure the effects of prayer; they do not explain how it can help the sick. In Jewish thought, prayer is more than just a matter of asking the Almighty to make the problem go away. The relationship between suffering and illness is bound up with the whole purpose of creation.

One of the secrets contained in the first verse in the Torah is that the word *Bereishis* (in the beginning) may be read as a compound of the words *Bara* (He created) and *shis* (a veil).[3] We are being taught that God created the universe with a veil that manifests itself as the forces of nature that make it difficult for us to perceive his existence. It is our task in life to seek out God in the world—to pull away the veil and glimpse the reality that underlies everything.

The Jewish concept of prayer is that by asking God for our physical needs, we thereby acknowledge that God is the only One who can fulfill them, that he is the source of life, and that anything else, including doctors and medicines, are only intermediaries. This

DID YOU KNOW?

- In a report for CBS News, Dr. Bernadine Healy wrote, "In scores of studies, medical research has shown that people who believe in God or in prayer generally fare better than those who do not."
- A Dartmouth Medical School study found that older people who underwent open-heart surgery and lacked social support from an organized group, or said they received no comfort from religion, were three times more likely to die within six months of their operation than those who said they did get solace from religion.
- Some studies indicate that prayer is effective, even though the patients were not even aware they were being prayed for.
- At St. Luke's Hospital in Kansas City, a yearlong study involving 990 coronary patients showed that after four weeks, the prayed-for patients had suffered about 10 percent fewer complications, ranging from chest pain to cardiac arrest, than patients that were not prayed for.

is the pulling away of the veil of nature for which we were given life in the first place. It is logical, therefore, that God should want to grant us more life with which to draw even closer to him.

But because so much depends on the level of clarity attained, prayer cannot be regarded as a cure-all. As in the biblical account, prayer, which represents our spiritual exertion and expression, needs to be used in conjunction with *hishtadlut*—efforts that we exert in the physical realm. In the matter of healing, this could manifest by tapping into any of hundreds of therapeutic approaches. Unlike some religious groups, Jewish tradition strongly discourages reliance on faith alone to the exclusion of medical treatment.

In our generation, however, the tendency is just the opposite. People often rely on the doctors of Mount Sinai Hospital, to the exclusion of the spiritual teachings of the original Sinai.

We are not the first to fall into this trap; as so often happens, the ancients were there long before us. The copper snake that Moses made was preserved for centuries as a testament to that extraordinary

> ### From the Sources
>
> There are eight things which in large quantities are harmful but in small quantities are beneficial. They are traveling, sexual relations, wealth, work, wine, sleep, hot baths, and blood-letting.
>
> Talmud, *Gittin* 70a.

event. In the passage of time, however, its meaning became distorted, and people began to say that the snake possessed power of its own. When it reached the point of becoming an image of idolatry, the Jewish King Chizkiyahu made the decision to destroy it.

The key in Jewish healing is to find a balance. We need to remind ourselves that God is the source of life and death, of health and illness. We must not make an idolatry of modern medicine, investing powers in the medical establishment far beyond its true capacity. Much as he may hold aloft the dazzling instruments of medical technology, of miracle drugs, laser surgery, and gene therapy, the doctor's power to heal is limited to that which God wills. In other words, Mount Sinai Hospital cannot be detached from Mount Sinai in the desert, where it all started.

ᕍ *Rabbi Yisrael Rutman*

Notes

1. "During your lifetime and during your days and during the lifetime of Rabbi Moshe ben Maimon."
2. Moses could also be tough when necessary. When he saw an Egyptian mercilessly beating a Jewish slave, he rose up and killed the Egyptian. And he stood up to Pharaoh, the leader of the superpower of that time, demanding to "let my people go."
3. Heard from Rabbi Asher Wade.

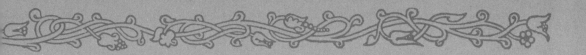

Chapter 5

The Healing Path of Jewish Tradition Is Entering Upon an Awakening

"My son, the doctor!"—a Jewish mother introduces her child with pride. Although we may laugh, this thinking is emblematic of the movement of Jews into the professions in modern times. It also has deep roots in Jewish history. We can trace interest in medicine to King Hezekiah's time (circa 700 B.C.E.), when a "Book of Remedies" was popular, and to the era of the Talmud (200–600 C.E.), when Mar Shmuel, the Talmudic sage, was also a well-known physician. In the Middle Ages, a number of rabbinic scholars were also doctors, the best known being the outstanding legalist and philosopher, Rabbi Moshe ben Maimon (1137–1204 C.E.), who served as the personal physician to the Sultan of Egypt.

Moshe ben Maimon is also known as Maimonides or, in Jewish sources, the Rambam. His magnum opus, *Mishneh Torah*, includes a section (*Hilchot Deot* 3) with useful suggestions for preserving and enhancing health, along with Torah wisdom and legal codes.

The early history of Jewish medical ideas was recorded in a great nineteenth-century German work by Julius Preuss, describing how the ancient sources viewed bodily organs and systems and the use of various types of remedies and healing practices. Yet from the Bible to Maimonides, there does not seem to be any established system of medicine or a distinctively Jewish way of approaching the body.

Given this strong concern for physical health in Judaism, why didn't a specific and distinctively Jewish approach to healing develop?

The reason goes as far back as King Hezekiah, who hid the Book of Remedies because people were depending on the book rather than on God. He believed that spiritual orientation was essential to Jewish healing. Because of this foundational principle, Talmudic attitudes to medical practice were not entirely positive. A Talmudic sage notes, "Even good doctors go to *Gehinnom* (Hell)."

According to this approach, God is the Healer of all flesh, not doctors, yet "permission is given" to physicians and other healers to assist the sick and prescribe remedies. In the view of the sages, a person might accept almost any current, reliable medical practices—for example, the natural herbal remedies that dominated most pre-modern cultures. The implication, though, was that complete healing demanded attention to one's relationship with God.

Now, in the early twenty-first century, emphasis on a spiritual approach to healing has resurfaced among a few Jewish health professionals and in some recent books on Jewish spirituality. Some have broken new ground by introducing the power of meditation in healing; others have developed profoundly effective methods of body awareness. Still others have found that acknowledging a world of spirit beyond death could help many of their patients.

Some of the most exciting work invites us to reexamine Jewish prayer as a resource in health and healing. Traditional Judaism always inserted a prayer for healing in every Torah service, and saying *tehillim* (psalms) in time of sickness has been a custom for many centuries. Now, however, some teachers are suggesting specific practices of prayer, movement, and meditation that can enhance physical vitality and spiritual focus at the same time. Insights from Jewish mysticism and Hasidic teachings are central in these new ideas, but classical sources are also used to demonstrate how the body is intended to be the "temple of the soul" and therefore must come to the forefront of our attention.

From the Sources

A sick person's prayers on his own behalf are more effective than the prayers of anyone else.

Genesis *Rabbah* 53:14.

DID YOU KNOW?

Rabbi Nachman was very interested in healing and, like many of his Hasidic contemporaries in the early nineteenth century, insisted that body and spirit are intimately interrelated.

In particular, the teachings of Rabbi Nachman of Bratslav have come to the fore in recent works.

In his teachings, joy is the foundation of healing, and prayer, song, and dance are part of a total spiritual practice to bring deep and lasting joy into one's life. Rabbi Nachman also focused on the saying of *tehillim* and selected ten psalms to be said for nighttime protection and in times of duress.

The healing path of Jewish tradition is entering upon an awakening. Further research in our rich tradition will undoubtedly uncover more treasures. In the near future, we can look forward to a deeper integration of all these insights about healing the body, mind, and soul.

Tamar Frankiel, Ph.D.

Taking Care of the Body

Chapter 6

Whose Body Is It Anyway?

An old stereotype suggests that we Jewish people are obsessed with our own health. Perhaps you already know the joke I recently heard from Rabbi Samuel Karff—the one about the German, the Frenchman, and the Jew, who were shipwrecked, tossed at sea for three days and nights, with no food and water, before landing on a barren, deserted island. The German said: "I'm hungry; I'm tired; I'm thirsty. I really need a beer." The Frenchman said: "I'm hungry; I'm tired; I'm thirsty. I could really stand a fine bottle of wine." The Jew said: "I'm hungry; I'm tired; I'm thirsty. I must have diabetes."

Yes, it's a stereotype but not an anti-Semitic one, or even quite false. The truth is that seeking appropriate health care is not just a Jewish obsession; it's a *mitzvah*—a religious obligation before God. One verse in Deuteronomy begins, *v'nishmartem m'od l'nafshote-ichem* (carefully guard your lives). The rabbis interpreted those words to mean that we are required to protect our health. When the Talmud declares: "Whoever is in pain should be led to the doctor," the rabbis conclude that Jews are commanded to live in proximity to available medical care.

But what is the basis for a commandment—a *mitzvah*—that we take care of our own health? Doesn't my body belong to me? Our modern society and culture would seem to suggest that I am autonomous and therefore free to behave as I please, as long as I don't hurt anybody else.

I recall a movie from some years ago in which Richard Dreyfuss plays a young man diagnosed with a terminal illness. I haven't seen the film recently, but as I recall, the man is encouraged to pursue significant medical treatment, which he ultimately refuses. The decision

31

From the Sources

You are not in any way allowed to weaken your health or shorten your life. It is only when the body is healthy that it is an efficient instrument for the spirit's activity. . . . Therefore, you should avoid anything which could possibly injure your health. . . . The law asks you to be even more careful when avoiding danger to life and limb than in the avoidance of other transgressions.

Rabbi Samson Raphael Hirsch, *Horeb*, chap. 62, sec. 428.

to eschew treatment may indeed be appropriate in this particular character's case. However, the premise on which he makes this decision is troublesome. The movie's point of view is embedded in the rhetorical question that is the movie's title: "Whose Life Is It Anyway?" The apparent answer to this question, for the film and for our modern world, is that each of our lives is our own.

Judaism would disagree. Our bodies, indeed our very lives, are merely on loan to us from God. When we die, our bodies will return to the earth; our souls will return to God. The ancient rabbis would make an analogy, which I will modernize a bit. Suppose that the president of the United States came to you with a highly fragile, original copy of the Declaration of Independence. Imagine that he asked you to guard it for safekeeping until he could come and retrieve it. Would you not invest a great deal of energy to ensure that the document remained safe, secure, and intact? Of course you would! How much the more so, then, should we guard our bodies—flesh and blood, not mere paper—on loan, not just from the president but from God.

Unfortunately, we Americans are doing a poor job as stewards of our own bodies. Although we spend enormous sums of money on

From the Sources

More people die from overeating than from hunger.

Talmud, *Shabbat* 33a.

> ### *From the Sources*
>
> Pay attention to the advice of the physician while you are still healthy.
>
> *Yurushalmi, Taanit* 3:6.

medical care, studies indicate that we follow doctors' orders 20 to 50 percent of the time, at best. Too many among us use and abuse mind-altering substances, including alcohol, engage in unhealthy sexual activity, drive without wearing seat belts, and smoke cigarettes, to name a few.

Obesity, in particular, has reached epidemic proportions. As we heard, to our shame, San Antonio has again been declared the fattest city in the nation. Now, I am certainly not one to lecture people about proper diet and exercise. Having struggled with my own weight for most of my life, I am well aware that obesity is a complex matter, not easily explained by gluttony and sloth. And yet the disastrous health consequences of being significantly overweight cannot be ignored. Nor may we minimize the negative role played by our cultural and societal attachments to fatty foods, sugar, supersized quantities, and fast-food franchises. We have a problem in the United States, and we have a special challenge in San Antonio, which threatens to be not just the obesity capital of America but also the center of diabetes, heart disease, and a host of other maladies. I am constantly in awe of the people I know who have conquered their long-standing weight problems through hard work, discipline, commitment to exercise, and even surgery. We must follow their brave example; we must do better, as individuals, as a city, and as a nation. Observing the *mitzvah* to care for our bodies is a matter of life and death.

Health care professionals bear a particular responsibility for the *mitzvah* of maintaining good health. The great Rabbi Moses Maimonides was also a leading physician of the Middle Ages. Although there may be no such thing as a medical doctor in the Torah itself, Maimonides interpreted several passages of the Torah as obliging the physician to heal the sick. The medieval Jewish law code, *Shulchan Aruch*, records a requirement that doctors reduce their rates for poor patients.

Physicians today work under terrible strain. Too many managed care companies offer rates that will not cover doctors' overhead costs. Often physicians are not paid promptly, and they must submit the same legitimate claims, over and over again, merely to receive what they are justly due. Adding insult to injury, managed care not infrequently directs doctors to practice medicine in ways they do not believe to be in the best interest of their patients. At the same time, the threat of lawsuits, both meritorious and frivolous, constantly hangs over even the very best practitioners. The high cost of malpractice insurance has left some communities with a dangerous lack of physicians, particularly in the border regions of Texas.

Our physicians must be permitted to continue fulfilling the *mitzvah* to heal. Their issues must be effectively addressed in our legislature and in our courts, without restricting the rights of those who have been injured or bereaved by very real medical error. At the same time, let us be grateful for those doctors who have not become cynical but have maintained their commitment to their patients, treating all with care, insured or not, able to pay or not. Even in difficult times, may our physicians continue to give thanks to God for the healing gifts that God has given them and for their ability to support themselves and their families in the practice of a profession that gives meaning to their lives.

Even patients and physicians, together with health care professionals at all levels, hospitals, and medical schools cannot preserve our nation's health on their own. Indeed, Judaism teaches that health care is the responsibility of our entire society. Maimonides listed medical care first on his list of the ten most important communal services that a city is required to provide to its residents. In ages past, Jewish communities established communal subsidies when doctors were overburdened with caring for patients who were too poor to pay for their services.

My friends, the United States of America is guilty. The State of Texas stands accused. Here, in the greatest nation on earth, with all the wealth our land possesses, more than forty-one million Americans lack any type of health care coverage, and more than eight million of them are children. Our fellow Americans are suffering, and we, as a society, are standing idly by.

In Texas, the situation is particularly dire. The state ranks near the bottom among the fifty, in terms of the amount of money

---

 DID YOU KNOW?

In his great Jewish law code, the *Mishneh Torah*, Maimonides quotes that famous passage from Leviticus: "You shall not stand idly by while your neighbor bleeds." His interpretation is that anyone who is able to save another and does not is guilty of sin.

---

the state allocates to cover the health care needs of the poorest among us. In many cases, Texans are specifically in violation of Maimonides' law, for we have the resources to save lives, but we choose not to use them. Time after time, Texas elects not to participate when the federal government offers to match health care spending, even more than dollar-for-dollar.

A particularly egregious example is something called the Medicaid Waiver for Women's Health Care. Today, a poor woman in Texas is offered basic preventive health care, including cancer screening, family planning, and the like, only if she is pregnant or has a baby less than four months old. What's unbelievable is that the federal government will supply fully 90 percent of the money needed, if Texas will elect to participate in a program for all women. We are able to save poor women in Texas, but some will die because we refuse to offer them the basic health care services they need.

Several years ago, Texas finally signed onto the Children's Health Insurance Program (CHIP)—another example of the federal government providing much of the money. Sadly, state leaders have failed to provide all the funds that are needed to cover the eligible children. Now they propose cutting out many of these poor kids. We will be guilty of sin, standing idly by while babies are denied adequate health care.

The legislature, at last, enacted a law to simplify the process for registering children for Medicaid. Instead of having to fill out the lengthy and complicated forms twice every single year, impoverished Medicaid recipients and their parents would only have to deal with that bureaucracy once a year. Now some state leaders propose saving money by going back to the old, more complicated and cumbersome way. They have cynically devised this plan, knowing that it means that fewer deserving children will receive the coverage they need. If we let them get away with this, we will have blood on our hands.

Each human being is responsible for the care of his or her own body. Preserving our health is service to God, for we are stewards of these bodies that our Creator has lent to us for life. That's not optional. It's a *mitzvah.*

Those God has endowed with the special skill of healing are obligated to care for the health of their fellow human beings, for they are God's agents in bringing divine healing powers to earth. Even when it's hard, it's compulsory. It's a *mitzvah.*

Every citizen of our nation is required to ensure that each and every one of our fellow Americans has access to the medical care that God has permitted to humanity. It's not a luxury. It's a *mitzvah.*

Rabbi Barry H. Block

Chapter 7

Jewish Stress Management

The stress-management experts correctly observe that chronic activation is hard on the body, and this is a matter of consensus. Accordingly, Dean Ornish's heart-repair program (see *Dr. Dean Ornish's Program for Reversing Heart Disease*) combines good meals with good meditating. Our bodies also deeply understand this need for downtime, as shown by everybody's natural heart-protection program. This most important muscle needs periods of profound rest even more than any other muscle. How does it get it? With precision: in between remarkably powerful thrusts projecting life into every cell of the body, the heart rests fully, having an astounding ability to completely relax between every beat.

THE DAVEN RESPONSE

The heart teaches the body what it needs, and the soul shows the way. Two gifts give us the right amount of downtime to avoid burnout. The wisdom of repetitive prayer provides the first of these. Three times a day, tradition provides fixed formulas for *davening*—the Yiddish word, with the Hebrew rendering of the same experience called *tefilah*. The closest translation of both words is "prayer," yet Jewish prayer, like the Torah itself, is intricate in nuance and subtly layered with endless depths of meaning.

Next are three of the dimensions involved when a Jew davens.

1. The most straightforward meaning: it is an opportunity to ask God for help. The formula of the typical sequence is that

individuals first present their credentials as the latest in the chain of merit that begins with the original fathers and mothers (Abraham, Sarah, Isaac, Rebecca, Jacob, Leah, and Rachel), extends through the Torah sages, who compiled the oral explanations, and includes all those who stood up to the ultimate test of early death. The next part in the sequence acknowledges the eternal love between God and Israel. Finally, sandwiched in the middle of the statements of praise and gratitude, people state their needs.

2. Others suggest that asking for help would imply that the Divine Energy would not know what to do without our direction, and that prayer really expresses both gratitude and acknowledgment that there is only one source for all the gifts involved in any life. Three times a day we stop to point out, especially to ourselves, that we know from where the fountain springs.

3. My favorite dimension, courtesy of the mystical brilliance of the Lubavitcher Rebbe, is that davening purifies the vessel of our lives to be a suitable conduit for heaven's blessings. The existence of both the world and the Torah shows that God wishes to bless us (see the chapter "Good Deeds" in *Simple Words* by Adin Steinsaltz). Our davening, as well as the other *mitzvot*, prepares us and the world to receive, with the least distortion, the continual light shining our way.

However you frame it, after practice makes davening familiar, it becomes repetitive, so that no strain is required to move through the formulas. It now qualifies for Herbert Benson's "relaxation response."

Benson's work on stress reduction at his Mind/Body Medical Institute, as published in his famous *Relaxation Response* (HarperCollins, 2000), was expanded in his recent *Timeless Healing*, after he saw that the repetitive prayer achieves profound stress reduction. He suggests various formulas for students of his methods to follow. Jewish prayer, repeated with attention, provides this in addition to its other benefits.

SABBATH WHOLENESS

As welcome as these mini-respites are throughout our day for those who taste them, there is another form of stress-vacation that is powerful enough to defy easy description. It is the Jewish Sabbath. A. J. Heschel, as always, does a splendid job of evoking this aspect of Jewish experience in his book *The Sabbath* (Farrar, Straus & Giroux, 1975). In Hebrew, this weekly transformation is called *Shabbat*. Yet this is one experience that crisp, modern Hebrew just cannot name adequately. Anyone who has drunk deeply of this spring will be tempted to call it by its intimate, Yiddish name, "*Shabbos*," as in "Hold on! Shabbos is coming!"

This is the day of stopping all creation, of making nothing, of resting our bodies as our souls literally double, according to tradition. If one has put the pedal-to-the-metal as the Jewish week urges, the mind and body has to crave cessation, and the Torah puts this right in the Big Ten Rules.

So, what is it like? How can people raised in a culture that sees such a break as imprisonment sense the sweetness that has inspired the saying, "It is not that Israel has kept the Sabbath, as much as the Sabbath has kept Israel."

We can get a quick hint from a very surprising source. The non-Jewish world has such a day, but it not their version of the Sabbath.

RESTING ON THE SABBATH

I came to having a Sabbath in small steps. Years ago, I read a discussion between poets Allan Ginsberg and Gary Snyder about the Sabbath. Snyder said that, from a Zen point of view, dividing between work and play was artificial. Ginsberg, interested in Buddhism himself, agreed with this ideal, but replied that he certainly experienced this distinction. He suggested that, if he ever transcended it, then a Sabbath would not be psychologically necessary, but in the meanwhile, stopping whatever he experienced as work one day a week was useful. Made sense to me, so that is how I started. For example, did going to the mall feel like work? As a matter of fact, going to stores and wrestling over what I could afford and which item to buy was squarely in the work column, so I stopped. Watching a movie without commercials seemed okay at the time.

Since then, the Sabbath came in and out of my life several times, until it grabbed me by the spirit. Now, I no longer have a sense of the Sabbath living in my week. My week lives inside the centering focus of *Shabbos Kodesh*, as it is called, "the Holy Sabbath." It must be holy since it makes life whole.

A SURPRISING SABBATH IN U.S. CULTURE

Every December, non-Jews have an experience similar to Sabbath rest, and they call it Christmas. I have watched it many times, as my Christian clients often build up a heady tension during the first few weeks of the last month of the sun-year. The pace becomes frenetic as people plan the day. Challenges abound: Where to be on Christmas Eve, Christmas Day, and Christmas Night; whom to have and how to manage the invitees who have issues between them? There are foods to plan, decorations and trees to purchase and set up. But, of course, the presents take the epicenter of the stress stage. Everyone needs to be remembered; the amounts have to be gauged according to the relationship so that no one is either embarrassed or offended, and funds need to be accessed. At my first counseling job, they would put an ad in the paper every year at this time: "Merry Stress-mas! Call 'Change Agents'—247-1912."

Now, my point is not to disparage these heroic preparations as much as to enjoy what happens when it is over. At some point on Christmas Eve, the stores close. That's it. Whatever is not bought is not going to be, and everything is as ready as it is going to get. The sounds on the radio no longer urge purchases but instead offer associations of peace. No point any more in banging one's head against the store window; the rest begins. I have believed for years that the joy of the holiday is connected to this phenomenon of a buildup toward a cessation of work. Finally, people just visit with loved ones, enjoy the warmth and smiles, and feast together. Even the presents become more spiritual once the stores close and they symbolize thoughtfulness and affection.

As a result, most of my clients do, in fact, have happy holidays. In short, they have every December what I experience every Friday night and Saturday. It is almost a guilty pleasure—a day when nothing has to get done except feel gratitude, get to learn what the week has prevented, read, and enjoy friendly feasts, uncluttered naps, and more gratitude. No wonder the world's blueprint, the Torah, places the command to rest on *Shabbos* in the central ten. We would never give ourselves such a gift without it.

Rick Blum, Ph.D.

Chapter 8

Nurturing the Nurturer

Be Good to Yourself

Women are the caretakers in our society. Many of us care for children, parents, friends, and pets, with little thought to ourselves. At the same time, we try to balance the often-too-thin ideal of beauty with the reality of daily temptation. We are nurturers who do not nurture ourselves.

Fortunately, there is something we can do. Lifestyle habits are one of the few things in life over which we have control, and we can use that to our advantage. We need to take care of our own needs, as well as those of the rest of the world. This means that what you eat, when you eat, how much you eat, and your activity patterns are critically important. To improve them, you do not have to start from scratch. Little changes work as well as, or even better than, big ones because you can sustain them over a longer period of time.

As a first step, it is important to be self-caring, which is very different from being selfish. We all need to nurture ourselves in the following ways:

- Physically
- Intellectually
- Nutritionally
- Spiritually
- Mentally

In order to do this, think about the internal messages that you give yourself. Are they positive or negative, supportive or destructive? Take the time to identify what obstacles get in the way of self-nurturing. List what self-changes are realistic and can be maintained. Ask yourself what you are willing to take on and what you would be willing to relinquish.

Think about how you see yourself and how you feel living in your body. Realize that you are more than body parts or a number on a scale. The health risks associated with a relentless quest for physical perfection can be quite devastating, and it is important to realize that being thin or having tiny thighs does *not* always equal success, happiness, or physical attractiveness.

When it comes to food, there are no bad foods, only bad attitudes. A slice of coffeecake is not the enemy, but if we berate ourselves for eating the coffeecake and use that as a reason to eat more, it is time to consider an attitude adjustment. Learn to separate the truth from the fiction when it comes to food. Give yourself permission to eat an amount that feels comfortable for you. And give yourself time to change. Improvements don't happen overnight.

Use food to your advantage. Dieting is *not* wellness! Do you wait to eat until you are famished? If you do, you will probably eat more than you want. Consider smaller, more frequent meals to prevent getting overly hungry and to keep your energy levels up throughout the day.

It is important to realize that a woman's caloric needs are different from a man's. We don't live in a portion-friendly world. This is not to say that we should avoid *kugel* altogether, but perhaps a slightly smaller piece would be a good idea. I always tell my clients, "never eat anything bigger than your head!"

Relish the foods you eat. If it doesn't taste good to you, why are you eating it? Enjoy a variety of tastes, textures, colors, and temperatures. Each one of us needs to eat carbohydrates such as fruits, vegetables, rice, pasta, bread, and cereal; we need the protein in meat, fish, poultry, eggs, soy products, nuts or seeds, and dairy foods, and we need the fats from oil, margarine, mayonnaise, salad dressing, butter, sour cream, and nuts or nut butters every day. Consider a meal where one-third of the plate is composed of a fist-sized portion of something starchy, one-third of the plate is a fist-sized portion of fruit or vegetables, and one-third of the plate is a palm-sized amount of protein. Include a thumb-sized amount of fat to add to the starch or vegetable.

> ### *From the Sources*
>
> When you are in pain, go to a physician.
>
> Talmud, *Baba Kammah* 46b.

Eliminating an entire group of foods is not going to make you healthier. If you find a particular food to be too tempting, consider a substitute, or look at the food label and eat the serving size. Make your eating environment conducive to success. If you find that it is too tempting to keep ice cream in the house, then when you want it, go out and have a cone. If you have a hard time leaving food on the plate at a restaurant, ask the server to bring half the entrée to the table and wrap the rest to bring home.

Make your personal health message one of inclusion, instead of exclusion. Take time to listen to your body:

- When it needs to rest or move
- When it is hungry or full
- What it is craving

Say something positive about yourself every day, and find something to smile about. Emphasize what you *can*, *did*, and *are going to do*, not what you *shouldn't*, *didn't*, and *will never* do! This is my nutrition prescription for your health and well-being.

  Leslie Bonci, M.P.H., R.D., L.D.N.

Chapter 9

The People of the Treadmill

When we think of the High Holy Days, many things come to mind: lots of praying, plenty of family, and, more than anything else, a plethora of food.

Distinctive delicacies grace the traditional Rosh Hashanah table, as we dip apples in the honey, experiment with new recipes, and generally eat to excess. Even Yom Kippur is preceded by a large and special feast and is usually followed by one as well, as though forgoing a day's worth of food requires some form of caloric compensation.

The challahs will be round; the kugels will be hot—oh, and please hurry up and pass some of that chocolate dessert.

But as much as food has come to play a central role in our celebration of the festivals, there is another key component of Judaism that seems to have gotten lost amid all the gorging.

It may sound odd, or even peculiar, but physical exercise is actually something that is valued, or is supposed to be, by the people who gave the world pastrami and corned beef.

Yes, I know what you are thinking. Jews are the "People of the Book," which necessarily implies a sedentary type of lifestyle rather than one that involves heavy lifting or even a moderate amount of sweat.

But put aside the stereotypes for a second, and consider the following: if you thought Richard Simmons was a big believer in exercise, you should hear what the rabbis have to say about it.

This is more than just a bit of useful advice from the early medieval scholar, who was himself a physician. For by including it in his work on Jewish law, Maimonides was signaling that the need to

> ### *From the Sources*
>
> "As long as a person exercises and exerts himself," writes Maimonides in his compendium of Jewish law known as the *Mishneh Torah*, "sickness does not befall him and his strength increases." But as for "one who is idle and does not exercise. . . . even if he eats healthy foods and maintains healthy habits, all his days will be full of ailments and his strength will wane."
>
> *Hilchot Deot* 4:15.

exercise is itself a form of religious obligation—one that is incumbent upon each and every one of us.

During these Days of Awe, it is especially interesting to note that Rabbi Abraham Isaac HaKohen Kook, who became the first Chief Rabbi of the Land of Israel in 1921, listed "bodily" or "physical" repentance as the first prerequisite to drawing closer to the Divine.

In his work *Orot HaTeshuvah* (chapter 1), Rabbi Kook stresses the need for man to recognize that "he himself through his bad conduct is responsible for that very same diminution of life that has come to him" and that only by correcting his indolence can "life return to him in all of its freshness."

Although there are different ways of understanding the text, its simple meaning is fairly clear: in order to truly enhance one's spirituality, a person must get active and take care of his (or her) body. For, as Maimonides put it centuries ago, "maintaining a healthy body is among the ways of serving God, since it is impossible for one who is not healthy to understand or know anything of the Creator."

> ### *From the Sources*
>
> The Torah says that it is necessary to "guard yourself and greatly guard your soul" (Deuteronomy 4), and the sages explain the words "guard yourself" as a reference to protecting one's health.

> ### *From the Sources*
>
> God's word calls to us, and limits our presumption against our own body. "Do not commit suicide!" "Do not injure yourself!" "Do not ruin yourself!" "Do not endanger yourself!" "Do not weaken yourself!" "Preserve yourself!"
>
> Rabbi Samson Raphael Hirsch, *Horeb,* chap. 62, sec. 427.

The significance of these words is far-reaching. Essentially, it means that being a loyal and faithful Jew constitutes not only sitting and studying but also jogging, running, or even a bit of kickboxing, too. The reason is fairly obvious: exercise is not only good for the body but for the soul as well, enabling it to better fulfill its purpose in this world.

Taken to its logical conclusion, then, it would seem that the "People of the Talmud" must also become the "People of the Treadmill." As silly as it might sound, it is time for us to ensure that all schools, *yeshivot,* and seminaries take steps toward adding work-out rooms, where students could periodically engage in physical exercise to keep themselves trim and fit.

There is no better way to hit the books than by first getting the adrenaline flowing and the heart pumping through a regular program of physical activity. It would not only improve the strength and concentration that is required for study, but it would also make for a healthier crop of students, who are less prone to exhaustion or illness.

Of course, we need to keep things in perspective. As far as Judaism is concerned, exercise is a means to an end rather than an end in itself. But it is important, nonetheless.

So at the time of the High Holy Days, when our focus is on improving ourselves and our behavior, we might want to consider adopting an additional resolution. Although engaging less in gossip and more in Torah study or being kinder to our neighbors will certainly make us into more spiritual beings, adding a few sit-ups or push-ups to our daily regimen might just work some wonders as well.

Michael Freund

Is There a Blessing for Exercise?

Dear Rabbi,

What would be an appropriate prayer to say upon the completion of exercise, such as jogging? The *Shehekianu* is the only prayer I could think of. Is there one that is more appropriate?

Answer: The Talmud says that someone who lets blood for health reasons should say a special prayer before and after. Before the procedure he should say, "May it be Your will, *Hashem* my God, that this procedure have a healing effect, for You are the free healer." Afterwards he should say, "Blessed are You, Who heals the sick."

The purpose of this prayer is to remind a person that it is *Hashem* who heals, not the medicine. So whether "letting-blood," taking medicine, or undergoing any medical treatment, one should say this prayer.

Similarly, if you jog for health reasons you can say a prayer such as, "It should be the will of *Hashem* that my exercise help me have good health." But one shouldn't say the version mentioned in the Talmud unless he is actually sick.

Ohr Somayach, "Ask the Rabbi" Archives.

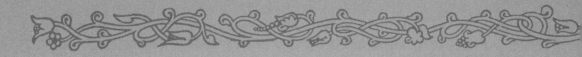

Chapter 10

Finally, Kosher Yoga

Yoga teacher Diane Bloomfield explains how she incorporates Judaism into her classes.

How did you initially make a connection between yoga and Judaism?

I've always been interested in my Judaism, but in my twenties I began to really want to know the Torah. I spent many years immersed in Torah text in a very traditional way, in Jerusalem, and I became quite observant. I've always been a mystically inclined person, so after five years, I began to sense that I wanted to understand the Torah with my body. My mind was just full of text. I felt like I needed to feel it more deeply, and I was very attracted to dance and movement. I came across a yoga teacher and took a class and deeply connected to it. It really spoke to me.

At that point I had a very solid Torah background and was teaching in different settings in Jerusalem. Yet suddenly I was feeling that I needed to understand this in a different way. I knew I needed to move and dance and do yoga. I could understand when I was practicing yoga that this was described in the Torah, that what was happening in yoga was something that had its equivalent in the Torah. So much of what I was experiencing, I translated just naturally into Torah because my mind very much thinks in Torah terms. It's just the way I'm wired—I translate into Torah.

When you say you translate yoga into Torah, do you mean the actual postures?

Not so much the postures or any particular shape, but the experience. There *are* people who work with the shapes of the (Hebrew) letter and the shape of the body, but that's not what I'm doing. There is a spiritual experience that comes with a yoga posture. It has a wisdom in it, and the wisdom in it is connected to wisdom from the Torah. Basically, I realized that I could teach them together, that they enhanced each other, that the practice of yoga could lead to a deeper understanding of Torah, and the study of Torah could lead to a richer experience of yoga. Rather than yoga just being a physical or spiritual experience, it could also be a Jewish spiritual experience.

Were you the first person to do this?

Yes, I was the first person as far as I know. It was 1991 when I started to teach the two together. It is popping up all over the place at this point.

How do people who insist on the purity of the yoga discipline, or see yoga as strictly a Hindu practice, react to your teaching?

I think you would get different answers to that from different people. Ida Unger, who does Jewish yoga in Los Angeles, isn't connected to the Hindu tradition, but she feels it's more important to keep it integrated within that tradition. I haven't ever really come across any resistance to it. In my understanding, the practice doesn't have to be connected to the tradition—to Hinduism or Buddhism. Traditionally, it very often is connected to Hinduism, but many yoga teachers in India tell their students to use yoga to deepen their own tradition. They themselves say that yoga can help you become more of who you are, and you don't have to become Hindu to be doing yoga.

There's one quote I have in my book by B.K.S. Iyengar—one of the foremost yoga teachers in the world: "Yoga was given for the human race, not for the Hindus." I firmly believe that there's a way to take the physical practice of the postures and the breathing practice and disconnect it from Hinduism. Some people would disagree with me, but there's a lot of support for saying that. Yoga is not integrally interwoven with a religion, and it is not a religion in and of itself. It's a very spiritual path. It's about God; it's about consciousness. That is one of the reasons why many Jewish people love the

Torah yoga class—they're really happy to do yoga extracted from the Hindu context. More and more, there's chanting in yoga classes, and Jewish people are not comfortable. They don't want to be chanting Sanskrit, or they don't understand it. They'd rather be chanting Hebrew and studying Torah.

About ten years ago, this older man who had been doing yoga for twenty years came to my class. After class he said, "Finally, kosher yoga." To me, that was a pretty good description.

Some people say, "I can't do yoga; I'm not flexible." It's not about that. It's learning to stretch in a way that you are so attentive to every stage of the posture. It's not about getting your head to your knee or doing the splits. It's how attentive you can be on each step of the way.

If you look at the book of Genesis and the description of the creation of trees, when God says, "Let there be trees," the way God says it is, "Let there be fruit trees, bearing fruit." That's God's command for the fruit trees. Well, Torah study looks at words very, very closely. So when you actually come to the passage where the trees come out, it says, "And there were trees bearing fruit" instead of "there were fruit trees bearing fruit." One understanding of that is that there should be a distinction between the actual tree and the fruit. The tree itself was full of fruit, which is a way of saying, "The whole thing is full of fruit." But often in our lives people are waiting for the fruit. They're waiting until they get somewhere before they enjoy or before they really taste something, instead of really feeling like every day, every moment, every breath has its particular taste, or its particular fruit.

Every posture is a possibility to bring you back to that consciousness of being in the moment and feeling the fruit of this particular moment, rather than someday, when you're finally able to do a headstand or a handstand or anything else. They're both very process-oriented.

So in your classes, you begin by teaching that example from the Torah first and then you could go into the postures?

Yes. In my classes, I always start with a few minutes of stretch and movement. I'm really emphasizing that the wisdom of the Torah is contained in the body, so we want to also really be connected to the body. As Jewish people, we spend a lot of time looking outside ourselves and looking at text and very little time looking at our bodies. So I always start the class with ten minutes of some kind of stretching so that people will immediately remember that we are also going to include our body. Then I'll do a Torah teaching in a traditional way, for ten or fifteen minutes. I've been doing this for fourteen years, so I have hundreds of teachings. The rest of the class, which would be about an hour after that—it's an hour and a half altogether—we will do yoga postures, and I will continually remind the class of the concept that we are focusing on and how to experience it in the body.

Do any non-Jews ever attend your classes?

Yes.

What do you think they get out of it?

I have one very loyal student right now—a woman who's Lutheran. I think it's very comforting for her because the roots are her roots. She can relate to the Jewish roots, or the Old Testament, more than the Far East or more than Hinduism. I really choose the aspects of the Torah that are universal for any spiritual seeker. There are certain parts of the Torah that are specific for the Jewish people, but much of it is universal. So on one hand, I think non-Jewish people enjoy it because it's comforting to stay closer to their tradition, or their roots, but any spiritual seeker can enjoy the powerful Jewish wisdom.

Have you ever gotten any adverse reactions from Jews?

I have not ever personally encountered anyone who has rejected yoga as being wrong for Jews to practice.

So for someone who has never done yoga before, is this a good way to begin?

Yes. It depends on what someone is looking for. Many of my students have never done yoga before. There's no reason not to begin with it, especially if you are interested in your Jewish spirituality and you want to stay within that context. It's not the only place to begin, but for many people it will be the most comfortable place to begin.

Jewish meditation classes are very popular right now. Is Jewish yoga related to meditation?

It's very related. Yoga, in my opinion, is meditation. In each chapter of my book I have an opening meditation. Yoga is sometimes called meditation in motion. It's obviously not just sitting-still meditation, but my understanding is that meditation is a focus practice—the practice of concentration. So yoga is definitely a cousin, or a sister or brother, to sitting meditation.

Returning to what you said about wanting to connect to Judaism with your body: it seems like there are other ways that Jews do that. Davening [praying] is a very movement-oriented practice for some people. Are there other ways Jews incorporate movement into their Jewish practice?

It's true that shuckling [moving back and forth while praying] is a natural way for Jews to kind of get their body moving, or get their body to wake up. The difference is they don't then stop and focus on the sensations of their body as an aspect of the prayer. It's not the same thing. What I'm saying is, you can listen to your body and feel something about the truth of the prayer right in your body.

So the way they move while praying is not exactly the same?

I think what's more similar is the Hasidic tradition of dance as a celebration. I mean the fact that they danced and they were joyful in their bodies—that experience is a little closer. But it's still not the same. Torah yoga is very intellectual, in a way, about the body. It says the body is smart. The body knows things, and you can learn things with the body.

Rebecca Phillips

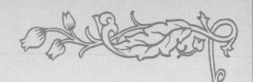

✎ Special Focus

Specific Health Care Issues

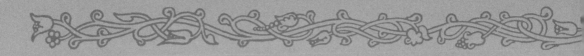

Chapter 11

How to Talk to Your Doctor

✍ *An Rx for M.D. Visits*

Why do even those women who run companies, litigate cases in court, or manage complex family households become intimidated when visiting a doctor's office?

The Healthy Women, Healthy Lives program, created and run by Hadassah, has found that few women prepare for a doctor's visit in the same way they might prepare for a professional or family-related event. The program, which offers materials on subjects ranging from breast cancer and osteoporosis to nutrition and exercise, suggests that careful homework and planning can help every woman make a visit to her doctor a success. Here are some tips for mastering your M.D. visits:

- *Compile and regularly update a family medical history, and take it to every visit.* Dr. Ellen Wolfson, a Greenwich, Connecticut internist and Hadassah member, even suggests sending this family history to your doctor in advance.
- *Ask a new doctor for a preliminary meeting.* "Not every doctor will do this," Dr. Wolfson admits. "But I think the degree of comfort on both sides is important to a good doctor-patient relationship, so I do it. During this visit, I tell patients how I run my office and when and how I can be reached; I answer any questions about my educational background and style."
- *Make a separate (also ongoing) list of all your medications and take it to your visit.* Include brand or generic names, as well as dosage amount and frequency. "Don't forget to include herbals and over-the-counter preparations," warns Dr. Wolfson. "Not

all interact well with prescription medications. And remember that eye drops and nose drops are also medicine; for some reason, many patients forget."

- *Take a friend or relative with you as your second set of ears.* Dr. Wolfson explains, "Sometimes, particularly if you're discussing a potentially serious or worrisome symptom or illness, anxiety can diminish your ability to take in information clearly. A trusted second person can listen carefully to the discussion and take notes."
- *Don't hide anything!* You're there for help. If you're hindered by embarrassment, or even denial, you will lessen your chances of being helped. "Before each visit, write down your symptoms, if any," Dr. Wolfson says. "Even if they are vague, note them as best as you can. Bring this written record to your visit, and refer to it as needed."
- *Be sure you understand your diagnosis.* Don't leave the office until you do! Ask questions, or have your "visit buddy" ask questions. "It's important that you know your diagnosis, the nature of your illness, and the treatment steps that will follow," advises Dr. Wolfson. If you've forgotten, call later and ask.
- *When necessary, go for a second opinion.* Bring all your notes with you. Both before and during an illness, learn all you can on the Internet or through other research. Speak to your doctor about this information, and understand that not everything you read is either appropriate for you or medically on target. Only a professional can help you sift through the data.

For information about Healthy Women, Healthy Lives, please call Women's Health at (212) 303-8094 or e-mail us at womenshealth@ hadassah.org.

ഏ *Fran Levine*

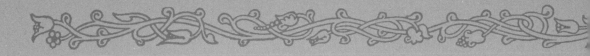

Chapter 12

Women and Heart Disease

The misconception that heart disease is mainly a male affliction has dominated the medical field for many years. Today we know that women, especially after menopause, are as prone to develop heart problems as men; nevertheless, most of the medical literature consists of data concerning men only. At the Heart Institute of the Hadassah Medical Organization, we decided to dedicate major resources to the study of women and heart disease on the level of clinical and basic research. Our goal is to further the understanding of what specifically has turned heart disease into the leading killer of women in the developed world.

The research is being carried out at the newly established Cardiovascular Research Center, located in the Heart Institute at the Hadassah-Hebrew University Medical Center at Ein Karem. Projects range from epidemiological studies to pure basic research—all having the same aim in common: to improve diagnosis, prevention, and treatment of women with heart disease. The following are examples of current epidemiological studies.

Understanding the factors that lead to coronary artery disease (CAD) in Israeli women of different ethnic backgrounds will help us tailor more specific preventive measures. To this end, we have initiated a project to compare risk profiles of CAD in Israeli and Arab women. Mortality rates from CAD are significantly higher among Arab residents of Jerusalem than among Jewish residents, and there are clear differences in diet, socioeconomic level, medical care, and stress between Arab and Jewish women in Israel. Results of this study may help to invest more effort in reducing the incidence of CAD through early detection, modification, and prevention of the appropriate risk factors among this ethnic group.

The major project in the Molecular Cardiac Research Facility is focused on women who suffer from a very aggressive form of breast cancer—the "Her-Neu positive" variant. These women are treated with Herceptin—a new and very effective drug. Unfortunately, up to one-third of patients develop mild to severe heart disease as a side effect of the treatment, the causes of which are not known. Could this be due to a genetic predisposition, or maybe some other reason, such as lifestyle? This question can only be answered by basic laboratory experiments; therefore, we study the effect of Herceptin in tissue culture and in rat hearts. Analysis of the molecular changes in heart tissue with and without the drug will give us an insight into the mechanism of this highly beneficial drug. This, in turn, may lead to significant improvements in the therapy protocol.

A combination of basic and clinical research is being conducted to explore the relationship between homocysteine levels and genetic predisposition to develop CAD in women. For this research we study patients who have come to the clinic with signs of heart disease. The women are asked to participate and to sign an informed consent form. For each patient a biochemical profile, including her homocysteine level, is determined. Next, the MTHFR gene, known to be involved in regulating homocysteine levels, is isolated from blood samples and analyzed, in order to determine whether it carries a mutation. Protective treatment, such as adding folic acid to the diet, can then specifically be targeted to women who have a genetic predisposition to develop high homocysteine levels.

We are establishing a computerized database based on our past research to assess risk factors in women with CAD. This will allow us to create the best possible primary and secondary prevention programs. At the Heart Institute of the HMO, we have been able to show that CAD in women is considerably more prevalent and serious than in men of the same age. In order to substantiate our findings, we are using our database to assess the risk factors that may be elevated or even unique in female patients. We have written a computer program that includes socioeconomic parameters, as well as the medical history of each patient, including any hormonal treatment received, for

Ask the Expert: High Blood Cholesterol Screening and Prevention

An expert answers your questions about cholesterol screening and prevention.

How often do I need to get my cholesterol checked?

Everyone age twenty and older should have his or her cholesterol measured at least once every five years. High blood cholesterol plays a major role in the development of heart disease and is a major women's health issue. A quarter of all American women have blood cholesterol levels high enough to pose a serious risk for heart disease.[1] An expert panel of the National Cholesterol Education Program (NCEP) recently issued new guidelines for cholesterol management, based on mounting evidence that deaths from heart disease—the number-one killer of American women—could be reduced with aggressive treatment of high cholesterol. The new NCEP guidelines spotlight LDL cholesterol—the type of cholesterol that injures blood vessel walls—as the primary target of therapy.

The new NCEP guidelines recommend a complete lipoprotein profile (a blood test that measures total cholesterol, LDL cholesterol, HDL cholesterol, and triglyceride levels) as the initial test to determine if your cholesterol levels are within normal ranges. This type of test, called a fasting lipoprotein test, is taken after not eating for nine to twelve hours. Older guidelines called for an initial nonfasting cholesterol test only. Be sure to ask your health care professional about the fasting-type blood cholesterol test, if you've never had one.

If my cholesterol levels are fine, does that mean I won't have a heart attack?

Even if your cholesterol levels are normal, you still need to think about other risks for heart disease. Smoking, having high blood pressure or diabetes, being overweight or physically inactive, and having a family history of heart disease all contribute to your risk for developing heart disease. Some, but not all, of these risk factors can be improved with dietary and lifestyle changes.

That's why it's so important to maintain a healthy diet and regular exercise habits as you age. And if your health care professional prescribes medication to lower your cholesterol or to control your blood pressure, be sure to take it as prescribed. Leading a healthful lifestyle and following your health care professional's instructions will go a long way in reducing your risks of heart disease.

 Margo A. Denke, M.D.

example, for prevention of pregnancy, in vitro fertilization treatment, and hormone replacement therapy. This allows us to concentrate on specific female aspects that are usually neglected.

The combination of research and clinical services carried out at the Heart Institute of the HMO as described here will help to lessen the disparity between men and women in all aspects related to the common enemy: heart disease.

 Chaim Lotan, M.D., and Thea Pugatsch, Ph.D., T.P.

Note

1. National Cholesterol Education Program, National Heart, Lung, and Blood Institute, National Institutes of Health. "Third Report of the Expert Panel on Detection, Evaluation, and Treatment of High Blood Cholesterol in Adults (Adult Treatment Panel III)." May 2001 [http://www.nhlbi.nih.gov/guidelines/cholesterol].

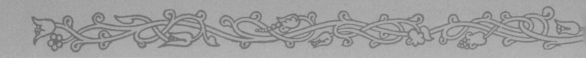

Chapter 13

Take Control of Your Heart's Health

In a recent survey on health concerns, when asked what they fear most, the number-one response from women was breast cancer. However, did you know that more women die from heart disease each year than from breast, ovarian, and uterine cancers *combined?* Long viewed as just a man's problem, heart disease is actually the leading cause of death and disability among women in the United States. In fact, heart disease kills more women than men each year. One in ten American women aged forty-five to sixty-four has some form of heart disease, and this increases to one in four women over the age of sixty-five. In addition, two million women have had a stroke, and 93,000 women die of stroke each year.

The good news: heart disease is, in large part, preventable. In the past, most research on cardiovascular disease was conducted in men only, but the findings were extrapolated to guide treatment and prevention decisions for women. Today, a new national focus on women's health is yielding important knowledge about these diseases in women.

This chapter highlights what every woman needs to know about heart disease, including its risk factors, diagnosis, and treatment. Steps you can take to keep your heart healthy and decrease your chance of developing cardiovascular diseases to ensure a healthier future are provided.

The author acknowledges the contributions of Om L. Lala in the preparation of this chapter.

60

WHAT CARDIOVASCULAR DISEASES ARE AND WHO GETS THEM

Both heart disease and stroke are known as cardiovascular diseases—disorders of the heart and blood vessel system. Coronary heart disease—the most common form of heart disease—affects the blood vessels of the heart, known as the coronary arteries. Disease takes many years to develop and can begin as far back as childhood. In a process known as atherosclerosis, fatty substances build up inside the walls of blood vessels. The vessels narrow and harden, becoming less flexible. The buildup and narrowing proceed gradually and result in decreased blood flow and, eventually, the development of symptoms. When blood flow to the heart is reduced, chest pain—"angina"—can result. When the blood flow is critically reduced, a heart attack may occur and cause muscle cells in the heart to die. Because the cells cannot be replaced, the result is permanent heart damage. About half the women who have a heart attack will be disabled with heart failure within six years. Heart failure is a life-threatening condition in which the heart cannot pump enough blood to meet the body's needs. A lack of blood flow to the brain or, in some cases, bleeding in the brain, causes a stroke.

About 6.7 million American women have heart disease. One in ten women ages forty-five to sixty-four has some form of heart disease. Each year about 88,000 women ages forty-five to sixty-four and 372,000 over the age of sixty-five have a heart attack. The average age for women to have a first heart attack is about seventy. About 35 percent of women who have had a heart attack will have another within six years. That increases to one in five for women over age sixty-five.

Some women have more risk factors for cardiovascular diseases than others. *Risk factors* are habits or traits that make a person more likely to develop a disease. Some risk factors for heart-related problems cannot be changed, but many others can. The major risk factors for cardiovascular diseases are behavioral factors that you can do something about, including smoking cigarettes, being physically inactive or poorly nourished, being overweight, and having high blood pressure or high cholesterol. Other risk factors such as diabetes, stress, heavy drinking, and use of birth control pills (especially if you smoke or are diabetic) are also conditions that you have some control over.

Some minority groups, including African Americans, Hispanics, and Native Americans, have a higher incidence and death rate from cardiovascular disease. Risk factors you can't change include being age fifty-five or older and having a family history of early heart disease. Although high cholesterol is a well-recognized risk factor for heart disease, an estimated 50 percent of people who have heart attacks have cholesterol readings within normal ranges. This poses some intriguing questions about what other factors may contribute to the development of heart disease. Researchers have discovered biological factors in the blood linked to chronic inflammation that appear to be associated with increased risk, including C-reactive protein (CRP), homocysteine, fibrinogen, and lipoprotein (a). Scientists used to think that clogged arteries were caused by the passive buildup of bad cholesterol (LDL—low-density lipoprotein). More recent studies, however, show that the body's response to LDL, in the form of inflammation, causes a significant part of this damage. More research is needed to better define the contributions of these substances to heart disease in women.

Also important to know is that the various risk factors for heart disease and stroke do not add their effects in a simple way. Rather, they multiply each other's effects. So, for example, if you smoke and have high blood pressure and high cholesterol, you're eight times more likely to develop heart disease than a woman with no risk factors. Even just one risk factor will raise your chances of having heart-related problems, but the more risk factors you have, the more likely you are to develop cardiovascular disease and the more concerned you should be about protecting your heart health.

SYMPTOMS OF HEART DISEASE

The most common symptom of heart disease is chest pain or pressure. Chest pain typically occurs behind the breastbone and may cause numbness or tingling in the left arm or up your neck and shoulders. Or it may be experienced as a squeezing or pressing sensation that does not change with breathing. The pain usually lasts two to five minutes. Reduced blood flow to the heart can also cause a lingering chest pain, occurring in a different location than behind the breastbone.

Women may exhibit different symptoms of heart attacks from those of men. For example, some women may experience shortness of breath, indigestion, nausea, lightheadedness, or significant fatigue. Other women will not have any of these symptoms before or during a heart attack. Likewise, symptoms can be either mild or severe and can subside and then return. Frequently, women and health care providers may mistake this pain signaling a heart attack as indigestion. If you should have such symptoms, talk with your doctor immediately. If treated, the outlook is good. Without treatment, however, the symptoms of heart disease may recur and worsen and can lead to a heart attack.

The symptoms of a stroke include sudden weakness or numbness of parts of one side of the body, usually the face, arm, or leg; sudden dimness or loss of vision, particularly in one eye; loss of speech or trouble talking or understanding speech; sudden severe headaches with no known cause; or unexplained dizziness, unsteadiness, or sudden falls.

DIAGNOSIS OF HEART DISEASE

Diagnostic tests are needed to confirm the presence and to assess the severity of coronary heart disease. Often more than one test is required because different tests supply different information. The main tests for coronary heart disease include blood tests, an electrocardiogram, stress test (or treadmill test), echocardiography, nuclear scan, and coronary angiography. New procedures, including electron beam computed tomography (EBCT), magnetic resonance angiography (MRA), and computer tomographic angiography (CTA), can provide important diagnostic information and are being studied for their effectiveness in detecting cardiovascular disease. Stroke is diagnosed by several techniques, including neurological examination, blood tests, CT and MRI scans, and arteriography.

TREATMENT OF HEART DISEASE

There are three main types of interventions for heart disease: lifestyle changes, medication, and special procedures for advanced atherosclerosis (a buildup of fatty substances inside the walls of the blood vessels). The Talmud says, "Do not mistake talk for action." If you have heart disease, several critical actions can reduce your risk of future complications and improve your overall health as well:

• *Stop smoking.* Smoking is the leading preventable cause of death for women in the United States. Smoking accelerates atherosclerosis and makes you two to six times more likely to suffer a heart attack. If you quit, the risk to your heart drops sharply, even in the first year, no matter what your age.

• *Lower high blood cholesterol.* The body makes all the cholesterol it needs. Extra cholesterol and fat in the diet cause the atherosclerotic buildup inside blood vessels, increasing risk for heart attacks. There are two types of cholesterol: low-density lipoprotein (LDL), which causes deposits and is termed the "bad" cholesterol, and high-density lipoprotein (HDL), which helps remove excess cholesterol from the blood and is termed the "good" cholesterol. Normal total blood cholesterol for women is less than 200, with an LDL of less than 100 and an HDL between 50 and 60 mg/dL. Blood cholesterol levels for women in the United States tend to rise from about the age of twenty and sharply increase at about age forty.

Today, about one-quarter of all American women have blood cholesterol levels high enough to pose a serious risk for heart disease. More than one-half of women over age fifty-five need to lower their blood cholesterol. High blood cholesterol can be lowered by lifestyle changes, including maintaining a healthy weight, being physically active, and consuming a diet low in saturated fat and cholesterol and rich in fruits, vegetables, and fiber. Medication such as statins may be required for some women to lower their cholesterol levels. All women over age twenty should have their blood cholesterol checked regularly.

• *Lower your triglyceride level.* Many people with high triglycerides have underlying diseases or genetic vulnerability to cardiovascular disease. A healthy triglyceride level is less than 150 mg/dL. Strategies to lower your triglycerides include maintaining a healthy body weight; eating foods low in saturated fat, cholesterol, and carbohydrates; and being physically active.

• *Lower high blood pressure.* High blood pressure (hypertension) is called the "silent killer" because most people who have it

Questions to Ask About High Blood Cholesterol

- When can I schedule a cholesterol test?
- What do the test results mean?
- What steps should I take to lower my cholesterol?
- When should I have a follow-up test?
- How can I determine my optimal caloric intake?
- My cholesterol is high. Should I be taking a cholesterol-reducing drug?
- What are the pros and cons of hormone replacement therapy in my situation? Could we consider a cholesterol-reducing drug instead of, or in addition to, HRT?
- What are the side effects of the medications I've been prescribed? Does it make any difference what time of day I take them?
- Do you know a good registered dietitian with a track record in helping women get their cholesterol down?
- I have diabetes. How does that change our approach to treating high cholesterol?

Hadassah Health Memo, Winter 2001.

do not feel sick. That's why your blood pressure must be checked regularly. About twenty-four million women age sixty and older have high blood pressure. Blood pressure is the amount of force exerted by the blood against the walls of the arteries. Depending on your activities, blood pressure may rise and fall in the course of a day. Blood pressure is considered high when it stays above 140/90 mm Hg over a period of time. High blood pressure makes the heart work harder and, uncontrolled, can lead to heart disease, stroke, heart failure, kidney problems, and other conditions. Many people can lower their blood pressure through lifestyle changes, including losing excess weight; increasing physical activity; eating a diet low in salt and sodium and rich in potassium, fruits, and vegetables; and limiting alcohol intake. Some women will also need medication to treat their hypertension.

• *Maintain a healthy weight.* Being overweight increases the risk of heart disease, even if no other risk factors are present. To lose weight, take it slow and steady, following a healthy eating plan. Even a small amount of weight loss can have a significant health benefit.

• *Become physically active.* Physical activity is critical to achieving and maintaining a healthy weight over the long term. Physical activity helps lower LDL and raise HDL levels, as well as decrease blood pressure.

Research shows that even a moderate amount of physical activity can improve your health. Incorporate physical activity into your daily routine, such as taking the stairs instead of the elevator or walking inside of driving. Aerobic activity and strength training are vital to your overall health. The federal guidelines recommend thirty to sixty minutes a day of physical activity, five days a week, but it doesn't have to be continuous.

 ## Dietary Suggestions to Reduce Blood Cholesterol Levels

• *Weight your diet toward fruits and vegetables*, as well as cereals, breads, rice, and pasta made from whole grains (such as rye bread or whole-wheat spaghetti).
• *Limit meat to 6 ounces of fish, poultry, or lean cuts of meat per day.* Remove fat and skin before eating; avoid processed meats or organ meats.
• *Drink skim or 1 percent milk instead of whole milk or cream.* Switch to low-fat or nonfat cheeses and yogurt.
• *Use as little fat and oil as possible.* Look for margarine and oil low in saturated fats. In general, the softer the margarine, the better.
• *Avoid egg yolks, but feel free to eat egg whites, which are fat- and cholesterol-free.* You can substitute two egg whites for one yolk in many recipes.
• *Avoid fried foods* in favor of broiled, baked, roasted, or poached alternatives.
• *Read product labels* to find foods low in saturated fat, total fat, and cholesterol. Keep an eye on total calories.

Hadassah Health Memo, Winter 2001.

• *Take medication.* Drugs may be required, especially if you have chest pain, high blood cholesterol, or hypertension that is not reduced by positive lifestyle changes. Medications for these conditions include blood-cholesterol-lowering agents such as the statins, digitalis, ACE inhibitors, beta-blockers, nitrate, calcium-channel blockers, and diuretics. Other drugs that reduce inflammation are also being explored in the treatment of heart disease. Low-dose aspirin is recommended if a person is having a heart attack and as a way to reduce the risks of a second heart attack.

Other interventions are available as well. The two main procedures used to treat severe blockage and improve blood flow to the coronary arteries are *angioplasty* (which stretches the artery by insertion of a tiny balloon, followed by placement of a stent) and *coronary artery bypass surgery* (where a piece of blood vessel from the leg or chest is used to bypass the blockage, resulting in increased blood flow).

PREVENTION OF HEART DISEASE AND STROKE

Prevention is the best way to reduce your risk of heart disease. You hold much of the future of your heart's health in your own hands. Lifestyle changes, plus early identification of risk factors and prompt medical attention when symptoms appear, can help to significantly reduce the risk of heart disease and stroke among women.

The major steps a woman can take to reduce her risk of heart disease are maintaining a healthy weight, not smoking, and getting at least thirty to sixty minutes of moderate physical activity most days of the week. Choose activities you like, such as brisk walking, dancing, biking, or gardening. Research has also shown a connection between stress and heart disease, so it is important to find activities that you enjoy and to take time for yourself every day. Not only do these lifestyle interventions help lower cholesterol, but exercise and weight loss also work to reduce inflammation in the fat cells and liver.

A diet rich in fruits, vegetables, whole grains, and omega-3 fatty acids helps reduce inflammation as well. Because the modern diet is often deficient in omega-3s, a fish-oil supplement, as well as daily vitamins, including folate, is recommended for many women. Avoid trans fats and limit your intake of high-glycemic-load foods such as sweets, refined-grain breads, pasta, and cereals. Drink alcohol in moderation or not at all. Women should have no more than one drink per day (one drink is 12 ounces of beer, 5 ounces of wine, or 1.5 ounces of spirits). The beauty of these lifestyle changes is that they are low-tech, affordable, and effective. It is estimated that as many as 70 percent of heart attacks and strokes could be prevented by lifestyle modifications.

Although studies have shown that low-dose aspirin is effective in reducing the risk of heart attacks in men, recent findings from the Women's Health Study—a ten-year study of forty thousand healthy women—revealed that aspirin did not prevent first heart attacks in women but did modestly reduce the risk of stroke in women over the age of sixty-five. These results were striking because they are the exact opposite of what occurs in men. Low-dose aspirin has, however, been found to reduce the chances that women who have already had a heart attack will have, or die from, another one. The study also found that vitamin E did not prevent cardiovascular disease.

In recent years there has been a sea change in the use of hormone replacement therapy (HRT) to prevent and treat heart disease. In the past, HRT had been thought to prevent heart attacks. However, recent results from the NIH-supported Women's Health Initiative—a fifteen-year study of 162,000 women aged fifty to seventy-nine, conducted in forty states nationwide—found that HRT actually increased the risk for heart attack, stroke, and blood clots. In addition, the study found that HRT should not be used as a treatment for heart disease.

Hadassah members understand the importance of relationships and community, so it should come as no surprise that emotionally supportive relationships may help improve the quality of life, as well as potentially prolong life following a heart attack. Family and friends are critical in prevention, too. It's more fun and easier to engage in healthy behavior if others join you.

Knowledge is power when it comes to your health. Enter into a partnership with your physician for your health. Know your family's medical history and share it with your doctor. Be alert for disease symptoms in order to detect health problems early. In order to get the best treatment, help your doctor by keeping a diary of your symptoms so you can describe them accurately, and inform your doctor of any past therapies and current medications. Put prevention into practice yourself and teach your parents, children, and grandchildren habits for a healthy heart. This knowledge will be a gift of life.

For more information, visit the National Heart, Lung, and Blood Institute's Web site on women and heart disease at http://www.hearttruth.gov and http://www.womenshealth.gov or call (800) 994-WOMAN.

Rear Admiral Susan J. Blumenthal, M.D., M.P.A.

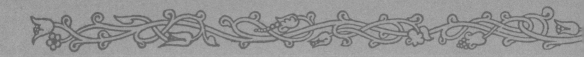

Chapter 14

Stress and Heart Disease

Heart disease is the leading cause of death in American women, accounting for more deaths than all cancers combined. A woman's lifetime risk of developing heart disease is less than 30 percent and rises each decade after age fifty. Only about 50 percent of heart disease can be explained by the traditional risk factors (smoking, abnormal cholesterol, hypertension, and inactivity). Recent studies have begun to explore the relationship between acute and chronic stress and the development of heart disease. The mechanism by which stress contributes to heart disease is not completely understood, but stress appears to play a role.

WHAT IS STRESS?

Stress results when you perceive a situation or event as threatening or overtaxing. The sympathetic nervous system is activated. Stress hormones (epinephrine and adrenaline) are rapidly released into the blood to prepare the body for action—often called the "fight or flight" response. There is an immediate increase in heart rate, blood pressure, breathing, and muscle tension. Examples of common stresses include sitting in traffic, waiting in long lines, having family conflicts, and running late.

HOW DO I MANAGE STRESS?

Stress does not have to negatively affect your life and health. By following this plan you can take control. The first thing to do is to recognize common stress warning signs:

- Tension headache
- Tight neck and shoulders
- Feelings of anxiety, irritability, or frustration
- Trouble remembering things
- Difficulty sleeping
- A run-down, tired feeling
- Cold hands
- Heart racing or palpitating

The Four-Step Model

1. *Stop!* Each time you encounter stress, stop—before your thoughts escalate into the worst scenarios:

   Oh no!
   Why me?
   Nothing will ever change.
   This always happens to me.
   I'll never get everything done.

2. *Breathe.* Breathe deeply and release physical tension.
3. *Reflect.* Focus on the problem at hand and appraise the situation. Ask these questions:

   What's going on here?
   Why am I so distressed?
   Am I jumping to conclusions?
   Am I blowing this out of proportion?
   How do I know it will happen?
   Can I handle it?
   Will worrying about it help?

4. *Choose.* How else can I think about this (restructure negative thoughts)? Here are some possibilities:

   It's just a bump in the road.
   I'm doing the best I can.
   One day at a time.
   It's OK to make a mistake.
   I can deal with this.

What can I do to cope with this?

Do I need to temper my emotional response before I can act responsively?

More steps that you might take include making time for relaxation each day:

- Try taking a mindful walk.
- Sit and focus on your breath (feeling the chest rise as you inhale and relax as you exhale); visualize yourself walking along a beautiful beach; feel the sand on your feet; hear the waves as they roll onto the shore; feel the breeze on your back.
- Listen to soothing music; light a candle; take a bubble bath.
- Read for pleasure.
- Rent a funny movie.
- Write (keep a journal).

Another step is this: avoid putting too much on your plate. Make a list of what needs to be done and then prioritize:

- A (must get done)
- B (can wait)
- C (not important; let go of)

By following the Four-Step Model and taking these further steps to manage your stress, you increase your ability to live a more serene and heart-healthy life.

Aggie Casey, R.N., M.S.

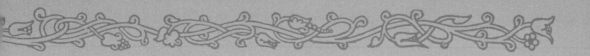

Chapter 15

Menopause and Hormones

As a member of the Food and Drug Administration (FDA) Office of Women's Health Task Force on Hormone Therapy, it is my pleasure to share with you the following fact sheet and questions to ask your doctor, nurse, or pharmacist about hormone therapy. This is the most current information available at press time. Women's Health will continue to monitor the research as it is presented and will inform you of changes through "What's New What's Hot," as well as the Hadassah Intranet.

What is menopause?

Menopause is a normal change in a woman's life when her period stops. That's why some people call menopause "the change of life" or "the change." During menopause a woman's body slowly produces less of the hormones estrogen and progesterone. This often happens between the ages of forty-five and fifty-five years old. A woman has reached menopause when she has not had a period for twelve months in a row.

What is hormone therapy for menopause?

Hormone therapy for menopause has also been called hormone replacement therapy (HRT). Lower hormone levels in menopause may lead to hot flashes, vaginal dryness, and thin bones. To help with these problems, women are often given estrogen or estrogen with progestin (another hormone). Like all medicines, hormone therapy has risks and benefits. Talk to your doctor, nurse, or pharmacist about hormones. If you decide to use hormones, use them at the lowest dose that helps and for the shortest time that you need them.

What are the symptoms of menopause?

Every woman's period will stop at menopause. Some women may not have any other symptoms at all. As you near menopause, you may have

Changes in your period (time between periods or flow may be different)

Hot flashes (flushing)—getting warm in the face, neck, and chest

Night sweats and sleeping problems that lead to feeling tired, stressed, or tense

Vaginal changes (the vagina may become dry and thin, and sex may be painful)

Thinning of your bones, which may lead to loss of height and bone breaks (osteoporosis)

Who needs treatment for symptoms of menopause?

For some women, many of these changes will go away over time without treatment.

Some women will choose treatment for their symptoms and to prevent bone loss. If you choose treatment, estrogen alone or estrogen with progestin (for a woman who still has her uterus or womb) can be used.

What are the benefits from using hormones for menopause?

Hormone therapy is the most effective FDA-approved medicine for relief of your hot flashes, night sweats, or vaginal dryness. Hormones may also reduce your chances of getting thin, weak bones that break easily (osteoporosis) and may reduce your risk of colon cancer.

What are the risks of using hormones?

For some women, hormone therapy may increase their chances of getting blood clots, heart attacks, strokes, breast cancer, and gallbladder disease. For a woman with a uterus, estrogen increases her chance of getting endometrial cancer (cancer of the uterine lining). Adding progestin lowers this risk.

Should hormone therapy be used to protect the heart or prevent strokes?

Do not use hormone therapy to prevent heart attacks or strokes.

To Learn More About Menopause and Hormones

National Women's Health Information Center
U.S. Department of Health and Human Services
http://www.4woman.gov
(800) 994-9662
TDD: (888) 220-5446

Food and Drug Administration
U.S. Department of Health and Human Services
http://www.fda.gov/womens
http://www.fda.gov/cder

National Institutes of Health
U.S. Department of Health and Human Services
http://www.NIH.gov/PHTindex.htm

Should hormone therapy be used to prevent memory loss or Alzheimer's disease?

Do not use hormone therapy to prevent memory loss or Alzheimer's disease.

Do hormones protect against aging and wrinkles?

Studies have not shown that hormone therapy prevents aging and wrinkles.

How long should I use hormones for menopause?

You should talk to your doctor, nurse, or pharmacist. Again, hormones should be used at the lowest dose that helps and for the shortest time you need them.

Does it make a difference what form of hormones I use for menopause?

The risks and benefits may be the same for all hormone products for menopause, such as pills, patches, vaginal creams, gels, and rings.

Questions to Ask About Women's Health Screenings

Discuss your screening and prevention options with your health care professional. Here are some questions to help start the conversation:

- Am I at risk for high blood cholesterol and high blood pressure?
- Am I at risk for breast, colorectal, or cervical cancer?
- What screenings are available for these conditions, and which one is best for me?
- How often should I be screened for high blood cholesterol; high blood pressure; and breast, colorectal, and cervical cancer?
- How should I prepare for the screenings?
- Do I need to see a specialist or go to a specialized medical facility for these tests or can my primary health care professional perform them in her or his office?
- Are there any risks associated with the screenings?
- When and how will I be informed of the test results?

Hadassah Health Memo, Spring 2002.

Are herbs and other "natural" products useful in treating symptoms of menopause?

At this time, we do not know whether herbs or other "natural" products are helpful or safe. Studies are being done to learn about the benefits and risks.

✑ Dale L. Mintz, M.P.A., C.H.E.S.; developed by the U.S. Department of Health and Human Services and the Food and Drug Administration

Nutrition

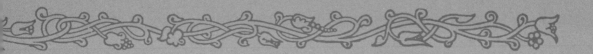

Chapter 16

You Are What You Eat

Our eating style reflects and affects who and what we are. It identifies our approach to life. If we examine various societies and cultures, we see that each has its traditional foods and food ceremonies. "I am Italian. I often eat spaghetti, lasagna, or pizza." Or somebody says, "I am a real American—I eat hamburgers, hot dogs, steak, Coke, and french fries." The French eat crepes, Belgians eat waffles, Chinese eat rice, Ethiopians eat teff, the Swiss eat chocolate, Israelis eat falafel, and Eskimos eat whale blubber. In short, the "way we eat" reveals how we identify ourselves. It reflects and often determines our worldview, our values, and our entire approach to life.

"You are the way you eat." Foods are much more than just a collection of nutrients; they are a wealth of influences and connotations. Rare foods and spices are treasured as special culinary delights. Some foods are worshiped in various cultures as having an unusual holiness or are avoided altogether. The type of food we choose can affect our moods. Hot, spicy, or stimulating foods may influence many of us toward hot-temperedness or nervousness. Cooling foods can relax us and give us peace of mind. Foods can help us celebrate and can comfort us when we mourn. They are a sign of love and are a means of uniting people on many occasions.

The "way we eat" as Jews is an important part of our heritage and spans from simple rules of common eating etiquette to complex kabalistic combinations of God's Divine Name concentrated upon while eating. We make a blessing over our food before and after eating and thank God for his wonderful kindness, which enables us to eat and to continue our lives for his service.

SAGELY ADVICE

Traditional Jewish dishes have developed that have many important cultural and religious connotations. Nevertheless, those of us choosing to follow a healthier, lighter style of eating can find a firm foundation for natural nutrition in the eight-hundred-year-old writings of Maimonides, the great Torah scholar and physician. One of the foremost preventive-health advocates of all time, he prescribes a synthesis of good health and a nutritional lifestyle, reflecting and deepening our connection to our own Jewish roots.

Maimonides' medical writings contain the Jewish roots of today's system of natural nutrition. Our modern approach is basically an extension of his main principles and teachings. He emphasized the importance of preventive medicine and disease prevention. He foreshadowed today's "discovery" of the effect of proper lifestyle, discussing the role of diet and exercise. Mind-body interaction was primary in his approach to illness and wellness.

To preserve health, Maimonides taught that we should eat only when genuinely hungry and drink when truly thirsty. Drinking during meals should be minimized to avoid diluting the digestive juices. The preservation of good health rests on the avoidance of overeating, which he refers to as "the poison of death" and the cause of most illness. He taught us that eating a little of bad foods is actually less harmful than eating a lot of good and healthy food.

He advocated some exercise before eating to warm the body for improved digestion and, in general, taught that exercise removes the harm caused by most of the bad habits people have. Meals should be eaten while sitting or reclining, and we should rest after meals for good digestion. Avoidance of constipation is essential for good health. Eating according to the seasons was also promoted, with cool foods and lesser quantities in the summer and warm, spicier foods in greater quantities in the winter.

Whole-grain bread was cited by Maimonides as "the best of food." The bread must not be made of refined flour and should consist of the rough grain, unchaffed and unpolished. He taught that white bread or bread made of refined flour was not a good food.

SPIRITUALITY OF EATING

When asked why they eat, people usually respond, "I eat because I'm hungry," "I eat when something looks or smells good," or "I eat because it's meal time." For many, the routine of eating is an agony to minimize or avoid by skipping breakfast or using instant powders or fast foods. Others snack through the day without ever sitting down to a meal!

To achieve historical perspective, we must go back in time to the beginning—to the Garden of Eden and the Tree of Knowledge.

God took the man and put him into the Garden of Eden to work it and keep it. God commanded the man, saying, "You may freely eat from every tree of the garden. But from the Tree of Knowledge of good and evil do not eat, for on the day you eat from it, you will surely die" (Genesis 2:15–17).

If only the first man, Adam, had kept on occupying himself with Torah and with guarding the way to the Tree of Life, he would have continued to stroll through the Garden of Eden like one of the guardian angels. Shortly after God created Eve, in the afternoon of the first Friday of Creation, the first couple in the world committed the first sin by eating the forbidden fruit of the Tree of Knowledge of good and evil. If they had only waited a few hours for Shabbos, they could have eaten the fruit with God's blessings (*Shaar ha-Kavanos*, Rosh Hashanah, Discourse A).

From the Sources

Since maintaining a healthy and sound body is among the ways of God—for one cannot understand or have any knowledge of the Creator, if he is ill—therefore, one must avoid that which harms the body and accustom himself to that which is healthful and helps the body become stronger.

Maimonides, *Mishneh Torah*, Book of Knowledge 4:1.

The FDA's Food Pyramid Guidelines

- Breads, cereals, rice, and pasta: 6 to 11 servings (1 slice of bread; 1 ounce of ready-to-eat cereal; 1/2 cup of cooked cereal; 1/2 cup of cooked cereal, rice, or pasta)
- Vegetables: 3 to 5 servings (1 cup of raw leafy vegetables; 1/2 cup of other vegetables; 3/4 cup of vegetable juice)
- Fruits: 2 to 4 servings (1 medium apple, banana, orange; 1/2 cup of chopped, cooked, or canned fruit; 3/4 cup of fruit juice)
- Milk, yogurt, and cheese: 2 to 3 servings (1 cup of milk or yogurt; 1-1/2 ounces of natural cheese; 2 ounces of processed cheese)
- Meat, poultry, fish, dry beans and peas, eggs, nuts, and seeds: 2 to 3 servings (2 to 3 ounces of cooked lean meat, poultry, or fish; 1 cup of cooked dry beans or 1 egg counts as 1 ounce of lean meat; 2 tablespoons of peanut butter or 1/3 cup of nuts count as 1 ounce of meat)

Hadassah Health Memo, Winter 2001.

Likewise, we read in the Torah: "The woman saw that the tree was good for food and desirable to the eyes, and the tree was attractive as a means to gain intelligence. She took some of its fruit and ate, and also gave some to her husband, and he ate" (Genesis 3:6).

The trees were real trees, the fruits were real fruits, and the eating was actual eating, but the fruits were fine and the eating was delicate. As Rabbi Moshe Chaim Luzzatto explains, the eating from the Tree of Knowledge introduced desire for all material, bodily pleasures, and for all sins.

In the beginning, good and evil had been separate, both in the fruit and in the entire world. But when the sin of the Tree of Knowledge corrupted the world, good became mixed with evil. Sparks of holiness fell into their husks, and the pure combined with the impure. Man was sentenced to work hard for his food and to die. The world became more coarse.

It is clear that the soul is not nourished by physical bread, as the body is. The food we eat is actually a combination of both a physical and a spiritual entity. The body is nourished by the physical aspects, or nutrients, contained in the foods we eat; the soul is nourished by the spiritual power—or sparks of holiness—that enlivens the physical substance of all matter, including food. Therefore, body and soul are united in the act of eating (Ruach Chaim on *Pirkei Avot* 3:3; Code of Jewish Law OC 6:1, with Magen Avraham).

We have seen that all of creation is composed of a mixture of good and evil. Likewise, in every food that a person eats, there is a combination of good and evil. Food physically consists of good counterparts, that is, nutrients, and bad aspects, that is, waste or indigestible matter. Likewise, spiritually, food contains sparks of holiness, or good components, and husks, or *kelipot*, which are the gross, bad components that encompass the sparks.

    Yaakov Levinson

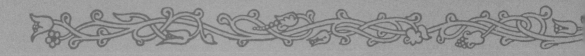

Chapter 17

Making Your Kitchen Healthy
✑ *Food, Halakhah, and Hygiene*

Each day we ask *Hashem* to cure us or our loved ones from illness ("*Refa'ainu Hash-m V'neirafeh*"). We also beseech him to protect us from the various causes of illness, such as those from bacterial infections, rough weather conditions, poverty, intemperance of food and drink, or the malfunctioning of a part of our body or mind. Yet we ourselves are obligated to make our own efforts to avoid dangers such as food spoilage or inappropriate safety precautions during food preparation.

People are tempted, at times, to take dangerous shortcuts in their kitchen, which may be tantamount, heaven forbid, to serving poisonous foods to the family.

We have to learn and then remind ourselves of the basic rules of Torah hygiene and to be careful that we do not become sloppy or lazy in our kitchen habits.

The Torah instructs us to guard our health and life (*Devarim* 4:9,15) and, as the Talmud explains (*Berachos* 32b), this refers to our physical safety.

Rabbi Yisroel Salanter has said that this *mitzvah* to protect one's health is, in a sense, the greatest *mitzvah* of the Torah because being healthy enables one to fulfill all of the other *mitzvot*.

When shopping, we are advised to buy the cold or frozen items last and to get them home in time to be refrigerated promptly. Food should not be left out when brought home or cooked more than two hours before refrigeration. Leftovers from a meal should be refrigerated promptly.

> ### *From the Sources*
>
> The following three are but a few examples of rabbinic wisdom in dealing with food preparation.
>
> - The Talmud (*Bava Metzia* 29b) teaches that one should not drink warm water without first boiling it.
> - It is a *mitzvah* to ensure that all eggs, meat, and poultry are thoroughly cooked in order to kill any salmonella bacteria that may be present.
> - Proper food handling begins with hand washing. The Mishnah *Berurah* (4:14) taught that one should be careful not to touch any food without first washing his hands. If the food was touched, it should be rinsed three times.

The Raavad said that one should not say, "Let me eat it; I can't throw it out. It is *bal tashchis.*" If the food is spoiled, then ingesting it would be destructive to his body (*"bal tashchis d'gufo"*), much worse than any waste of food might be.

> ### *From the Sources*
>
> The rabbis even prescribed the kind of food men should eat and that from which they should abstain.
>
> - Wheat bread, fat meat, and old wine are recommended as the most wholesome (*Pesachim* 42a).
> - Salt and hot soup are pronounced to be essentials of a meal (*Berachot* 44a).
> - "After all solid food eat salt, and after all beverages drink water" is the advice of the rabbis (*Berachot* 40a).

Food that was inadvertently left out must be discarded, even if it does not smell spoiled, for someone still might become ill. "When in doubt, throw it out."

As kosher consumers, it is our duty to realize that our kitchens are actually frontiers of *mitzvah* opportunities, including making sure that the food we share is both kosher and healthy.

෧ *Rabbi Moshe Goldberger*

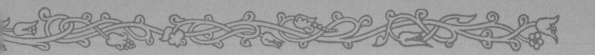

Chapter 18

Vegetarianism and Judaism: Frequently Asked Questions

What is Jewish about vegetarianism?

All the reasons for becoming vegetarian can be connected to important Jewish values. These include taking care of our health, showing compassion to animals, protecting the environment, conserving resources, helping hungry people, and seeking and pursuing peace. As later responses indicate, many teachings in the Torah, the Talmud, and other sacred Jewish texts can be used to argue that vegetarianism is the diet most consistent with Jewish values.

Why did God give people permission to eat meat?

People are not always ready to live up to God's highest ideals. By the time of Noah, humanity had degenerated greatly. "And God saw the earth, and behold it was corrupt; for all flesh had corrupted their way upon the earth" (Genesis 6:12). People had sunk so low that they would eat a limb torn from a living animal. As a concession to people's weakness, permission to eat meat was then given: "Every moving thing that lives shall be food for you; as the green herb have I given you all" (Genesis 9:3).

Weren't people given dominion over animals? Didn't God put them here for our use?

Dominion does not mean that we have the right to conquer and exploit animals. Immediately after God gave people dominion over

> ### From the Sources
>
> Rabbi Huna said, "No scholar should dwell in a town where vegetables are unobtainable."
>
> Talmud, *Eruvin* 55b.

animals (Genesis 1:26), he prohibited their use for food (Genesis 1:29). *Dominion* means guardianship or stewardship—being coworkers with God in taking care of and improving the world.

The Talmud interprets *dominion* as the privilege of using animals for labor only (*Sanhedrin* 59b). It is extremely doubtful that the concept of dominion permits breeding animals and treating them as machines designed solely to fulfill our needs.

Rav Kook (1865–1935), the first chief rabbi of prestatehood Israel, stated that dominion does not imply the rule of a haughty despot who tyrannically governs for his own personal selfish ends and with a stubborn heart. He rejected the idea that such a repulsive form of servitude could be forever sealed in the world of God whose "tender mercies are over all His work" (Psalms 145:9).

Rabbi Samson Raphael Hirsch (1808–1888) stressed that people have not been given the right or the power to have everything subservient to them. In commenting on Genesis 1:26, he stated,

> The earth and its creatures may have other relationships of which we are ignorant, in which they serve their own purposes. Thus, above people's control over nature there is a divine control to serve God's purposes and objectives, and people have no right to interfere. Hence, people, according to Judaism, do not have an unlimited right to use and abuse animals and other parts of nature.

If God wanted us to have vegetarian diets and not harm animals, why were the Temple sacrificial services established?

During the time of Moses, it was the general practice among all nations to worship by means of sacrifice. There were many associated idolatrous practices. The great Jewish philosopher Maimonides (1135–1204) wrote that God did not command the Israelites to give up and discontinue all these manners of service because "to obey such a commandment would have been contrary to the nature of man, who generally cleaves to that to which he is accustomed." For this reason, God allowed Jews to make sacrifices, but "He transferred to His service that which had served as a worship of created beings and of things imaginary and unreal." The elements of idolatry were removed. Maimonides concluded:

> By this divine plan it was effected that the traces of idolatry were blotted out, and the truly great principle of our Faith, the Existence and Unity of God, was established. This result was thus obtained without confusing the minds of the people by the abolition of a service they were accustomed to and which was familiar to them.

The Jewish philosopher Abarbanel (1437–1502) reinforced Maimonides' argument. He cited a *Midrash* that indicated that the Jews had become accustomed to sacrifices in Egypt. To wean them from these idolatrous practices, God tolerated the sacrifices but commanded that they be offered in one central sanctuary: "Thereupon the Holy One, blessed be He, said 'Let them at all times offer their sacrifices before Me in the Tabernacle, and they will be weaned from idolatry, and thus be saved.'" Rabbi J. H. Hertz, former Chief Rabbi of England, stated that if Moses had not instituted sacrifices, which were admitted by all to have been the universal expression of religious homage, his mission would have failed and Judaism would have disappeared. After the destruction of the Temple, Rabbi Yochanan Ben Zakkai stated that prayer and good deeds should take the place of sacrifice.

Rashi indicated that God did not want the Israelites to bring sacrifices; it was their choice. He bases this on the haftorah (portion from the Prophets) read on the Sabbath when the book of Leviticus, which discusses sacrifices, is read: "I have not burdened thee with a meal-offering, nor wearied thee with frankincense" (Isaiah 43:23).

Biblical commentator David Kimchi (1160–1235) also believed that the sacrifices were voluntary. He ascertained this from the words of Jeremiah:

> For I spoke not unto your fathers, nor commanded them on the day that I brought them out of the land of Egypt, concerning burnt-offerings or sacrifices; but this thing I commanded them,

saying, "Obey my voice, and I will be your God, and ye shall be my people; and walk ye in all the ways that I have commanded you, that it may be well unto you (Jeremiah 7:22–23).

Kimchi noted that nowhere in the Ten Commandments is there any reference to sacrifice, and even when sacrifices are first mentioned (Leviticus 1:2), the expression used is "when any man of you bringeth an offering"; the first Hebrew word *ki*, being literally "if," implies that it was a voluntary act.

Sacrifices, especially animal sacrifices, were not the primary concern of God. As a matter of fact, they could be an abomination to God if not carried out together with deeds of loving kindness and justice. Consider these words of the prophets, the spokespeople of God:

"I desire mercy, not sacrifice." (Hosea 6:6)

"To what purpose is the multitude of your sacrifices unto Me?" says the Lord. "I am full of the burnt offerings of rams, and the fat of fed beasts; and I delight not in the blood of bullocks, or of lambs or of he-goats. Bring no more vain oblations. Your new moon and your appointed feasts my soul hates; . . . and when you spread forth your hands, I will hide my eyes from you; yes, when you make many prayers, I will not hear; your hands are full of blood." (Isaiah 1:11–16)

"I hate, I despise your feasts, and I will take no delight in your solemn assemblies. Though you offer me burnt-offerings and your meal offerings, I will not accept them; neither will I regard the peace-offerings of your fat beasts. Take thou away from me the noise of thy song; and let Me not hear the melody of thy psalteries. But let justice well up as waters, and righteousness as a mighty stream." (Amos 5:21–24)

Deeds of compassion and kindness toward all creation are of greater significance to God than sacrifices: "To do charity and justice is more acceptable to the Lord than sacrifice." (Proverbs 21:3).

Why were the laws of kashrut (the kosher laws) given?

Along with permission to eat meat, many laws and restrictions (the laws of kashrut) were given. These laws were designed to sanctify the act of eating and to keep people from taking the everyday act of eating for granted.

Rav Kook believed that the regulations related to the consumption of meat implied a reprimand and is an elaborate apparatus designed to keep alive a sense of reverence for life and to lead people away from their meat-eating habit. This is echoed by Torah commentator Solomon Efraim Lunchitz in *K'lee Yakar,* his commentary on the Torah:

> What was the necessity for the entire procedure of ritual slaughter? For the sake of self-discipline. It is far more appropriate for man not to eat meat; only if he has a strong desire for meat does the Torah permit it, and even this only after the trouble and inconvenience necessary to satisfy his desire. Perhaps because of the bother and annoyance of the whole procedure, he will be restrained from such a strong and uncontrollable desire for meat.

During the messianic period, when the Temple in Jerusalem is rebuilt, won't the sacrificial services be restored, and won't people have to eat meat?

Rav Kook and Joseph Albo (fl. 15th cent.) believed that in the days of the messiah, people will again be vegetarians. Rav Kook stated that in the messianic epoch, "the effect of knowledge will spread even to animals . . . and sacrifices in the Temple will consist of vegetation, and it will be pleasing to God as in days of old." He believed that

---

From the Sources

Accordingly, the laws of kashrut come to teach us that a Jew's first preference should be a vegetarian meal. If however one cannot control a craving for meat, it should be kosher meat, which would serve as a reminder that the animal being eaten is a creature of God, that the death of such a creature cannot be taken lightly, that hunting for sport is forbidden, that we cannot treat any living being callously, and that we are responsible for what happens to other beings (human or animal) even if we did not personally come into contact with them.

Pinchas Peli, a modern rabbi, in *Torah Today.*

at that time human conduct will have advanced to such high standards that there will no longer be need for animal sacrifices to atone for sins. Only nonanimal sacrifices (grains, for example) to express gratitude to God would remain.

There is a *midrash* (teaching based on Jewish values and tradition) that states: "In the messianic era, all offerings will cease except the thanksgiving offering, which will continue forever." Rav Kook based his view on the prophecy of Isaiah:

> And the wolf shall dwell with the lamb, And the leopard shall lie down with the kid; And the calf and the young lion and the fatling together; And a little child shall lead them. And the cow and the bear shall feed; Their young ones shall lie down together, And the lion shall eat straw like the ox. They shall not hurt nor destroy in all My holy mountain (Isaiah 11:6–9).

Wasn't Genesis 1:29 (the first dietary law) overridden by later biblical commandments and teachings?

Although God's original intention was that people be vegetarians, God later gave permission for meat to be eaten as a reluctant concession to people's weakness. Many biblical commentators regard vegetarianism as the ideal diet, and modern science has verified that our body structure and digestive system are most consistent with this type of diet.

In a *teshuvah* (response to a question related to Jewish law), Rabbi Moshe Halevi Steinberg expressed his belief that the fact that meat was initially forbidden and later permitted indicates that each person is thereby given a free hand to either be a vegetarian, as was the first human, or to eat meat, as Noah did.

The question is then on what basis should that choice be made? Should it be on the basis of convenience, habit, and conformity or on considerations of basic Jewish values and teachings?

Rabbi Alfred Cohen wrote that "the Torah does not establish the eating of meat as a desirable activity, only as something which is not forbidden to do."

Inconsistent with Judaism, doesn't vegetarianism elevate animals to a level equal to that of people?

Concern for animals and a refusal to treat them brutally and slaughter them for food that is not necessary for proper nutrition (indeed, is harmful to human health) does not mean that vegetarians regard animals as equal to people.

The test of our behavior toward animals should be, as the British philosopher Jeremy Bentham (1748–1832) put it, "not can they reason, nor can they talk, but can they suffer?" And the great Jewish philosopher Maimonides felt that animals are like people in fleeing from pain and death.

If Jews don't eat meat, won't they be deprived of the opportunity to do many mitzvot *(commandments)?*

There are other cases where laws were provided to regulate things that God would prefer people not to do. For example, God wishes people to live at peace, but he provides commandments related to war, because he knows that human beings quarrel and seek victories over others. Similarly, the laws in thc Torah related to slavery are a concession to human weakness.

As indicated before, by not eating meat, Jews are acting consistently with many *mitzvot,* such as showing compassion to animals, preserving health, not wasting, feeding the hungry, and preserving the earth. Also, by not eating meat, a Jew cannot violate several prohibitions of the Torah, such as mixing meat and milk, eating nonkosher animals, and eating blood or fat.

Judaism considers it an averach *(sin) not to take advantage of the pleasurable things that God has put on the earth. As he put animals on the earth, and it is pleasurable to eat them, is it not an* averach *to refrain from eating meat?*

Can eating meat be pleasurable to a religious person when he or she knows that, as a result, health is endangered, grain is wasted, and animals are being cruelly treated? There are many other ways to gain pleasure without doing harm to living creatures. The prohibition against abstaining from pleasurable things only applies when there is no plausible basis for the abstention; vegetarians abstain because eating meat is injurious to health, because their soul rebels against eating a living creature, or because they wish to have a diet that minimizes threats to the environment and that best shares resources with hungry people.

There are other cases in Judaism where actions that some people consider pleasurable are forbidden or discouraged, such as using tobacco, drinking liquor to excess, having sexual relations out of wedlock, and hunting.

Don't the laws of shechitah *provide for a humane slaughter of animals so that we need not be concerned with violations of* tsa'ar ba'alei chayim *(undue suffering of animals)?*

It is true that *shechitah* has been found in scientific tests conducted in the United States and other countries to be a relatively painless method of slaughter. But can we consider only the final minutes of an animal's life? What about the tremendous pain and cruelty involved in the entire process of raising and transporting animals? When the consumption of meat is not necessary and is even harmful to people's health, can any method of slaughter be considered humane? Is this not a contradiction in terms?

Some animal rights advocates have been critical of *shechitah* because of the practice of shackling and hoisting, a very painful process in which the animal is raised off the ground by its hind leg prior to slaughter. It is important to recognize that shackling and hoisting is not a necessary part of *shechitah*. It was instituted by the U.S. Department of Agriculture in 1906 in order to avoid the blood of diseased animals contaminating other animals when they were cast on the floor.

Fortunately, an alternative, more humane method that is acceptable to Jewish law has been developed and put into practice in many slaughterhouses. Holding pens have been developed that meet the requirements of ritual slaughter and also U.S. Department of Agriculture requirements, while avoiding the use of shackling and hoisting. These pens have been endorsed by the Jewish Joint Advisory Committee on *shechitah*, the Rabbinical Council of America, and prominent Orthodox rabbis.

Several animal rights groups have pushed for legislation banning shackling and hoisting. Unfortunately, some anti-Semitic groups have used the issue to try to attack *shechita*. The Jewish community must work to extend the use of humane alternatives to shackling and hoisting, primarily to avoid *tsa'ar ba'alei chayim*, but also to reduce criticism. Of course, as indicated earlier, the best way to be consistent with Jewish teachings concerning animals is to be a vegetarian.

Won't a movement by Jews toward vegetarianism mean less emphasis on kashrut (the Jewish kosher laws) and eventually a disregard of these laws?

Quite the contrary. One of the underpinnings of the laws of kashrut is reverence for life, which is consistent with vegetarianism. Another is to avoid pagan practices, which often involved much cruelty to animals and people. This too is consistent with vegetarian ideals.

In many ways, becoming a vegetarian makes it easier and cheaper to observe the laws of kashrut; this might attract many new adherents to keeping kosher and eventually to other important Jewish values. As a vegetarian, one need not be concerned with using separate dishes; mixing milchigs (dairy products) with fleischigs (meat products); waiting three or six hours after eating meat before being allowed to eat dairy products; storing four sets (two for regular use and two for Passover use) of dishes, silverware, pots, and pans; and many other considerations that must concern the nonvegetarian who wishes to observe kashrut strictly. In addition, a vegetarian is in no danger of eating blood or fat, which are prohibited, or the flesh of a nonkosher animal. It should be noted that being a vegetarian does not automatically guarantee that one will maintain the laws of kashrut as, for example, certain baked goods and cheeses may not be kosher. When in doubt, a trusted rabbinic authority should be consulted.

Some people today reject kashrut because of the high costs involved. Since a person can obtain proper nourishment at far lower costs with a vegetarian diet, this may prevent the loss of many kashrut observers.

There are several examples in Jewish history when a change to vegetarianism enabled Jews to adhere to kashrut. As indicated in the Book of Daniel, Daniel and his companions were able to avoid eating nonkosher food by adopting a vegetarian diet (Daniel 1:8–16). The historian Josephus relates how some Jewish priests on trial in Rome ate only figs and nuts to avoid eating flesh that had been used in idol worship. Some Maccabees, during the struggles against the Syrians, escaped to the mountains, where they lived on only plant foods to avoid "being polluted like the rest" (by eating nonkosher foods).

Isn't a movement toward vegetarianism a movement away from Jewish traditions with regard to diet? Isn't there a danger that once some traditions are changed, others may readily follow, and little will be left of Judaism as we have known it?

Jewish law is based on a two-part structure: written law (the Jewish Bible) and oral law (Talmud, responsa literature, and other rabbinic writings). Although the written law remains the unchanging base, the oral law has components that are constantly adapting to current conditions. This system has kept Judaism as alive and applicable today as it was centuries ago. In contemporary times, the vast responsa literature of this century has enabled new traditions to form within halakhic bounds.

A move toward vegetarianism is actually a return to Jewish traditions, to taking Jewish values seriously. A movement toward vegetarianism can help revitalize Judaism. It can show that Jewish values can be applied to help solve current world problems related to hunger, waste, and pollution. Hence, rather than a movement away from Jewish traditions, it would have the opposite effect.

Weren't the Jewish sages aware of the evils related to eating meat? If so, why does so much of Talmudic literature discuss laws and customs related to the consumption of meat? Are you suggesting that Judaism has been morally wrong in not advocating vegetarianism?

Conditions today differ greatly from those in biblical times and throughout most of Jewish history. Only recently has strong medical evidence linked a meat-centered diet to many types of disease. Modern intensive livestock agriculture results in conditions quite different from those that prevailed previously. As indicated, to produce meat today, animals are treated very cruelly; they are fed tremendous amounts of grain (and chemicals) while millions of people starve, and much pollution and misuse of resources result. When it was felt that eating meat was necessary for health and the many problems related to modern intensive livestock agriculture did not exist, the Jewish sages were not morally wrong in not advocating vegetarianism.

By putting vegetarian values ahead of Jewish teachings, aren't vegetarians, in effect, creating a new religion, with values contrary to Jewish teachings?

Jewish vegetarians do not place so-called vegetarian values above Torah principles. They are saying that Jewish values mandate that we treat animals with compassion, guard our health, share with hungry people, protect the environment, conserve resources, and seek peace and hence point to vegetarianism as the ideal diet for Jews today, especially in view of the many problems related to modern methods of raising animals on factory farms. Rather than rejecting Torah values, Jewish vegetarians are challenging the Jewish community to apply Torah values to their diets in a daily meaningful way. They are respectfully challenging Jews to live up to Judaism's splendid teachings.

Aren't vegetarians being more righteous than God, since God gave permission to eat meat?

There is no obligation to eat meat today. God's first dietary law (Genesis 1:29) was strictly vegetarian; also, as discussed before, according to Rav Kook and others, the messianic epoch will be vegetarian.

Jewish vegetarians believe their diet is most consistent with God's desires that we protect our health, be kind to animals, share with hungry people, protect the environment, and conserve resources. Rather than being more righteous than God, they are urging people to live up to God's highest ideals.

This viewpoint is conceded by Rabbi Alfred Cohen: "If a person tends toward vegetarianism because he sees it as a lifestyle consonant with the way the All-Mighty really wanted the world to be, there can be no denying that he has a valid point of view."

How can you advocate making changes in Judaism?

What is really advocated is a return to Jewish values of showing compassion, sharing, helping the needy, preserving the environment, conserving resources, and seeking peace. Also, rabbinic enactments to meet changing conditions have historically been part of Judaism. Of course, changes must be consistent with Jewish values and teachings.

Finally, global threats today—pollution, hunger, resource scarcity, violence—are so great that a new thinking or rethinking about values and new methods is necessary. Albert Einstein's statement, "The unleashed power of the atom has changed everything except our ways of thinking; hence we drift toward unparalleled catastrophe," has a parallel to the effects of our diets today.

Jewish vegetarians are not advocating that changes be made in the Torah but that the Torah be used to master present world conditions, as it has in the past. Global survival today requires the application of Torah values to our diets, as well as other aspects of our lives.

Because the majority of Jews will probably continue to eat meat, isn't it better that they do so without being aware of the Jewish principles such as bal tashchit *(the mandate not to waste resources),* tsa'ar ba'alei chayim *(the mandate to avoid causing unnecessary harm to animals), and* pikuach nefesh *(the mandate to protect human life) that are being violated? Shouldn't a Jewish vegetarian abstain from meat quietly and not try to convert others to his or her type of diet?*

This is a common attitude. Many people feel that if there are benefits to vegetarianism and if some people want to have such a diet, fine. But they should keep it to themselves and not try to convert others.

The question really becomes one of how seriously we take Jewish values. Are we to ignore Torah mandates to preserve our health, show compassion for animals, not waste, help feed the hungry, preserve the earth, and many others that are violated directly or indirectly by meat-centered diets? Is it proper that people be kept uninformed about the many violations of Torah law so that they can continue their eating habits with a clear conscience?

Judaism teaches that one should try to teach others and assist them to carry out commandments. A Hasidic teacher asserts: "Man, the master of choice, shall say: 'Only for my sake was the whole world created!' Therefore every man shall be watchful and strive to redeem the world and supply that wherein it is lacking, at all times and in all places."

Given that Rav Kook felt that a vegetarian period would come later, after people had moved to a more ethical level and there was much progress in solving problems affecting people, shouldn't we refrain from promoting vegetarianism today?

Because many problems related to modern intensive livestock agriculture have become far worse since Rav Kook passed away in 1935, one can only wonder what his view would be today if he were aware of the epidemic of disease, the soaring medical costs that result in cuts in other essential social services, the increasing environmental threats, the widespread hunger, the cruel treatment of animals, and other negative effects of animal-centered diets.

As indicated previously, a consideration of vegetarianism is not a retreat from concern about improving people and their lives and is not focusing on issues that can wait for human improvement. It is, arguably, the most important thing that can be done to improve the lot of the world's people and our imperiled planet, as well as to show that the Torah has a message that can help combat today's many threats.

How would a Jewish vegetarian celebrate Pesach (Passover)?

Today there is no need to cook or eat meat on Passover. The eating of the Pascal lamb is no longer required now that the Temple has been destroyed. One is required to commemorate this act, not to participate in it. The late Dayan Feldman stated that mushrooms, which have a fleshy appearance, can be used on the Seder plate to commemorate the Pascal lamb. The Talmud indicates that a broiled beet can be used.

The proper celebration of Passover requires the absence of leaven and the use of unleavened bread, which we are commanded to eat "throughout your generations." There are many vegetarian recipes that are appropriate for Seders and other Passover meals, a number of which can be found in some of the books listed in the bibliography at my Internet site.

Because Passover is the celebration of our redemption from slavery, we should also consider freeing ourselves from the slavery to harmful eating habits. As our homes are freed from leaven, perhaps we should also free our bodies from harmful foods. Because Passover is a time of regeneration, physical as well as spiritual, the maximum use should be made of raw fruits and vegetables, which have cleansing properties.

There are other Passover themes related to vegetarian ideas. The call at the Seders for "all who are hungry to come and eat" can be a reminder that our diets can be a factor in reducing global starvation. The Passover theme of freedom is related to the horrible conditions of slavery under which animals are raised today (see http://www.jewish veg.com/schwartz).

In Jewish literature, it is stated that with the advent of the messiah, a banquet will be given by God to the righteous in which the flesh of the giant fish—leviathan—will be served. Isn't this inconsistent with the idea that the messianic period will be vegetarian?

These legends concerning the leviathan are interpreted as allegories by most Jewish scholars. According to Maimonides, the banquet is an allusion to the spiritual enjoyment of the intellect. Abarbanel and others consider the expressions about the leviathan to be allusions to the destruction of the powers that are hostile to the Jews.

Isn't much of Judaism today related to the use of animals for teaching and ritual purposes? Consider the Sefer Torah, tefillin, the shofar (ram's horn used on Rosh Hashanah and at the end of Yom Kippur), and so forth.

The number of animals slaughtered for these purposes is minute compared to the billions killed annually for food. The fact that there would still be some animals slaughtered to meet Jewish ritual needs shouldn't stop us from doing all we can to end the horrible abuses of factory farming. Also, most problems related to animal-centered diets—poor human health, waste of food and other resources, and ecological threats—would not occur if animals were slaughtered only to meet Jewish ritual needs. Our emphasis should be on doing a minimum amount of harm to other people, the environment, and animals. In addition, for *hiddur* (enhancement of) *mitzvah*, it would be better if ritual objects were made from animals who at least led cruelty-free lives. Also, *tefillin* can be made from the leather of animals that were raised without cruelty and died a natural death.

Some people believe that vegetarians are supposed to aspire to become vegans (people who don't use milk, eggs, leather, honey, or any product from an animal). How can an orthodox Jew be a vegan, since he would not be able to use tefillin, a shofar, a Sefer Torah, and other ritual items?

If a person became a vegetarian but not a vegan, he or she would still do much good for animals, the environment, hungry people, and the preservation of his or her health. If a person embraces veganism except in cases where specific *mitzvot* require the use of some animal product, even more good will be done.

Once again, it is important to emphasize that the religious items mentioned can be made from animals that were raised compassionately and died natural deaths.

What would happen to butchers, shochtim, *and others dependent for a livelihood on the consumption of meat?*

There could be a shift from the production of flesh products to that of nutritious vegetarian dishes. In England during World War II, when there was a shortage of meat, butchers relied mainly on the sale of fruits and vegetables. Today, new businesses could sell such food products as tofu, miso, falafel, soy burgers, and vegetarian *cholent* (stew).

The change to vegetarianism would probably be gradual. This would provide time for a transition to other jobs. Some of the funds saved by individuals and groups because of lower food and health costs should be used to provide incomes for people during the retraining period.

The same kind of question can be asked about other moral issues. What would happen to all the arms merchants if we had universal peace? What would happen to doctors and nurses if people took better care of themselves, stopped smoking, improved their diets, and so on? Immoral or inefficient practices should not be supported by pointing out that some people earn a living from them.

What if everyone became vegetarian? Wouldn't animals overrun the earth?

This concern is based on an insufficient understanding of animal behavior, both natural and under present factory conditions. There are not millions of turkeys around at Thanksgiving because they want to help celebrate the holiday but because farmers want them to exist. The breeders, not the animals themselves, control the breeding behavior and thus the number of stock. Recent studies have shown that animals, in natural conditions, adjust their numbers to fit their environment and food supply. An end to the distortion of the sex lives of animals to suit our needs would lead to a decrease, rather than an increase, in animals.

We are not overrun by the animals that we do not eat, such as lions, elephants, and crocodiles. The problem often is that of the extinction of animals rather than their overrunning the earth. There are many meat-bearing animals today because they are raised under rigid, breeding-controlled environments.

Instead of advocating vegetarianism, shouldn't we try to alleviate the evils of the factory-farming system so that animals are treated better, less grain is wasted, and fewer health-harming chemicals are used?

The breeding of animals is a big business, whose prime concern is profit. Animals are raised the way they are today because it increases profits. Improving conditions, as suggested by this question, would certainly be a step in the right direction, but it would be strongly resisted by the meat industry and, if successful, would greatly increase already high prices.

Here are two counterquestions: (1) Why not abstain from eating meat as a protest against present policies while trying to improve them? (2) Even under the best of conditions, why take the life of a creature of God, "whose tender mercies are over all His creatures," when it is not necessary for proper nutrition?

Isn't it important that we keep our priorities straight? How can we be so concerned about animals when there are so many critical problems related to people today?

Certainly, many critical issues face the world today. I have written two other books, *Judaism and Global Survival* and *Mathematics and Global Survival*, which address current world problems.

There is an ecological principle that "everything is connected to everything else." This means that every action has many ramifications. Hence, adopting vegetarian diets not only reduces brutal treatment of animals; it also improves human health, reduces stress on threatened ecosystems, conserves resources, and provides the potential to reduce widespread hunger. In view of the many threats related to livestock agriculture, next to attempting to reduce the chance of nuclear war, working to promote vegetarianism may be the most important action one can take for global survival.

While it is true that some people who love animals are cruel to people, the reverse is more often the case: those who are cruel to animals are also cruel to human beings. Some of history's greatest humanitarians were vegetarians or strong advocates of vegetarianism, or both. These include Plutarch, Leonardo da Vinci, Sir Isaac Newton, Jean Jacques Rousseau, General William Booth, Ralph Waldo Emerson, Henry David Thoreau, Percy Bysshe Shelley, J. H. Kellogg, Horace Greeley, Susan B. Anthony, Leo Tolstoy, Upton Sinclair,

H. G. Wells, George Bernard Shaw, Albert Schweitzer, and Mahatma Gandhi. Among Jewish vegetarian humanists are Isaac Bashevis Singer, Shmuel Yosef Agnon, Franz Kafka, and Isaac Leib Peretz, as well as several chief rabbis.

How can an Orthodox Jewish vegetarian pray for the restoration of the Temple sacrificial services?

This response is based on an essay by Rabbi David Rosen, former chief rabbi of Ireland. He reminds us that Maimonides believed that the sacrifices were a concession to the times and that Rav Kook felt that the messianic period in which the Temple would be rebuilt will be a vegetarian period and that the Temple service can be maintained without animal sacrifices, as is indicated by the previously mentioned teaching that states that "in the future all sacrifices will be abolished, except for meal offerings." He argues that the liturgy in the Sabbath and festival *musaph* (additional) service need not be understood as expressing a hope for the restoration of animal sacrifices. Rather, it can be interpreted as a recognition on our part of the devotion and dedication to God that our ancestors showed and an expression of our hope that we may be inspired to show the same spirit of devotion in our own way.

If vegetarian diets are best for health, why don't doctors recommend them?

According to Julian M. Whitaker, M.D., author of *Reversing Heart Disease and Reversing Diabetes,* there seem to be three aspects of modern medicine that work together to discourage the use of diet and exercise as primary tools of treatment:

1. *Modern physicians are taught to prescribe.* Medical schools teach that prescription drugs are the most powerful tools available for treating disease. Unfortunately, nutrition is barely taught in medical schools, and many doctors lack information about the relationships between food and health. The accepted approach today seems to be to prescribe first and, perhaps, recommend a diet as an afterthought.

2. *There has recently been an explosion of technology in medicine, from which many alternative diagnoses and treatments have sprung.* For example, in the heart disease treatment field, physicians

can call on such diagnostic techniques as the CAT scan, the angiogram, the echocardiagram, and the thallium scan. Based on this diagnostic power, patients are increasingly funneled into increasingly more aggressive therapies, such as bypass surgery.

3. *There are many pressures to conform in the medical field.* Conforming to medical norms provides a degree of safety during various phases of the physicians' education and medical practice. Hence the current enthusiasm for drugs and technology that is promoted by medical training is perpetuated by conformity in professional practice.

Why don't medical and governmental authorities recommend vegetarianism?

There have been some medical and governmental indications of the benefits of vegetarian diets. For example, as long ago as June 1961, an editorial in the *Journal of the American Medical Association* indicated that a vegetarian diet can prevent 90 percent of strokes and 97 percent of heart attacks. The U.S. Senate Select Committee on Nutrition and Human Needs recommended in February 1977 that Americans decrease their consumption of meat and increase their consumption of fruits, vegetables, and whole grains. Also, the 1988 report of the U.S. Surgeon General indicated the many negative health effects of meat-centered diets and recommended an increase in the consumption of plant-based foods. Perhaps more will be done in the future, but the factors given in the previous answer still have to be overcome.

Doesn't humane legislation ensure the welfare of farm animals?

On both state and federal levels, the raising of animals for food is specifically exempted from every piece of humane legislation. Strong opposition from the powerful farm lobby has defeated every legislative effort to even study the treatment of farm animals.

Since animals kill each other in nature, why should we be concerned about killing animals for food?

Predator animals have no choice. They must eat other animals in order to live. Perhaps this is the way that nature takes care of old and weak animals that would not be able to survive much longer anyway. But human beings do have a choice, and we now know that we can be very healthy on a vegetarian diet, in fact, far healthier than on a meat-based diet. Hence there is no good reason to raise and slaughter animals for food.

Do you believe that flesh should not be served at Jewish functions and that all Jews should be vegetarians?

Because the realities of livestock agriculture are inconsistent with basic Jewish values, Jews should ideally be vegetarians, and flesh should not be served at Jewish functions. But since the Torah does give permission for people to eat meat (as a concession to human weakness), people have been given the free will to make a decision. The purpose of these questions and answers is to give Jews and others the information to help them make a decision that is informed and is based on Jewish teachings.

Doesn't the Torah mandate that we eat korban Pesach *(the Passover sacrifice) and other* korbanos *(sacrifices)?*

Without the Temple, the sacrificial requirements are not applicable today. And, as indicated, Rav Kook felt, based on the prophecy of Isaiah, that there will only be sacrifices involving vegetarian foods during the messianic period.

Aren't people who abstain from eating meat but who consume eggs and milk being hypocritical?

Many of the arguments made for not eating meat are valid with regard to eggs and milk. Factory farming also cruelly treats egg-laying chickens and dairy cows, wastes resources, and pollutes the environment.

The vegan diet (which uses no animal products) is a more humane diet. However, an estimated 90 percent of vegetarians today are lacto-ovo vegetarians. Many hope to become vegans eventually.

Rather than looking at vegetarians who consume eggs and milk as hypocrites, I prefer to look at them as people who have made an important ethical decision but who have not yet gone as far as they can in terms of a humane, sensible diet. One can become a vegetarian by degrees. What is important is to take the first step and then progress toward your goal.

Isn't it hypocritical for a vegetarian to wear leather shoes and use other leather products?

It depends on one's reasons for being a vegetarian. If it is based on health rather than concern for animals, for example, it would not be inconsistent. Some vegetarians use leather products because these are by-products of slaughter rather than prime causes of it. Many vegetarians have changed to shoes of natural or synthetic, nonanimal materials. It has become easier to get such products recently, as the demand for them has increased. Some vegetarians continue to wear leather products until they wear out and then purchase nonleather products.

Wasn't Hitler a vegetarian?

Is it really relevant what Hitler ate or did not eat? Would anyone cite Hitler's abstinence from smoking to discredit nonsmokers? However, Hitler's alleged vegetarianism is often brought up and hence this response.

Because he suffered from excessive sweatiness and flatulence, Hitler occasionally went on a vegetarian diet. But his primary diet included meat. In his definitive biography, *The Life and Death of Adolph Hitler*, Ralph Payne mentions Hitler's special fondness for Bavarian sausages (p. 346). Other biographers, including Albert Speer, point out that he also ate ham, liver, and game.

I enjoy eating meat. Why should I give it up?

If one is solely motivated by what will bring pleasure, perhaps no answer to this question would be acceptable. But Judaism is motivated by far more: doing *mitzvot*, performing good deeds, sanctifying occasions, helping feed hungry people, pursuing justice and peace, and so on. I believe that people who take such Jewish values seriously should be vegetarians.

Even if one is primarily motivated by considerations of pleasure and convenience, the negative health effects of animal-centered diets should be taken into account. One cannot enjoy life when one is not in good health.

Richard H. Schwartz, Ph.D.

Chapter 19

Tips on Fasting

Fasting is no fun. It isn't supposed to be. Nevertheless, fasting is said to have salutary effects and is therefore held in high esteem by many religious traditions and health regimens. In the Jewish tradition fasting is taken quite seriously, so we find that on a major holy day like Yom Kippur, even Jews who wouldn't think of entering a synagogue will nevertheless fast because they believe fasting to be good for either the body or the spirit, or both.

In the Jewish religious tradition, the discomfort that is produced by fasting is thought to have instructional value and is intended to help us reflect on our human frailty. This does not mean that Jews are intended to make themselves as miserable as possible on Yom Kippur, only that they not eat or drink. The discomfort some people experience during a fast is so extreme that they forget the appropriate agendas for the day. It is possible to diminish that discomfort without losing awareness of the fast.

Not only is eating wisely tricky, so is fasting wisely. Here are some strategies that may make the fast a little easier.

• *Drink lots of water.* This may be hard to believe after one is twenty or so hours into a fast, but most healthy adults can survive well over a month without eating. Most of the unpleasantness associated with a fast does not come from lack of food but from lack of fluid. The solution therefore is to super-hydrate beforehand. "Camel up" before a fast, drinking a great deal the prior afternoon, perhaps two quarts well in advance of your final pre-fast meal. At the time you may feel you are going to float away; before the fast is over, you will be glad you did it. Diluted orange juice is a good drink; so is water. Beer or other alcoholic beverages will dehydrate you.

• *Eat meat and potatoes.* Though you should drink a lot before a fast, you do not need to stuff yourself with food. Eat a normal meal but emphasize carbohydrates like potato or noodle dishes, not proteins or fats. Carbohydrates bond with water, which your body can "drink" when it needs to during your fast. Proteins do not. Most of the dramatic but limited weight loss that people on high-protein diets experience is lost water that protein molecules cannot hold onto or bring into the system—water that you want to have around during a fast. I have heard of grandmothers in Europe who fed their families immense starch meals for the better part of the week before a fast and then, at the final meal encouraged everyone to eat heavy meat dishes. The carbohydrates taken early would provide the necessary water reservoir. The last-minute meat meal would give the comfort of a full stomach for a number of hours. What people who still eat this way before a fast have to consider is whether they really want to take on all those calories. This kind of pre-fast diet might have been suitable for a culture in which meat was a rarity and people were close to involuntary fasting through much of the year. It is not clear that it makes sense in ours. Fast food does not need to be hopelessly bland, but go easy on the salt, which may make you thirsty. Season with nonirritating spices and herbs.

• *Can the caffeine.* The nausea and headaches that many people who are fasting report have nothing to do with either food or fluid. They are usually the result of caffeine withdrawal. If you are a heavy coffee or cola drinker, start tapering off a week or so before the fast. Unless you drink a great deal of caffeine, one cup less a day, with the day before the fast being caffeine-free, will usually do it. Using decaffeinated coffee during this period may help you fool your system. Caffeine withdrawal symptoms are less of a problem when you are eating and drinking than when fasting.

A brief fast is not a quick weight-loss scheme. An average adult burns 2,000 to 2,500 calories—about two-thirds of a pound—during a twenty-four-hour fast. It doesn't take long at all to put that back on again. A couple of pieces of cheesecake and you will be just about even. Most of the weight loss that you see on the scale for the day or two after a fast is fluid that you will quickly replace.

After the fast, be careful not to gorge yourself. Because the body protects itself from starvation when you are not eating by slowing down the rate at which it burns food, the calories you take on right after a fast will stay with you a lot longer than those acquired when your metabolism is once again functioning at full speed.

These suggestions will not prevent you from experiencing the fast. If you are not eating or drinking for twenty-four to twenty-six hours, there is no chance you will forget that you are fasting. But it is important for you to be able to focus on some soul searching and praying, rather than on your complaining stomach.

So prepare yourself for fasting, both physically and spiritually, and in the words of one of the traditional pre-fast greetings, "Have an easy fast!"

Rabbi Richard J. Israel

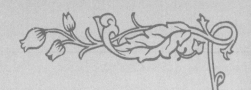

✍ Special Focus

Health Habits for Kids

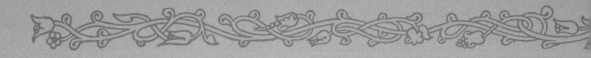

Chapter 20

Children and Exercise
A Lifelong Habit Starts Young

It is common knowledge that physical activity is good for you and is an essential part of healthy living. Regular physical activity reduces the risk for obesity, high cholesterol, coronary heart disease, osteoporosis, and certain cancers. Regular physical activity can also be used as a therapeutic and preventive tool for enhancing physical and mental health, increasing positive feelings about body image, and improving self-esteem and self-confidence.

Remember when we were children? We were always told to eat all our vegetables and do our homework on time and clean our room. Great advice, but teaching children what is beneficial to their future adult health is more challenging than saying, "Turn off the TV and go outside and play." According to research, American children today are more obese than ever. The fitness bug may have bitten the parents, but it certainly has not carried over to the younger generation.

There has been a dramatic, negative change in the lifestyle habits of our children, which has increased the fitness gap in America. Studies have shown that the average child, age six to eleven, watches twenty-five hours of television a week, which, coupled with computers and video games, is keeping our youth sedentary. Only about one-half of young Americans from ages twelve to twenty-one years participate regularly in vigorous physical activity. Inactivity is higher among females; males are more likely to participate in vigorous physical activity or strengthening activities such as walking or bicycling.

Inactive children grow up to be inactive adults. The best time to foster the enjoyment of healthy activity is in childhood, when lifelong habits are more likely to develop.

112

Helping Your Child Lose Weight the Healthy Way

Do
- Provide information
- Make observations
- Ask questions
- Offer suggestions
- Be honest
- Tread lightly
- Provide support
- Praise their attributes
- Provide encouragement

Don't
- Lecture
- Be judgmental
- Have all the answers
- Reprimand
- Be manipulative
- Nag
- Threaten
- Criticize
- Push

Judith Levine, R.D., M.S., and Linda Bine

As schools' physical education programs are being cut, it is a challenge to find ways to keep children physically active. The U.S. Surgeon General's Report on Physical Activity and Health[1] proposes that young adults engage in a total of at least thirty to sixty minutes of physical activity each day. The report stresses the importance of children participating in a variety of activities that work different parts of the body, as well as engaging in at least one ten- to fifteen-minute period of vigorous, pulse-raising, exercise per day.

Parents don't have to leave this up to the schools. Children are more likely to pursue physical activities if a parent participates with them. Find activities that all of you can do together: ride a bike, walk in the park, go ice skating. If your child wants to pursue something that you can't or don't want to do, encourage her by showing your support and interest that she does it safely and consistently. A child doesn't have to be a member of the track-and-field team to be active. He or she can learn and participate in such activities as dancing or fencing, or playing tennis or soccer. And keep in mind that regular daily activities can be active and efficient at the same time. Take the stairs instead of elevators or have the children help in the garden.

Active children tend to be active adults. Start now for a lifetime habit of physical activity.

Lisa Hoffman, M.A.

Note

1. U.S. Department of Health and Human Services, Centers for Disease Control and Prevention, National Center for Chronic Disease Prevention and Health Promotion, and President's Council of Physical Fitness and Sports. *Physical Activity and Health: A Report of the Surgeon General.* Washington, D.C.: Government Printing Office, 1996.

Chapter 21

Healthy Children Today, Healthy Adults Tomorrow

A Formula for Heart Health

When I was a young girl, the typical American family sat down to dinner together. Most mothers exhorted their children to eat their vegetables, drink their milk, and go outside to play. Suburban children walked reasonable distances to school, and in school they had gym class almost every day. In today's rushed, busy culture, many families cannot organize schedules so that they eat together. High-fat fast foods have become an easy substitute for home-cooked meals; suburban children are driven to school; gym classes are few and far between; and TV, video games, and the computer keep children sitting indoors for hours a day instead of playing outside.

We are seeing a generation of youngsters whose health may be in danger because of these unhealthy habits. The percentage of young people who are overweight has doubled since 1980. Of children aged five to fifteen who are overweight, 61 percent have one or more cardiovascular disease risk factors.[1] This is of particular concern, because adult diseases, such as heart disease, take years to develop and may actually have their origins in childhood.[2] This is borne out by a study in England that found that high cholesterol levels in children had a harmful effect on their arteries.[3] Although we can't guarantee that our children will grow to be healthy adults, there is a lot we can do to decrease their risk of developing heart disease.

If there were a magic pill that we could take every day to help our children and ourselves achieve good health, we would gladly take it. Well, there is a formula for good health that's available to all of us, but it's not magic. The formula is this:

Heart-Healthy Diet + Exercise = Better Health

This formula is promoted by such health agencies as the American Heart Association, the National Institutes of Health, the American Dietetic Association, and the U.S. Department of Agriculture.

According to a report in the National Heart, Lung and Blood Institute (NHLBI) *Health Memo:*

> Home-based interventions can change children's behavior and pro-mote a lifestyle that will reduce their risk of heart disease. An NHLBI-funded trial found that children can learn to eat and live heart healthy where they live and learn in an environment that encourages a healthy lifestyle.[4]

The first element in "The Formula" is diet. Children over the age of two can benefit from low-fat eating. The place to start imple-menting this is, of course, the supermarket. Learn to read nutrition labels. Look for foods that are low in fat, particularly saturated fat. Buy skim or 1 percent milk, low-fat or fat-free cheeses, and yogurt. Buy the softer tub margarines rather than the stick choices. In the oil section, opt for olive, canola, or peanut oils. Ask the butcher for the leanest cuts of meat. Serve fish at least once a week. Buy tuna packed in water instead of oil.

When you buy grain products, such as bread and rice, look for whole grain choices. In the produce section, choose a colorful variety of fruits and vegetables, including red, green, yellow, and orange. Buy enough produce to feed each member of the family a combination of at least five fruits and vegetables daily. Avoid prepared foods, partic-ularly baked goods such as cakes and cookies. These products are high in saturated fats and contain partially hydrogenated fats that are not healthy for the heart.

Serve chicken without the skin and avoid cream sauces. Include a fruit and vegetable with lunches and dinners and fruit with breakfast. Keep healthy snacks readily available. Leave a bowl of fruit on the table. Have a bowl of raw vegetables, such as carrots, broccoli, cauliflower, and soy beans, in the refrigerator. Have low-fat cheeses and yogurts available. Baked chips with a low-fat dip, such as salsa, make a good snack.

The second element in "The Formula" is exercise. Karen Donato, coordinator of the NHLBI Obesity Education Initiative, said, "Regular physical activity and heart-healthy eating habits are keys to preventing and controlling overweight and obesity, high blood pressure, and high blood cholesterol."

Promote an active family lifestyle. Be role models for your children and find activities that the family can do together. Try to find ways that your children can exercise for at least thirty to sixty minutes a day. Walks or hikes on weekends, jogging, dog walking, bike riding, swimming, and ice skating are just a few activities that the whole family can enjoy. Encourage your children to play outside after school rather than watch TV or play computer games.

Provide children with opportunities to participate in after-school sports programs. Soccer, tennis, track, gymnastics, and baseball, as well as dancing, skiing, and swimming, are good options that most communities, schools, or recreation departments offer. Participation in these activities is good for heart health and allows children to socialize and build self-esteem. Encourage your child's school to participate in the President's Challenge—a physical fitness awards program of the President's Council on Physical Fitness. There are awards for achieving different levels of physical fitness, and this can be a terrific incentive for children to participate in exercise.

These are a few suggestions to help our children decrease their risks of heart disease. If you and your family follow "The Formula," you should all be on the road to good health. Remember that the eating habits you teach your children today and the healthy lifestyle that you encourage them to develop now will benefit them always.

∾ *Rickie M. Haas, M.S., R.D., C.D.N.*

Notes

1. National Center for Health Statistics [http://www.cdc.gov/nchs].
2. D. S. Freedman, W. H. Dietz, S. R. Srinivasan, and G. S. Berenson. "The Relationship of Overweight to Cardiovascular Risk Factors Among Children and Adolescents: The Bogalusa Heart Study." *Pediatrics*, 1999, *103*, 1175–1182.

3. C.P.M. Leeson, P. H. Whincup, D. G. Cook, M. J. Mullen, A. E. Donald, C. A. Seymour, and J. E. Deanfield. "Cholesterol and Arterial Distensibility in the First Decade of Life: A Population-Based Study." *Circulation*, 2000, *101*, 1533–1538.

4. National Heart, Lung and Blood Institute, Cardiovascular Health Promotion Project. *Heart Memo* (spec. ed.) Bethesda, Md.: National Heart, Lung and Blood Institute, 1996.

Jewish Genetic Diseases

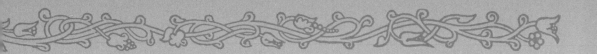

Chapter 22

Genetic Diseases Among Individuals of Ashkenazi Jewish Heritage

Barely a generation ago, infections were the major health threat to children in the developed world. Today, thanks to advances in medicine, we no longer fear childhood illnesses. Inherited diseases now account for an increasing proportion of children living with disability and shortened life spans. Although strides have been made toward finding treatments for these children, so far only a few children can be restored to good health and the ability to function well.

Even though the science of genetics offers hope for the future, today many families opt for an ounce of prevention in the form of prenatal testing and diagnosis. In order to understand how this works, it is important to understand that every human being normally carries forty-six chromosomes—twenty-three from the mother and twenty-three from the father. These chromosomes are the genetic material that contains the blueprint for our physical make-up. If a person inherits one disease gene from one parent and a matching healthy gene from the other, she is said to be a carrier of that disease, although not afflicted with it herself. This person has a recessive, or hidden, gene. If this person marries a man who carries a matching recessive gene, the couple has a one-in-four chance with each birth that their child will inherit two recessive genes and become ill. Prenatal testing, usually done by amniocentesis, can often let them know whether their child has inherited two recessive genes and, therefore, the disease.

121

Other genetic diseases do not require two recessive genes. One dominant disease gene is all it takes to predispose someone to certain illnesses. Some of these illnesses don't show up until adulthood; examples are Huntington's chorea and early-onset Alzheimer's disease. Scientists do not yet know the role of all our genes. It is estimated that everyone carries from five to ten defective genes, and not all of them do harm.

In some populations, such as Ashkenazi Jews, certain genes that cause diseases are more common. These diseases also occur in the rest of the population but not as frequently. This may be because of a phenomenon called the "founder effect." Before humans could travel with the ease and frequency they do today, small groups often lived in geographic or cultural isolation and intermarried. Because such people often shared a common ancestry, the risk for certain diseases was passed down from one generation to another by the "founders" of the group.

 ## Hadassah Policy Statement on Genetic Testing

Hadassah, the Women's Zionist Organization of America, Inc., an international health care provider and the largest women's and largest Jewish membership organization in the United States, applauds the joint National Institutes for Health and Hadassah Hospital study, which found a particularly high incidence of a mutation of the "BRCA1" breast cancer gene in Ashkenazi Jewish women. We believe that this important discovery will be essential in the early treatment of the disease in our community.

Hadassah is nonetheless concerned that this new genetic information or individuals' requests for genetic counseling services may result in higher health insurance premiums, changes in terms or conditions, or outright denial or cancellation of coverage. Hadassah opposes such insurance discrimination and strongly supports legislative efforts like H.R. 2748, the Genetic Information Nondiscrimination in Health Insurance Act of 1995.

For these reasons, many Jewish adults favor genetic testing when planning a family. It's almost standard practice for Jewish couples to be tested for Tay-Sachs disease, as well as several other inherited disorders. Although it may be frightening to discover that someone in your family has inherited a genetic disease, there is hope. There is now a specific therapy for Gaucher's (go-shayz) disease, which has the symptoms of bone pain, anemia, and enlarged liver and spleen. These medical problems result from an enzyme deficiency. Advances in genetic techniques have enabled production of the deficient enzyme that can be given intravenously to patients. This treatment has been shown to be safe and effective in reversing the symptoms of Gaucher's disease and preventing complications.

Although genetic testing can help couples make difficult decisions regarding their own and their future children's health, it is voluntary and no one should feel compelled to be tested. It is best to make informed decisions, and trained professionals such as genetics counselors can help people understand what is involved in testing and the significance of the findings. A genetics counselor or geneticist can also help ensure access to updated information. With this information, couples can draw strength from their beliefs and tradition and come to a decision regarding what is appropriate for their situation and their family.

Gregory M. Pastores, M.D., G.M.P.

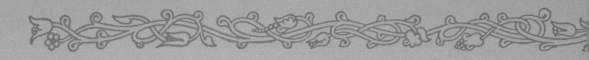

Chapter 23

Therefore Choose Life

Should we fear the knowledge that the science of genetics is making available to us? The popular media, which views genetic testing as a way of divining the future, often portrays this science as a kind of Pandora's Box. The truth is that genetics is only predictive in diseases like Huntington's chorea, when the prognosis is unavoidable. For most diseases, breast cancer among them, genetic testing provides a kind of weather map. The science tells us that there will be storms of varying frequency due to current conditions, but testing is limited in its ability to predict exactly when, where, and how severely the storms will strike.

For a woman with a history of breast cancer in her family, this means that the knowledge that she carries the mutation for breast cancer tells her little other than the fact that she's at increased risk for getting the disease. It doesn't tell her whether she will actually get breast cancer or what form it may take.

This raises the dilemma of whether she will be aided by the knowledge of her own risk. Obtaining knowledge may prompt some women to try different courses of treatment that may reduce risk. Others may feel a false sense of security when they find out their test was negative and become lax in having regular mammograms and examinations. Still other women may find that this knowledge opens a world of mental anguish. For them, having this knowledge creates feelings of constant anxiety over the fear of getting the disease or having passed on the gene to the next generation.

The Jewish tradition is very mindful of the need for medical knowledge and the compassionate dissemination of that knowledge. Judaism teaches us not to fear knowledge. The *Midrash* remarks

124

about the Torah that it begins with the letter *bet*, whose shape suggests that we should not inquire what is behind us, above us, or beneath us, only what lies ahead. This means that we shouldn't waste our time with things over which we have no control or influence; rather, we should use this knowledge to plan ahead for the future.

Embracing this knowledge, although it may be frightening, gives us opportunities to be nearer to God. According to Jewish tradition, to know God's creations is to come closer to knowing God. This notion runs like a thread through the work of Moses Maimonides—Judaism's great philosopher, physician, and codifier of Jewish law. Because of this belief, science and the gathering of knowledge are considered to be divinely ordained. Perhaps this is why so many Jewish scientists come from backgrounds in which study and learning are emphasized.

But with knowledge comes responsibility. Judaism also teaches that a patient's emotional health must be considered. If learning that she is at increased risk of getting breast cancer will cause a patient severe mental distress, this must be discussed with the physician. Doctors and patients can work together in this instance to decide what and how much information the patient wishes to have. It would be irresponsible to inform the patient without these considerations.

Hadassah has been instrumental in bringing these considerations to public debate. Because it has become known that Ashkenazi women carry a higher risk of getting breast cancer than the general population, Hadassah has advocated education and the protection of the rights of the individual through legislation.

The need for legislation was clearly illustrated by the health insurance discrimination experienced by Americans with the gene for sickle cell anemia. As we continue to decode the human genome, more and more people will find themselves in similar circumstances. As a result, all of the surrounding issues—discrimination in insurance and employment hiring, ethics, and psychosocial factors—will become increasingly important.

In Deuteronomy, God says: "I have put before you today the blessing and the curse; therefore choose life." With genetic testing the blessing is that we can choose; the curse is that, given the possibilities, we have to choose, even if that choice is to forego genetic testing. Choosing life requires that we continue to study and to learn, with the hope that we will one day be able to use this knowledge reliably to perfect God's world. Then we will have fulfilled the commandment: "therefore choose life."

   Rabbi Avis Dimond Miller and
Dale L. Mintz, M.P.A., C.H.E.S.

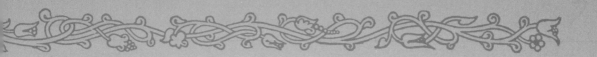

Chapter 24

Testing Genetic Tests for Jewish Values

For many religions, the idea of "playing God" with genetics is abhorrent. Not so for Judaism. Instead, the appellation "a partner with God in the work of creation" (Babylonian Talmud, *Shabbat* 10a) is one of the highest compliments that can be paid to a human being. With the remarkable recent advances in genetics, including genetic testing and the possibility of genetic engineering, new and vast vistas for such partnership with God are emerging. The moral test will be how we use these technologies. Would God want *us* as a partner in these endeavors?

Focusing specifically on genetic testing, we have a source of potentially important information, but we must use the information appropriately. Unfortunately, as with all technologies that are powerful tools for good, the potential for bad exists as well and must be guarded against.

Judaism does not have a legal principle of "the right to know." Information, for us, is value-neutral until we determine how the information will be used. That is the paradigm with which we must approach the question of genetic testing. For this reason proper counseling and education must accompany any testing protocol so that the information obtained will be used in the best possible way.

TESTING FOR GENETIC DISEASES

One of the many possibilities created by the new genetics technology is testing for possible genetic anomalies that might occur in children not yet born. Parents, prospective parents, or anyone contemplating marriage can be tested for genetic abnormalities. Or the fetus in utero can be tested through amniocentesis or other procedures to ascertain whether genetic illnesses are present.

Most Ashkenazi Jews are particularly concerned with Tay-Sachs disease.[1] A child born with two Tay-Sachs genes (one from each parent) will suffer from the disease and will die before the age of five. A child born with one Tay-Sachs gene will not become ill but might transmit the gene to an offspring. And someone with no Tay-Sachs genes will neither become ill nor transmit the gene to an offspring. To determine the likelihood of bearing a child with one or two Tay-Sachs genes, one must test the genetic makeup of both parents. If two carriers of the gene procreate, there is a one-in-four chance that any child born to them will contract the disease. There is a one-in-two chance that their child will be a carrier.[2]

From the perspective of Jewish law, the decision to seek or not seek information about genetic diseases depends on the use to which that information will be put. For this reason, amniocentesis for purposes of aborting a fetus carrying two Tay-Sachs genes is a problem. Rabbi Eliezer Waldenberg, a contemporary Israeli scholar and former president of the Rabbinical Court of Jerusalem, wrote in a 1975 responsum that abortion is permitted in these circumstances until the seventh month. However, Rabbi Moshe Feinstein, considered to be one of the most important contemporary halakhic scholars, did not permit it. The many Orthodox Jews who follow the opinion of Rabbi Feinstein therefore consider testing for this purpose forbidden.

But what if a couple wanted to test their fetus for Tay-Sachs— or Down syndrome, Gaucher's disease, or any other genetic disease— simply to prepare mentally and emotionally for what is to come? That might well be a different story. Some Orthodox authorities are concerned that because abortion is so readily available, there is a strong likelihood that the parents will ultimately turn to abortion if their fetus is genetically diseased. These authorities, then, refuse to grant permission under any circumstances for prenatal testing. However, some Orthodox rabbis do grant permission to the couple after discussing the issue thoroughly with them.

If fetal testing is a troublesome area within Jewish law, then doesn't it make sense for the married couple to get tested themselves before they procreate? The answer is no. After all, what use will the couple make of the information? Abortion of a fetus with genetic abnormalities, as we have seen, is forbidden by some halakhic experts—a position I adhere to. And according to Jewish religious law, the couple is obligated to have children. Besides, how will the information affect the relationship itself? Relationships are fragile; finding a flaw in one's partner, or even in oneself, might upset the delicate balance. Thus I do not advocate for the husband and wife to be tested at this point in their marriage until we have more advanced developments of reproductive technologies, such as the ability to identify and separate sperm and egg cells lacking the abnormal gene so that they can be used to produce the couple's children.

The best time to be tested is during the college-age years, before one has chosen a marriage partner. I myself, as a freshman at Yeshiva University, was tested for Tay-Sachs in a schoolwide program. I tested negative, which was a great relief, but I wondered what was done for those who tested positive. Any genetic testing program must be accompanied by counseling, so that anyone who tests positive can deal with the issues raised by this finding, learn how to use the information, and discuss when and how to inform a dating partner and how to deal with the person's reactions. The community at large, too, must be responsible for ensuring that no stigma will be attached to the carrier.

Frankly, some authorities are opposed to such testing because of the concern of community stigma. My own view is that the knowledge is valuable in and of itself. As long as we have genetic counseling and community education, we should encourage such testing. I do feel that, at the present time, there should perhaps be no testing in communities without the resources to eliminate the stigma.

TESTING FOR DISEASE MARKERS

Now let us examine a different purpose for genetic testing: to ascertain if an individual has a propensity to develop a certain disease. Let us take the example of a woman being tested for the breast cancer gene, particularly one who has relatives who have suffered or have even died from the disease.[3] The woman comes to the test with much trepidation. If she tests positive, it will seem to her that her

The Role of the Genetics Counselor

This is an exciting time in genetics and health. New gene discoveries are helping us to gain better understanding of many diseases, both common (heart disease) and rare (cystic fibrosis). One of the early applications of gene discovery is genetic testing—the ability to test an individual or unborn baby for a disease gene. The availability of genetic testing raises questions that many of us will have to answer at some time in our lives: For whom is testing appropriate? What kind of information can be learned from the results? Will the information gained be beneficial or burdensome? With whom should results be shared? How will the results of genetic testing affect one's choices about reproductive, health, or life-planning issues?

Fortunately, there is a health care professional who can help patients understand their options—the genetics counselor. Genetics counselors explain complex genetic conditions and testing options to families to facilitate informed decision making. With specialized master's-level training in medical genetics and counseling, genetics counselors provide information and support to individuals and families concerned about the risk or presence of a birth defect or inherited condition. By collecting detailed family, medical, and reproductive histories, genetics counselors are able to identify genetic risk factors. They translate this complex medical information regarding diagnosis, inheritance patterns, risks, and prognosis into language that can be understood and considered by families.

There are many different genetic-testing scenarios that genetics counselors can help patients understand. They may be considered in three broad categories: diagnostic, presymptomatic and predispositional testing.

Diagnostic testing can be used to screen a newborn for disorders that respond to early treatment, to confirm a diagnosis, to test for an inherited disorder, or to find out whether a fetus is at risk for a particular disease. Significant advances have been made since the first Tay-Sachs screening program was offered in the Jewish community in 1970. Today there are nine diseases for which carrier screening can be offered to individuals of Ashkenazi Jewish descent.

With *presymptomatic* testing, a healthy individual opts for testing to learn whether she carries a gene that will someday result in disease (for example, Huntington's chorea).

Testing for the breast cancer gene, BRCA1, is an example of a *predispositional* gene test. Women with a BRCA1 gene mutation face a 50 to 85 percent lifetime risk of breast cancer and a 20 to 40 percent lifetime risk of ovarian cancer. However, this does not mean they will actually get breast cancer. In predispositional testing, the identification of an altered gene in a healthy person indicates that individual is at increased, but not certain, risk.

In the future we can expect an increasing number of diagnostic and predictive tests, as well as genetic testing, to predict the effectiveness of medication. What remains unchanged from the early days of genetic testing is the importance of being an educated health care consumer. Learn about your family's health history and discuss it with your physician. If appropriate, request a consultation with a genetics counselor for an in-depth discussion of your concerns and options. You don't have to face the complex and often confusing world of genetics alone.

To find a genetics counselor near you, contact the National Society of Genetics Counselors at http://www.nsgc.org or (610) 872-7608, ext. 7.

Elaine Sugarman, M.S.

worst fears have been realized. It may be very difficult for her to understand the implications of what she has been told.

Genetic markers do not indicate the presence of the disease, only a propensity to acquire it. A woman who carries such markers must be especially careful to minimize other risk factors such as smoking and maintaining a poor diet. She must frequently conduct breast self-exams and have mammograms. Responding in this way would be in keeping with the Torah's imperative, "You shall be extremely diligent in caring for your souls" (Deuteronomy 4:9)—understood by the Rabbis, particularly by Maimonides, to require us to engage in healthful and life-preserving activities.

However, given the painful emotions that will, in all probability, be evoked by the positive test results, we must get this message across: *a person who has a particular genetic marker may never contract the illness at all.* It would be tragic if such test results led people to engage in high-risk behaviors or to avoid proper examinations on the assumption that their fate has been sealed.

In this regard, a prophylactic mastectomy (or other extreme measure) would be acceptable only under these circumstances: (1) that the woman is extremely likely to contract a fatal form of the disease, (2) that a mastectomy would prevent her from becoming ill, and (3) that frequent testing and early detection and treatment would be significantly less effective in combating the disease.

I doubt that many cases can meet these criteria, given the present state of our technology. As such, Jewish law is very reluctant to allow surgery that, as with all such procedures, comes with risk and involves mutilation of the body, except when absolutely necessary. One must be concerned, then, that inappropriate use of a positive test result may lead to unfortunate and irreversible consequences.

Now, what if the woman receives a negative test result? We would need to be concerned that she does not misinterpret this to mean that she will not contract the disease. If she did come away with such a false understanding and then did not guard her health, we would have done her a grave disservice with our new technology. This, too, must be taken into consideration in developing an educational program to accompany genetic testing.

GENETIC DISCRIMINATION

We must also be concerned with the use of genetic testing information by people other than the one who is tested. Confidentiality and privacy are important Jewish values that might be compromised in this context. Certainly, insurance companies will want this information, as will prospective employers and, possibly, even a prospective spouse.

Judaism has very strict rules regulating the use of personal information by third parties. These rules generally fall under the broad rubric of *lashon hara* (evil speech), but the term is used for all types of gossip. Although one can reveal information about a third party to prevent loss or harm to a potential spouse or business partner, this is acceptable only when such information is believed to be determinative. As genetic testing yields only an increased statistical probability, it hardly meets the test of being determinative. Hence confidentiality must be maintained, even against the inquiries of interested parties.

Among third parties, the strongest claim would come from the potential spouse. The *Shulchan Aruch* (Code of Jewish Law) recommends against marrying into families that tend to produce members who contract certain illnesses. Obviously, when it comes to marriage, some measure of genetic concern is allowed, even understandable. Nonetheless, we must also educate our singles population to view a potential partner as a total person and not as someone who meets a checklist created to suit imagined needs and concerns.

Finally, we must worry about the broader effect on people and families. Genetic testing can stigmatize people. We must be vigilant that it not have this effect. It may uncover evidence of illegitimacy or infidelity which, according to Jewish law, must never be revealed or even intimated if discovered in this way. Further, the tests, because they are expensive, might also serve to exacerbate the differences between high-quality health care for the rich and lower-quality health care for the poor. We must, therefore, ensure that access to the tests be available to members of all social and economic groups.

Judaism reveres the sanctity of life. Ultimately, if used correctly, genetic testing can and will save lives. No greater value can be given to any technology than this simple statement. There are some cautionary flags that need to be negotiated, but if saving a life is equal to the saving of an entire world, then genetic testing will, if used correctly, preserve galaxies of human worlds to shine as precious jewels in God's universe.

Rabbi Barry Freundel

Notes

1. Although only 3.7 percent of Ashkenazi Jews are carriers of the Tay-Sachs gene, that low percentage is ten times higher than among the general population.

2. This genetic pattern is typical of all autosomal-recessive genetic diseases, not just Tay-Sachs.

3. In 1994, scientists isolated genes known as the BRCA1 and BRCA2 genes. A mutation on these genes (which is often inherited) indicates a susceptibility to breast and ovarian cancer in women and to prostate, colon, and breast cancer in men. A woman with mutated BRCA1 or BRCA2 genes and a family history of breast cancer may stand as much as an 85 percent chance of developing breast cancer in her lifetime, in contrast to the average woman's 12.5 percent chance. Among Ashkenazi women, the mutation accounts for 16 percent of breast cancers and 39 percent of ovarian cancers diagnosed before age fifty.

Chapter 25

Ethics and Genetic Testing

The mastery of the human genome is recognized as possibly the greatest achievement of mankind. When the function of the proteins engineered by each gene is identified, both the cause and potential cure for most diseases will be known. However, this mastery of biochemistry and molecular biology, as well as the accompanying technology, presents society with a plethora of ethical, moral, and legal dilemmas that demand resolution.

Genetic probes can now identify hundreds of genes, many of them associated with specific disease syndromes. Some of these "disease genes" are found in higher incidence in certain racial or ethnic groups. For example, the "Jewish" genetic diseases—Tay-Sachs, Gaucher's, Fanconi's anemia, familial dysautonomia—are called carrier diseases; they are carried on a recessive gene and are manifested only when both parents are carriers. Other genetic diseases are found on a dominant gene, which means that afflicted people need only one copy. These diseases do not reveal their presence at birth but in the fourth decade of life, like Huntington's chorea, or even later, as in the case of Alzheimer's. A genetic probe can reveal the presence of these genes before birth by amniocentesis. This knowledge raises important questions. Is knowledge an absolute good? Is it sometimes better not to know? Here are the dilemmas raised by genetic testing.

TO TEST OR NOT TO TEST

It behooves anyone considering marriage to be tested for the presence of the known "carrier" genetic diseases. If found to be a carrier,

tragedy can be avoided by not marrying someone with the same carrier disease gene. For Jewish couples, such testing for the presence
of Jewish genetic disease genes has become routine. The incidence of
babies with Tay-Sachs has been greatly reduced because of this testing program. But what about diseases like Huntington's, which manifest themselves in adulthood without any available therapeutic
potential? The psychological trauma of knowing will surely have a
great impact on the quality of life of that individual for years before
the disease appears.

FEAR OF EUGENICS

The proliferation of genetic probes raises the specter of eugenics—
the "science" of improving the human race through selective breeding. The German medical community gave its scientific stamp to the
racist laws of the Third Reich during the Holocaust, based on dis-
credited eugenic principles. But we can now prove the existence of
"bad genes" in an individual or even a racial or ethnic group. Will
this lead us into the darkness and degradation of eugenics through a
back door? Putting a "price tag" on a specific genotype based on
genetic testing or screening threatens the very basis of an egalitarian
democratic social order. It is a real danger that must be overcome by
education and legislation.

DOES BIOLOGY EQUAL DESTINY?

The proliferation of psychological research studies on the interrela-
tionship of genes and behavioral traits has presented us with a dramatic challenge: the claim of predetermined behavior. Both the
American legal system and the ethical and moral biblical precepts
are based on the principle of personal responsibility for acts done voluntarily, without coercion. If genes are being implicated as coercive
forces in such behavioral traits as aggressiveness, or even criminal-
ity, how can society punish such individuals, whose genes determined their criminal behavior?

It is instructive to note that the Bible, in the Book of Genesis,
relates to this question. When Cain, who had just murdered his

brother Abel, responds to God's query with the well-known question "Am I my brother's keeper?" he introduced the "Cain defense": it wasn't me; it was my genes! Cain became the accuser: "You, God, made me this way. You gave me the genetic makeup to be a murderer."

But the Creator of mankind had previously deflected such a claim. In Genesis (4:7) God had warned Cain: "Evil inclinations are part of the human personality, but you have been given the moral strength to overcome these inclinations."

Genes do not determine behavior. Every individual has unique inclinations and predispositions that require moral effort to control and convert to productive forces. No one is compelled to do evil by a genetic master. God gave us a moral code of conduct—his Torah—to teach us how to control our actions so that they are pleasing to God and humanity.

Rabbi Moshe David Tendler, Ph.D.

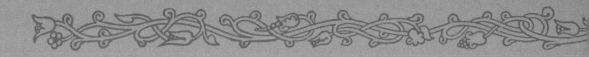

Chapter 26

Hadassah Policy Statement on Genetic Testing

Advances in genetic science are creating a paradigm shift in medicine, from symptomatic to presymptomatic diagnoses, thus potentially leading to a disease-free future. Researchers are currently racing to map the whole human genome and identify genetic "markers" that may be predictive of the onset of disease. Genetic tests, both those used in research and those available commercially, may be able to demonstrate whether an individual holds such a marker. The availability of such tests raises some very important ethical, legal, and social issues.

Recently, scientists have isolated two genes (BRCA1 and BRCA2) that are closely linked to breast and ovarian cancer if they are mutated, or altered. Further research has indicated that *certain* mutations of these genes have a higher-than-expected frequency in women of Ashkenazi (Eastern European) Jewish descent than in other population groups. (Some other BRCA1 and BRCA2 mutations are also found in higher-than-expected frequency in other population groups, and it is expected that more will be identified. The Ashkenazi Jewish population was chosen simply as a useful, early sample because of coherent population patterns.) It is now believed that 1 in 50 Ashkenazi Jewish women may carry one of these mutations, which may account for a slight (1 percent) increased lifetime risk for breast or ovarian cancer. It is important to note in this context that hereditary links account only for an estimated 5 to 10 percent of all cases of breast cancer.

Because at this time there are few preventive measures and no cure for breast cancer, the availability of genetic tests to determine the presence of mutations, and the corresponding degree of risk for the disease, raises some extremely important issues for Jewish women and their families. Imprecise press accounts and other forms of misinformation have raised the specter that Jewish women have a unique and greatly heightened predisposition to breast cancer, with implications for potential discrimination in employment and insurance. The most obvious way the discrimination may occur is through the use of genetic information by insurance carriers or employers.

Genetic tests for breast cancer cannot be 100 percent predictive of the onset of the disease. If an individual is found to have one of the mutations, he or she may have up to a 65 percent chance of eventually developing breast cancer. However, one in three individuals with a mutation will never have the disease. Conversely, an individual who tests negative for the mutations may still get breast cancer (all women have a 1 in 8 chance of having the disease if they live to age eighty-five). Moreover, a test may yield inaccurate results. The reproducibility, sensitivity, specificity, and predictive value of the tests are not fully known.

Nevertheless, information from these tests and research studies may be utilized by insurers or employers to discriminate. Discrimination based on genetic information has a long and well-documented history in other population groups with diseases such as sickle-cell anemia and hemachromatosis. Fear of discrimination is currently dissuading members of the Jewish community from participating in potentially important research projects or from getting a genetic test even where it is appropriate.

The Jewish community has long supported individuals' rights to determine the course of their own medical care and has actively participated in medical research. Hadassah believes that there should be ample opportunities for individuals to participate in promising research studies. However, legitimate tension exists between the Jewish community's interest in abating fear and avoiding stigmatization or discrimination and the scientific community's interests in furthering its knowledge in the quest to understand, prevent, and cure cancer. There is also the need to protect against the potentially aggressive and fear-based marketing techniques of those who stand to profit from commercially available genetic tests.

Hadassah is committed to the following courses of action:

1. Initiating a community-wide discussion nationally on the issue of breast cancer, hereditary and otherwise—its causes and risks, facts, and myths. In order to combat misinformation, Hadassah will disseminate public health materials to help Jewish women and their families assess their risk and their appropriateness for genetic testing or involvement in university-sponsored research protocols. It will also continue to advocate for measures aimed at identifying prevention strategies and finding a cure for breast cancer.

2. Advocating for legislative measures, at both federal and state levels, that will complement the "Kennedy-Kassebaum" law and prevent genetic-based discrimination in insurance and employment, and ensure the confidentiality of medical records.

3. Supporting widely available and appropriately administered research studies aimed at providing more information on this topic. Such research studies must be accompanied by proper informed consent procedures and comprehensive genetic counseling.

4. Working with the genetic testing companies, the oncological community, and others to combat fear-based and stigmatizing marketing techniques and inappropriate uses of genetic tests in the Jewish community, while reiterating that current knowledge does not provide a mandate for broad-scale testing of individuals outside of a controlled research setting.

5. Continuing to promote the study of the usefulness of genetic tests in the breast cancer context, the potential need for government regulation, and the impact of test results on members of the Jewish community.

Hadassah is hopeful that genetics research will play a major role in life-saving disease prevention and cures for all people, regardless of gender or ethnic heritage. However, it is essential that our country's public policy provide the needed safeguards with regard to these important findings.

Additional Resources and Contacts

National Breast Cancer Coalition: (202) 296-7477, http://www.stop
breastcancer.org

National Cancer Institute's Cancer Information Service:
(800) 4-CANCER

National Coalition for Health Professional Education in Genetics:
http://www.nchpeg.org

National Human Genome Research Institute: http://www.nhgri.
nih.gov

National Organization for Rare Disorders: http://www.rare
diseases.org

National Society of Genetic Counselors: (610) 872-7608

Nation's Investment in Cancer Research: http://plan2001.cancer.gov

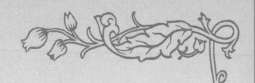

✑ Special Focus

Specific Genetic Conditions

Chapter 27

Gaucher's Disease, Type 1

Gaucher's disease, Type 1, is the most prevalent Jewish genetic disease, occurring in 1 in every 1,000 Ashkenazi Jews. Gaucher's Type 1 is an inherited disorder in which the body cannot break down a lipid called glucocerebroside.

Symptoms: Symptoms range from mild to severe and can appear at any time, from infancy to old age. Gaucher symptoms may include anemia, fatigue, easy bruising, and a tendency to bleed. An enlarged spleen and liver may also occur in Gaucher's disease, as well as bone pain, degeneration, and fractures. Bone disease may lead to neurological problems, such as compression of the spinal cord. Brown spots at the edges of the cornea (the front surface of the eye) are also a feature of Type 1.

Cause: Gaucher's Type 1 is inherited in an autosomal-recessive pattern, which means two copies of the gene must be altered for a person to be affected by the disorder. Mutation of the GBA gene leads to deficiency of an enzyme—glucocerebrosidase—that is needed to break down glucocerebroside. This fatty substance then accumulates in "Gaucher cells," which are found particularly in the liver, spleen, and bone marrow. Damage in these organs causes the symptoms of the disease.

Treatment: Enzyme replacement therapy has recently been shown to safely and effectively reverse most of the clinical manifestations in people affected by Gaucher's Type 1 disease. It is important to begin treatment before there is significant organ or bone damage.

Disease frequency: This disease is seen in 1 in 50,000 to 100,000 people in the general population. Type 1 Gaucher's disease is more common in people of Ashkenazi (Eastern and Central European) Jewish heritage than those with other backgrounds. The disorder affects 1 in 500 to 1,000 people of Ashkenazi Jewish heritage.

Carrier frequency: The carrier rate for the mutations that cause Gaucher's disease may be as high as 1 in 14 Jewish people of Eastern European ancestry and 1 in 500 in the general population.

Diagnosis: Gaucher's disease can be detected through a simple blood test. The testing process can be done at a hospital or a Gaucher specialist's office, or through your family physician. Your physician can draw blood that would then be sent to a specific laboratory for DNA-based diagnostic testing.

Screening: Carrier status can be detected through a simple blood test.

History: In 1882, a French physician named Philippe Charles Ernest Gaucher first described a clinical syndrome in a thirty-two-year-old woman whose liver and spleen were enlarged.

Future: The future offers much promise for Gaucher patients and their families. Currently, enzyme replacement therapy has replaced the bone marrow transplantations as the preferred method of treatment. The enzyme is regularly, frequently, and chronically infused into the bloodstream intravenously; the cost is significant.

Future treatments might include replacement therapy with manufactured longer-acting enzymes that could be given by injection into the fat layer of the skin instead of into the veins. Another future possibility is gene transfer therapy. A patient's immune cells would be removed and corrected in the laboratory, placed into cells with normally functioning enzyme-producing genes, then transplanted back into the patient.

Lisa Katz

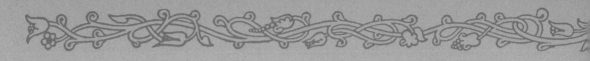

Chapter 28

Living with Gaucher's Disease

۞ A Guide for Patients, Parents, Relatives, and Friends

If you have just learned that you, your child, a relative, or a friend has Gaucher's disease, the odds are that this is the first time you have ever heard of this disorder. Gaucher's disease is not very common, and until recently it has received very little public attention.

Uncertainty can breed concern, and the anxiety many individuals have about the disease is due, in part, to a lack of information. In fact, since Gaucher's disease was first identified over one hundred years ago, much has been learned about the nature of the disease, as well as how the symptoms and psychological effects can be managed. Research conducted over the past thirty years has also led to new approaches to treatment, including the recent development of the first pharmaceutical that can reverse the major symptoms of the disease.

Gaucher's disease is an inherited disorder. People with this disease lack sufficient amounts of an important enzyme. This enzyme deficiency results in the accumulation of a fatty substance that is normally produced during the recycling of cells in the body. Symptoms of the disease can vary from very mild to severe, and they can appear at any time, from infancy to old age. In affected individuals, however, the genetic cause is present from the time of conception.

Fewer than 1 in 40,000 people in the general population have Gaucher's disease. The incidence is significantly higher among Jews of Eastern European (Ashkenazi) descent (in the range of 1 in 400 to 1 in 600 people). The higher frequency of Gaucher's disease among this population has led to the mistaken notion that it is a "Jewish genetic disease." In fact, individuals of any ethnic or racial background, including blacks and Hispanics, may be affected. Although Gaucher's disease is not very common, it is nonetheless as common as sickle-cell anemia in the black population or hemophilia in the general population.

What is the history of Gaucher's disease?

Gaucher's disease is named after the French physician Philippe Charles Ernest Gaucher, who first described this disease in 1882 in a thirty-two-year-old person whose liver and spleen were enlarged. In 1924, the German physician H. Lieb isolated a particular fatty compound from the spleens of people with Gaucher's disease. Ten years later, the French physician A. Aghion identified this compound as glucocerebroside—a component of the cell membranes of red and white blood cells. In 1965, the American physician Roscoe O. Brady and coworkers demonstrated that the accumulation of glucocerebroside results from a deficiency of the enzyme glucocerebrosidase. Dr. Brady's research provided the basis for developing enzyme replacement therapy, using glucocerebrosidase to replace the missing enzyme in Gaucher patients.

What is the basis of Gaucher's disease?

The human body contains specialized cells called macrophages that remove worn-out cells by degrading them to simple molecules for recycling. This process is analogous to eating and digesting food. The macrophages "eat" worn-out cells and degrade them inside cell compartments called lysosomes that serve as the "digestive tracts" of cells. The enzyme glucocerebrosidase is located within the lysosomes and is responsible for breaking down glucocerebroside into glucose and a fat called ceramide.

People with Gaucher's disease lack the normal form of the glucocerebrosidase enzyme and are unable to break down glucocerebroside. Instead, the glucocerebroside remains stored within the lysosomes, preventing the macrophages from functioning normally. Enlarged macrophages containing undigested glucocerebroside are called Gaucher cells. These cells are the hallmark of this disease.

What happens when Gaucher cells accumulate?

Gaucher cells most often accumulate in the spleen, liver, and bone marrow. However, they may also collect in other tissues, including

HEALTH FACTS

Gaucher's disease is the most common of ten so-called "storage" disorders. The most widely known of these disorders is Tay-Sachs disease.

the lymphatic system, lungs, skin, eyes, kidney, heart, and, in rare instances, the nervous system. Frequently, an organ that contains Gaucher cells becomes enlarged and does not function properly, resulting in clinical symptoms associated with the disease. The type and severity of symptoms can vary widely among individuals. Some individuals experience no symptoms; others may develop life-threatening conditions.

Gaucher cells in the spleen: One common site for the accumulation of Gaucher cells is the spleen. Typically, the effect of Gaucher cell accumulation in this organ is that it becomes enlarged and overactive. The enlargement may cause the abdomen to become distended so that a person appears overweight or looks pregnant. Normally, the spleen breaks down old blood cells at the same rate that new ones are produced in the bone marrow. When the spleen becomes overactive, it tends to break down red cells more rapidly than they can be produced, and a deficiency develops. The deficiency in red blood cells results in anemia. Red cells carry oxygen from the lungs to all cells in the body. Because anemic patients lack sufficient red cells, they suffer from the effects of insufficient oxygen. As a result, muscle cells cannot produce the energy they need, and the tendency is to become easily fatigued.

Overactivity of the spleen can also cause a deficiency of white blood cells, which may reduce the body's ability to fight bacterial infections. Or an overactive spleen can reduce the number of blood platelets. A reduction in platelets lowers the body's ability to form blood clots, increasing the tendency for bleeding and bruising. As a result, frequent and heavy nosebleeds are common in people with Gaucher's disease.

Gaucher cells in the liver: The liver is another frequent site for Gaucher cell accumulation. The liver can become enlarged and function abnormally. In some individuals, the liver enlarges along with the spleen. In patients who have had their spleens removed, the liver may become dramatically enlarged due to the displacement of Gaucher cell accumulation from the spleen to the liver. The effects of abnormal liver function are usually minor, although a few people may develop cirrhosis. In cirrhosis, the liver develops scar tissue.

Gaucher cells in the bone marrow: The other common site where Gaucher cells collect is the marrow inside bones of the skeleton. The accumulated Gaucher cells reduce normal bone marrow function in the areas where the Gaucher cells are most concentrated. This can lead to the variety of bone problems commonly found in people with Gaucher's disease. For example, Gaucher cells in the bone marrow can interfere with the production of blood cells (the marrow is one of the normal sites in the body where blood cells are formed), compounding the deficiencies caused by an overactive, enlarged spleen.

Bones affected by Gaucher's disease may be more prone to infection. The bones may be thinner or weaker than normal, or they may be deformed. In addition, "bone crises" can occur when there is a sudden lack of oxygen in an area where Gaucher cells have interfered with normal blood flow. These episodes can be extremely painful; they feel like a "heart attack of the bone." The restriction in blood flow can also result in destruction of bone tissue (called aseptic necrosis) and lead to permanent mobility problems.

In addition, the bones may become brittle and subject to spontaneous fractures. If these fractures occur in the spinal column, they are called compression fractures and can cause nerve damage. Individuals with Gaucher's disease often complain of general bone and joint pain. This pain is probably due to inflammation in the skeletal system caused by the presence of Gaucher cells.

Is there a typical Gaucher individual?

Although all people with Gaucher's disease lack normal levels of glucocerebrosidase activity, there is a variation from person to person. As a result, the timing and severity of symptoms vary greatly. At present, Gaucher specialists divide the disease into three classifications: Types 1, 2, and 3, based on the particular symptoms and course of the disease. In general, the later in life the first symptoms appear, the less likely it is that the disease will be severe.

Signs and Symptoms of Type 1 Gaucher's Disease

- Generalized fatigue: lack of energy and stamina
- Abdomen: enlarged spleen, enlarged liver
- Pain
- Compression of the lungs
- Skeletal system: growth retardation in children, pain and degeneration of joints and bone-covering tissue
- Loss of bone density, leading to widening of bones along the knee joint, curvature of the bones, spontaneous fractures, acute bone infarctions ("bone crises"), bone necrosis (death of tissue)
- Lungs: decreased ability to provide oxygen to the blood
- Kidneys: disruption of normal function
- Skin: yellow-brown pigmentation; nonraised, round, purplish-red spots, especially around the eyes
- Blood: increased bleeding tendency such as nosebleeds and bruising; subnormal levels of blood platelets, red blood cells, and white blood cells; elevated levels of acid phosphatase, plasma proteins
- Digestive system: loss of appetite, intestinal complaints

Most people with Gaucher's disease do not develop all of the possible symptoms. In addition, the severity of the disease varies enormously.

What is Type 1 Gaucher's disease?

Type 1 Gaucher's disease—the most common form—is often, but misleadingly, referred to as "adult Gaucher's disease." Individuals of all ages can be affected. The defective genes are found in fewer than 1 in 40,000 people in the general population. The defective genes are more common among Ashkenazi Jews, occurring in 1 out of every 400 to 600 births within this population. Because Type 1 Gaucher's disease does not affect the nervous system, it is sometimes referred to as nonneuronopathic Gaucher's disease.

Type 1 Gaucher's disease has a particularly wide variation in clinical signs, symptoms, and disease course. Many people with Type 1 disease have no clinical symptoms and lead normal lives. In some cases, however, the disease may become life-threatening. In general, the later in life the first symptoms appear, the less likely that the disease will be severe.

Perhaps the most common sign of Type 1 Gaucher's disease is an enlargement of the spleen or liver, or both. Overactivity of the enlarged spleen may result in an increased tendency for bleeding due to decreased platelets or fatigue related to anemia. Spleen enlargement is often the most frequent initial finding and may be first recognized when the child is as young as six months. The spleen may become sufficiently enlarged to affect the child's mobility and to attract attention. A child with severe disease may be shorter than average and may adopt a swayback posture to support the weight of an enlarged abdomen.

Skeletal symptoms of bone involvement can occur at any time in life: in children as young as two years of age or in adults as old as seventy. In more than half of the people with Type 1 Gaucher's disease, X-rays reveal a characteristic deformity called the "Erlenmeyer flask deformity" in the thigh bones. The thigh bones have a flaring at the knee (resembling an Erlenmeyer flask), instead of having a normal rounded shape. Some of the signs and symptoms that may be experienced by people with Type 1 Gaucher's disease are shown in the box on page 150.

What is Type 2 Gaucher's disease?

Type 2 Gaucher's disease is a very rare, rapidly progressive form of the disease that affects the brain, as well as the organs affected by Type 1. Formerly called "infantile Gaucher's disease," Type 2 is characterized by severe neurological involvement in the first year of life. Thus it is also called "acute neuronopathic Gaucher's disease." Fewer than 1 in 100,000 newborns have Type 2 disease. This form of Gaucher's disease does not appear to be concentrated within any particular ethnic group.

Infants with Type 2 disease typically appear normal during the first few months of life before developing neurological symptoms, along with many of the symptoms associated with Type 1. An afflicted child usually does not live past the age of two, due to the severe involvement of the nervous system.

What is Type 3 Gaucher's disease?

Formerly called "juvenile Gaucher's disease," Type 3 is characterized by a slowly progressive neurological disease. Type 3 Gaucher's disease is also very rare (an incidence of fewer than 1 in 100,000 people). As in Type 2, it does not appear to be concentrated in any particular ethnic group, although a number of cases with Type 3 symptoms have been reported in Scandinavia, particularly Sweden.

      The signs and symptoms of Type 3 Gaucher's disease appear in early childhood. Other than the nervous system involvement, Type 3 Gaucher symptoms resemble Type 1. Type 3 individuals who reach adolescence may survive into the third or fourth decade.

How does someone get Gaucher's disease?

Gaucher's disease is inherited. Much of a person's makeup is a result of what is inherited from each parent. Certain characteristics, such as eye color, height, and genetic disease, are passed from parents to children. The genes for these characteristics are organized on twenty-three pairs of chromosomes. Genes contain the blueprints that the body's cells use to produce proteins—the building blocks of life. Each chromosome contains thousands of genes. An individual normally inherits one copy of each gene from each parent.

      The genes for glucocerebrosidase are also passed on from parents to children. In Gaucher's disease, the blueprint for the glucocerebrosidase enzyme (a type of protein) is defective. As a result, the glucocerebrosidase produced from the defective genes is unable to perform its normal function.

Is the risk of inheriting Gaucher's disease the same for males and females?

Copies of the gene for glucocerebrosidase are carried on a chromosome that is not involved in determining an individual's sex. As a result, the defective glucocerebrosidase gene can be passed on to either males or females. One pair of chromosomes, called the sex chromosomes, differs between men and women in a way that determines their sexual identities. The other twenty-two pairs of chromosomes are called autosomes. The gene for the glucocerebrosidase enzyme is on one of the autosomal chromosome pairs. Gaucher's disease is referred to as an autosomal-recessive disorder. "Recessive" refers to the fact that in order to develop the disease, an individual must inherit two defective copies of the gene, one from each parent.

Who are Gaucher carriers?

A person with one normal gene and one defective gene for glucocerebrosidase is a carrier of Gaucher's disease. (Approximately 1 in 10 people in the Ashkenazi population are carriers.) Such individuals will not develop the disease because as long as one of the two genes for glucocerebrosidase is normal, enough glucocerebrosidase can be produced to prevent glucocerebroside from accumulating. Although a Gaucher carrier will have no symptoms of the disease, the odds are 50:50 that the "Gaucher gene" will be passed on to each of his or her children. A child will only develop Gaucher's disease if he or she inherits a defective gene from both parents.

What are the odds of having children who have Gaucher's disease or who are Gaucher carriers?

If both parents have normal genes for glucocerebrosidase, each child will inherit two normal genes, one from each parent, and will neither have Gaucher's disease nor be a carrier.

If one parent is a carrier of Gaucher's disease and the other parent is not, there is a 50:50 chance of having a child who inherits

 HEALTH FACTS

If one parent has Gaucher's disease and the other parent is a Gaucher carrier, there is a 50:50 chance of having a child who inherits a "Gaucher gene" from each parent and thus has the disease. There is also a 50:50 chance of having a child who only inherits the "Gaucher gene" from one parent and becomes a carrier. If both parents have Gaucher's disease, all their children will inherit two "Gaucher genes" and will have the disease as well.

the "Gaucher gene" from the carrier parent and becomes a carrier of the disease. None of the children will have Gaucher's disease, because they will have one normal gene inherited from the other parent.

If both parents are carriers of Gaucher's disease, with each pregnancy there is a 25 percent chance of having a child who inherits one "Gaucher gene" from each parent and thus has Gaucher's disease. There is a 50:50 chance of having a child who inherits a "Gaucher gene" from one parent and a normal gene from the other parent and becomes a carrier of the disease. Finally, there is a 25 percent chance for each pregnancy of having a child who inherits two normal genes (one from each parent) and who neither has Gaucher's disease nor is a carrier.

It must be emphasized that the odds, for each pregnancy, of inheriting Gaucher's disease are totally independent of whether or not a previous child has the disease. Having one child with Gaucher's disease does not mean that the next three children cannot inherit the disease.

If one parent has Gaucher's disease and the other parent neither has the disease nor is a carrier, all children will inherit the "Gaucher gene" from the parent with the disease and will become carriers. None of these children will have the disease themselves.

Who should be tested for Gaucher's disease for carrier status?

Because Gaucher's disease is a genetic disorder, all close blood relatives of patients are at risk of having the disease or are potential carriers of the "Gaucher gene." Families with a history of Gaucher's disease may want to discuss the possibility of genetic testing with their physicians. To screen for the disease, a blood sample is taken to measure glucocerebrosidase activity. Depending on the level of activity found, a person may be diagnosed as having Gaucher's disease or being a Gaucher carrier. For detecting carriers, the blood test is not always accurate, due to the variation in enzyme levels. Amniocentesis and chorionic villus sampling (CVS) can be used to diagnose Gaucher's disease early in pregnancy. Genetic counseling is available to couples who are found to be carriers or who have a family history of Gaucher's disease.

How is the disease diagnosed?

The process of diagnosing many diseases, especially Gaucher's disease, is not always straightforward. Often the patient initially visits the physician for another problem such as the flu, for nonspecific pain, or for a routine physical. Although making a diagnosis of Gaucher's disease is not difficult, some symptoms may resemble other diseases. The physician may first perform other tests to eliminate from consideration more common disorders. For example, in cases where patients have low platelet counts, physicians may first test for leukemia. If a patient complains of joint pain, the physician may first suspect arthritis. Sometimes a specialist physician, like a geneticist or hematologist, may be helpful in distinguishing the symptoms of Gaucher's disease from other diseases with similar symptoms.

Gaucher's disease might be suspected in a person who has an unexplained enlargement of the spleen, a tendency toward bleeding, bone or joint pains, or spontaneous fractures. A pediatrician might make the diagnosis in a child complaining of abdominal discomfort or of frequent nosebleeds. A hematologist might make the diagnosis in a person with low blood or platelet counts. An orthopedist might diagnose Gaucher's disease in the course of treating someone suffering from frequent, unexplained fractures. Gaucher's disease would be particularly suspected in people with blood relatives who have the disease. Physicians should be notified if there is a family history of genetic disease.

Indications of Gaucher's disease that are not noticed by the patient but are very apparent in laboratory analysis include elevated levels of acid phosphatase or of angiotensin-converting enzyme in the blood serum, and characteristic skeletal features, as revealed by X-ray examination.

When Gaucher's disease is strongly suspected, the diagnosis can be established by a blood test showing a significantly decreased activity level of glucocerebrosidase in white blood cells. If there is a question about the diagnosis, the physician may want to obtain a bone marrow sample to check for Gaucher cells in the marrow, or a skin sample. Certain skin cells called fibroblasts can be grown in culture and then used to measure glucocerebrosidase activity levels.

What about the uncertainty?

One of the most common emotional concerns posed by Gaucher's disease relates to the feelings of isolation and ignorance about the disease. There is often a feeling of great uncertainty because the symptoms and their severity may vary widely, and they may occur at any time. Some people remain symptom-free for many years; others may begin having symptoms very early in life. This uncertainty can add considerably to the usual difficulties in making short- and long-term plans and in setting goals. In addition, people with Gaucher's disease and Gaucher carriers face difficult decisions, with no easy answers, about marriage and children. For example, if they have the disease, will they have the physical stamina to raise children, or will their children be affected by the disease? However, this uncertainty sometimes adds to the development of an exceptional inner strength that many people with chronic illnesses often possess.

Is the disease painful?

Some people with Gaucher's disease go through periods of severe skeletal pain known as "bone crises." Joints swell, become shiny, red, and inflamed, and actually feel warm to the touch. Sometimes the slightest movement can elicit excruciating pain. If the pain becomes sufficiently severe, it may prevent people from moving about comfortably or make it difficult to sleep.

Adults and the parents of children with Gaucher's disease work with their physicians to learn which analgesics or pain-relieving techniques work best for them. In addition, they learn how to manage their lives to minimize the pain.

Is fatigue a problem?

Another challenge faced by some people with Gaucher's disease is fatigue that may occur as a consequence of anemia. People who are severely anemic may feel tired, even after a full night's sleep. Some children may lack the energy and stamina to play with other children. They may have difficulty staying alert in the classroom or concentrating on their homework. It is important for many people with Gaucher's disease to include naps in their daily schedules to help combat bouts of fatigue. Ordinary activities that a healthy person can do easily may require more effort for a person with Gaucher's disease. Many people find that they can do what they please if they are careful to pace themselves and ask for help when it is needed.

HEALTH FACTS

The pain associated with Gaucher's disease can range from very mild to severe. Coping with the pain, if it does become severe, can be a major challenge for people with Gaucher's disease. At times, painful episodes may occur involving enlarged organs or affected bones. These episodes usually resolve within a week or two, but they can last longer. Sometimes, potent medication may be necessary to control the pain during these episodes.

How does the disease affect mobility?

At different times, the effects of Gaucher's disease can impair mobility for some people. Walking can become tiresome and difficult, especially for long distances or up and down stairs. A decrease in mobility may occur as a response to a bone crisis or as a result of a bone fracture. The use of ambulatory aids such as a wheelchair, crutches, cane, or walker may be helpful in these situations. In rare instances, the lack of mobility may become so severe that a person requires hospitalization or confinement to bed. For children, this can result in missed days from school. Adults who are working may require extra time off from work. Lifestyle changes can help to conserve energy and minimize the strain on bones and joints.

How does Gaucher's disease affect appetite?

Pronounced liver or spleen enlargement can frequently affect a person's appetite because of the pressure exerted on the stomach. People with Gaucher's disease often report a sensation of feeling full, even after having only a few bites of food. The enlarged organs leave little room in the body cavity for a full stomach. People with Gaucher's disease may take longer to eat because their stomachs fill up so quickly. The fact that they may not eat much can become distressing for themselves and for family members. In these situations, empathy about the difficulties associated with mealtimes is helpful. People with digestive difficulties will also discover which foods or eating habits should be avoided in order to minimize digestive complaints.

How does Gaucher's disease affect appearance?

Body image can be a difficult challenge for Gaucher patients who suffer from pronounced spleen or liver enlargement, or both. Children and adults may be teased or ridiculed and accused of being fat, looking pregnant, or otherwise of being "different."

For children, who can be very conscious of their appearance, such treatment can be particularly unpleasant and can hurt their self-image. In addition to dealing with the inherent problems of Gaucher's disease, they have to contend with unjust comments focused on their appearance. In these situations, shopping for clothes that fit properly and are comfortable becomes important for children and adults. Individuals with pronounced abdominal protrusions may find that clothes that are loose-fitting or made of stretch fabrics are often the most comfortable. Jeans and other clothes with more defined waistbands may put too much pressure on the enlarged organs.

What happens to children with Gaucher's disease?

They may grow more slowly than other children, and they may be smaller and shorter because more of their energy is used to cope with the disease, and less is available for the growth process. Children may be below the normal percentile in growth and in weight for others of their age. These children may also appear clumsy and off-balance because of their enlarged organs. Parents and teachers may have the tendency to baby children with Gaucher's disease because sometimes they appear younger than their peers.

Teenagers with Gaucher's disease frequently experience a delay in the onset of puberty. By their late teens, most children with Gaucher's disease catch up with the rest of the population. They generally obtain their genetically programmed height and experience normal sexual development. However, the delayed onset of changes may cause some psychological difficulties during adolescence.

Depending on the severity of the disease, Gaucher children with reduced agility, with a tendency toward bleeding or bone fractures, or with enlarged spleens may be advised by their physicians to avoid contact sports. Instead they may be encouraged to take up non-contact sports, such as swimming, bicycle riding, or dancing. If their physical endurance is low because of breathing difficulties or anemia,

HEALTH FACTS

Body image can be a difficult challenge for Gaucher patients who suffer from pronounced spleen or liver enlargement or both. Children and adults may be teased or ridiculed and accused of being fat, looking pregnant, or otherwise of being "different."

nonaerobic activities may he preferable. More severely affected children should be careful about playing sports if they are susceptible to bone breaks, bruising, and fractures. However, less affected children can certainly participate in all but the most aggressive contact sports. A child who is strong enough to be actively interested in sports should be encouraged to participate and to learn to gauge the limitations of his or her own body.

It is important to encourage other activities to help the more severely afflicted group of children with Gaucher's disease to develop outside interests and healthy socialization skills. Children often compensate for the things they cannot do by excelling in other areas of their lives. Physicians and families can work together to determine which activities are most appropriate for children with Gaucher's disease. Schools are often willing to develop alternate activities and programs for children with physical limitations.

What are some issues that may face parents of children with Gaucher's disease?

Being the parent of a child with Gaucher's disease can involve difficult decisions that other parents do not have to face and for which there is often no clear advice. Gaucher parents must decide, with their physicians, if their child's activity should be restricted. They must balance the physical risks with their child's need to fit in with other children. Gaucher parents must choose how and when to inform their child of his or her condition. They must decide whether to inform others, such as school officials or friends. Parents must offer emotional as well as practical relief if their child suffers episodes of pain.

Family dynamics and relations among siblings may shift, as attention becomes focused on or away from the child with Gaucher's disease. Marriages can come under stress; siblings and parents may feel guilty or resentful.

The emotional issues associated with Gaucher's disease can become especially upsetting for children who are at an age when it is so important "to be like" other children and to "fit in" with their group. They may become frustrated if they do not look like other children and cannot always do the same things that other children can do. By understanding their child's emotional needs, parents can help the child deal with the hurt that he or she may be experiencing. Physicians and other community resources can often bring invaluable support to families with chronically ill children. Sometimes just sharing these concerns with others can be very helpful.

What are some of the issues that face adults with Gaucher's disease?

For individuals with Gaucher's disease who first experience disabling symptoms in adulthood, the psychological impact can be great. Adults may feel that they used to have much more stamina to be able to enjoy the varied pleasures of life. They were busy with their families, careers, and social lives. They were independent and mobile. An abrupt onset of severe symptoms may suddenly interfere with career and life plans. For other adults who experience mild-to-minimal symptoms, the disease may have only minor effects on their lives. Sometimes they forget about Gaucher's disease altogether. As the disease progresses, some adults may feel drained and burdened by their limitations. They are forced to make lifestyle changes, to pace themselves, and to learn to adapt to their new situation.

Is there treatment for Gaucher's disease?

Until recently, patient care and therapy for Gaucher's disease was directed at managing (relieving) the symptoms resulting from the accumulation of Gaucher cells in the various organs. Careful monitoring of the liver and spleen size and blood counts by a patient's physician helps to determine the appropriate therapy.

Depending on symptoms, therapy includes the following measures, either alone or in combination: bed rest, non-aspirin analgesics (aspirin inhibits the blood from clotting and is not advisable for people with Gaucher's disease), and anti-inflammatory drugs for acute and chronic pain, biofeedback techniques for pain management, hyperbaric oxygen therapy for the treatment of bone crisis, splenectomy (either complete or partial) for severe anemia, low platelet counts, and mechanical obstruction. Sometimes bleeding from a minor wound may require medical intervention to avoid a major blood loss. Oxygen therapy may be necessary for people who have reduced blood supply to the lungs.

Low blood count resulting from overactivity of a Gaucher-cell-containing spleen is sometimes treated by blood or platelet transfusions, or both, or by iron therapy to alleviate the anemia. In the case of a severe and persistent lowering of the blood count, physicians may decide to remove all or part of the spleen. Neither of these approaches is totally satisfactory. Iron therapy increases the risk of hemochromatosis (an iron surplus disease), whereas spleen removal increases the susceptibility to bacterial diseases and may lead to increased liver and bony symptoms. For these reasons, spleen removal is usually delayed as long as possible, and partial spleen removal (which may be more difficult to perform) may be recommended over total removal.

Orthopedic evaluation and intervention may be required for many of the bone complications associated with Gaucher's disease. These procedures include orthopedic surgical techniques to relieve pressure from damaged bony areas or the insertion of prosthetic devices (such as hip replacements) in joints that have been destroyed by the disease process.

Bone marrow transplantation has been tried as a treatment for severely ill people with Gaucher's disease. Because it is such a high-risk procedure, and it requires carefully matched donors, bone marrow transplantation is not performed often. The procedure is generally reserved as a treatment option for terminally ill patients.

What is enzyme replacement therapy?

Recently, progress has been made in the development of a safe and effective technique that promises to go beyond management of symptoms caused by the accumulation of Gaucher cells. Because people with Gaucher's disease are deficient in glucocerebrosidase enzymatic activity, the most direct and logical therapeutic approach to this inherited disease is to supplement or to replace the missing enzyme.

Dr. Roscoe Brady pioneered the development of this therapy at the National Institute of Neurological Disorders and Stroke. Initial research on the natural glucocerebrosidase enzyme showed that it was not particularly effective when administered by infusion to people with Gaucher's disease. The majority of the enzyme did not reach the "Gaucher cells" in the body. Dr. Brady developed a form of the glucocerebrosidase enzyme that was modified to increase targeting and uptake in the macrophages—the cells where the enzyme is needed. Modified glucocerebrosidase enzyme has been evaluated in clinical trials, which showed that repeated infusions of the enzyme reduced the signs and symptoms of the disease and reversed the disease progression. Specialists in Gaucher's disease believe that this development is a very exciting one and represents the first true therapeutic breakthrough. The administration of macrophage-targeted glucocerebrosidase will be required at regular intervals throughout an individual's lifetime. As such, the enzyme is an effective therapy rather than a cure.

What is the state of other research on Gaucher's disease?

Researchers are currently pursuing avenues of genetic investigation that may point to a possible cure for the disease. Currently, research is under way in three main areas: (1) production of the glucocerebrosidase enzyme using a recombinant cell line, (2) location of genetic predictors for clinical severity, and (3) attempts to do gene therapy.

The production of the glucocerebrosidase enzyme using a recombinant cell line has been achieved on a research scale. Development is under way, and clinical testing is planned.

Scientists have already identified some of the particular genetic differences in the glucocerebrosidase gene among people with Gaucher's disease. Scientists may be able to correlate the particular defects with the course that Gaucher's disease follows in an individual with those genes. Based on this research, physicians may one day be able to predict disease progression with more improved accuracy in prognosis than is available now.

Efforts are also under way to develop gene therapy. This approach involves introducing normal genes for glucocerebrosidase into cells of the affected person. These cells would then produce sufficient normal amounts of active glucocerebrosidase. Approaches to gene therapy are highly experimental at present, and major technical hurdles have to be overcome to demonstrate that this technology is safe and effective, as well as whether it can be applied in Gaucher's disease.

What support is available for Gaucher's disease?

The majority of people with Type 1 Gaucher's disease—even those with severe symptoms—are able to lead productive, happy lives. Just as each case of Gaucher's disease is unique, each person with the disorder draws on a unique combination of inner and outer resources to meet life's challenges. These resources certainly include family, friends, others with Gaucher's disease, physicians, and genetic counselors. They may also include religious faith and support groups such as the National Gaucher Foundation.

What is the National Gaucher Foundation?

The National Gaucher Foundation (NGF) is a nonprofit, tax-exempt organization whose primary objective is to assist in finding a remedy and viable treatment program for Gaucher's disease. Founded in 1984, the NGF supports medical research and clinical programs that enhance the current understanding of Gaucher's disease. The foundation also provides information and assistance to individuals and families affected by the disease and conducts education and outreach activities to increase public awareness of this disorder.

The research funded by NGF is conducted in the United States and abroad. The NGF is supported primarily through grants and contributions received from individuals, corporations, and foundations. The organization publishes a bimonthly newsletter that disseminates information to individuals, medical practitioners, and organizations interested in Gaucher's disease. Through the Gaucher's Disease Family Support Network, the NGF will place a contact person who has experience with Gaucher's disease in touch with others in need of assistance.

 Robin Ely Berman, M.D., and
 Roscoe O. Brady, M.D.

Chapter 29

Hadassah Saved My Daughter

I often tease my children that when I gave birth to them, the hospital gave me a third arm to help carry all of the extra items a mother has to carry and a third eye that could see what they were doing, no matter where they are. While I did not receive a third arm or eye, as useful as they would be, I, like many mothers, discovered my mother's instinct, unknown to me before I had children.

Prior to becoming a mother, I often watched mothers who seemed to know when a child was in trouble or needed their help. I witnessed mothers who would grab a child's hand before he ran into the street or seemed to stop in mid-activity to attend to a child who was in trouble. Once I became a mother, I learned to rely on that feeling I got on occasion that made me think that something was not right with my children. My mother's instinct, along with a little help from Hadassah, played a crucial role in my daughter Michelle's life in 2001.

When Michelle was born, she seemed to bring a ray of sunshine into our lives. She was a sweet child and loved to play and be with other children. When she was four, we enrolled her in one of the local Jewish day schools, where she quickly made friends.

In January 2001, she began to get sick. In the beginning, I thought she might be getting sick because she was in a new school with new children. She seemed to barely get better before she came down with another illness. Her pediatrician monitored her but felt she was just more susceptible to illnesses than other children and that as she got older, she would not get sick as often.

In April, while playing with her brother, she broke her arm. It was a typical childhood injury. In fact, the nurses at the hospital told us hers was the third broken arm they had seen that day. Again we were reassured that this was a typical childhood accident. Fortunately, a little bell began ringing in the back of my head, telling me something was not right.

As the summer progressed, Michelle continued to get colds and viruses. One day in July, I received a call from the head of the camp Michelle was attending. Michelle was not feeling well and was complaining of a bad stomachache. Her doctor suspected appendicitis, and we quickly rushed her to the hospital. After many tests, we were assured that Michelle's appendix was fine but were told that she had an enlarged spleen and liver and that her platelet count was low—around 95,000. Again, my mother's instinct bothered me; I wanted to find out why my daughter felt so bad.

Over the next two months, the pediatrician monitored Michelle, sending her from specialist to specialist and ordering one test after another. Michelle started feeling bad all the time. She became pale, had constant stomachaches, and fatigued easily. Her platelets continued to drop, and it was difficult to get her to eat more than three or four bites of food before she would complain of a stomachache. At night, Michelle would wake up crying from pain, and we would rock together for comfort. My heart was breaking as I saw my little girl fading right before my eyes. I felt so helpless.

Unfortunately, we became regulars at the local children's hospital. I learned the nurses' names and kept a special bag all packed to take each time Michelle was sent for tests. In it were magazines to distract me while I waited.

One morning in late August, Michelle was having an MRI to rule out cancer. She had just been transported to radiology when I saw a doctor approach the family in the next curtained area. The doctor told the parents that their daughter had a rare form of cancer, and my eyes filled with tears. The child was a beautiful, twelve- or thirteen-year-old girl with a sparkle in her eyes. I knew that Michelle was having the same test, and I prayed that she did not have cancer. I felt as though I could handle just about anything else but cancer.

Through my tears, I glanced down at the magazine that I was flipping through; it was my monthly *Hadassah Magazine.* I had stopped at a page with an advertisement for a disease I had never heard of: Gaucher's disease. The advertisement listed the symptoms, and I was amazed at how many my daughter had. She was fatigued; she had a low platelet count, a rounded stomach, and an enlarged spleen and liver; and she was very small for her age. I was surprised when I read that one in ten Jews of Ashkenazi descent are carriers. At the bottom of the advertisement it said that Gaucher's disease could be detected by a simple blood test. I wondered why I had never heard of a disease that my husband and I had a 25 percent chance of passing on to our children with each birth. I couldn't imagine why I had never heard of such a common disease.

My mother's instinct could not let it rest. I decided to contact my daughter's doctor and ask to have Michelle tested for Gaucher's disease. On Yom Kippur, the pediatrician called; Michelle did have Gaucher's.

As a mother, I cannot tell you that I am thrilled for my child to have Gaucher's. It is difficult to think that your child has a disease that she will have to live with for the rest of her life. What I can tell you is that had it not been for my mother's instinct and a little help from Hadassah, my daughter might have gone through a lot more tests and suffering before the disease was detected. Most individuals living with Gaucher's are not even diagnosed until they are adults.

Michelle is now in her eleventh month of treatment. In May, she celebrated her sixth birthday. I am amazed every time I look at her and see how healthy she is. Her last platelet count had increased to over 200,000, and her spleen and liver had shrunk from 13.5 times normal size to 6 times normal size. She has grown almost three inches and no longer complains of constant fatigue. Michelle doesn't like receiving intravenous treatments every two weeks but has come to accept them. We have a wonderful nurse who comes to our home and plays with her while she is receiving her IV. When I look at pictures of Michelle before her treatment, I am amazed at how sick she looks, and I am hopeful that she will live a full and productive life.

I am thankful that I was able to learn about Gaucher's disease. My hope is that you will share Michelle's story with friends and family. One in every 450 individuals of Ashkenazi Jewish descent has Type 1 Gaucher's disease, yet only some 1,300 of the estimated 17,000 individuals with the disease in the United States are diagnosed and treated for the disorder. It is up to each of you to spread the word. Maybe then affected people will take the time and have the blood work done. They could be leading happier, healthier lives. Just like Michelle.

_D.C._

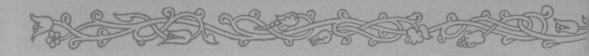

Chapter 30

Niemann-Pick Disease, Type A

Niemann-Pick disease, Type A, is a severe neurodegenerative disorder of infancy. By six months of age, affected babies experience feeding difficulty, recurrent vomiting, and enlargement of the spleen and liver, which causes the abdomen to appear distended. Some children with the disease have a cherry-red spot in the retina of the eye. Death usually occurs between ages two and four. One in seventy-five Ashkenazi Jews are carriers of Niemann-Pick Type A.

Niemann-Pick disease (NPD), Type A, is characterized by the following symptoms:

- Abdominal distention
- Coordination and motor-skill difficulties
- Feeding problems
- Progressive spasticity
- Blindness
- Enlarged liver or spleen, or both
- A cherry-red spot in the eye, visible by special eye exam

The child may present with jaundice in infancy, with progressive liver failure following. Usually, a baby with Niemann-Pick Type A dies by the second year of life.

Cause: NPD is inherited in an autosomal-recessive manner. When both parents are carriers of the gene mutations, there is a one-in-four (25 percent) chance in each pregnancy of having an affected child. The specific biochemical defect in this disease is the deficiency of an enzyme—acid sphingomyelinase (ASM)—that normally degrades a fatty substance known as sphingomyelin. The enzyme defect leads to the accumulation of sphingomyelin, primarily in the liver, spleen, lymph nodes, and brain.

Treatment: There is currently no treatment or cure for Niemann-Pick Type A.

Disease frequency: There are approximately 1,200 Type A or Type B cases diagnosed worldwide. It has been estimated that approximately two-thirds of all infants with Niemann-Pick Type A are of Ashkenazi Jewish descent.

Carrier frequency: Approximately 1 in 75 Ashkenazi Jews is a carrier of Niemann-Pick Type A.

Diagnosis: Diagnosis of people affected with Niemann-Pick Types A and B can be achieved by testing blood and measuring the ASM activity in the white blood cells.

Screening: Carrier screening requires a sample of blood to determine whether or not a gene change is present in the gene for Neiman-Pick. Prenatal screening, via chorionic villus sampling (CVS) or amniocentesis, can be performed early in the pregnancy.

History: The first case of infantile-onset NPD was described in 1914 by the German neurologist Albert Niemann. Niemann described a young child with an enlarged liver and spleen, enlarged lymph glands, swelling, and a darkening of the skin of the face. The child had brain and nervous system impairment and died before the age of two. Later, in the 1920s, Luddwick Pick studied tissues after the death of such children and provided evidence of the new disorder.

Future: In 1997, the gene responsible for NPD was discovered. This discovery has helped focus research for treatments. Gene therapy has shown effectiveness in mice for Niemann-Pick Type A.

Lisa Katz

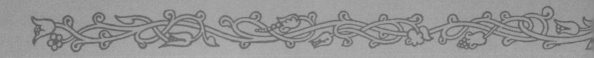

Chapter 31

Information from the National Niemann-Pick Disease Foundation, Inc.

The National Niemann-Pick Disease Foundation, Inc. (NNPDF) is an international, voluntary, nonprofit organization made up of parents, medical and educational professionals, friends, relatives, and others who are committed to finding a cure for NPD.

Its primary goals are as follows:

- To promote medical research into the cause of NPD in order to eventually find a cure
- To provide medical and educational information to assist in the correct diagnosis and referral of children with NPD
- To provide support to families of NPD patients
- To facilitate genetic counseling for parents who are known carriers of NPD
- To encourage the sharing of research information among scientists
- To support legislation that positively affects patients and families with NPD

Is a child you know experiencing some of these symptoms?

- Abdominal enlargement
- Enlarged spleen or liver
- Jaundice following birth

- Unusual shortness of breath
- Repeated lung infections
- Cherry-red spot inside the eye
- Vertical eye movement difficulties
- Progressive loss of early motor skills
- Feeding and swallowing difficulties
- Learning problems
- Sudden loss of muscle tone
- Slurred speech
- Seizures
- Hypersensitivity to touch

These symptoms may be an indication of Niemann-Pick disease.

What is Niemann-Pick disease?

Niemann-Pick disease is actually a term for a group of diseases that affect metabolism and are caused by specific genetic mutations. The three most commonly recognized forms of the disease are Types A, B, and C.

Niemann-Pick Types A and B are both caused by the deficiency of a specific enzyme activity—acid sphingomyelinase (ASM). This enzyme is ordinarily found in special compartments within cells called lysosomes and is required to metabolize a special lipid—sphingomyelin. If ASM is absent or not functioning properly, this lipid cannot be metabolized properly and is accumulated within the cell, eventually causing cell death and the malfunction of major organ systems.

Types A and B are both caused by the same enzymatic deficiency, and there is a growing consensus that the two forms represent opposite ends of a continuous scale. People with Type A generally have little or no ASM production (less than 1 percent of normal), whereas those with Type B have approximately 10 percent of the normal level of ASM.

Although both Types A and B have ASM activity that is significantly lower than normal, the clinical prognosis for these two groups of patients is very different. Type A Niemann-Pick is a severe neurological disease that leads to death by two to four years of age.

In contrast, patients with Type B generally have little or no neurological involvement and may survive into late childhood or adulthood. Type B individuals usually have enlarged livers and spleens, and respiratory problems are common. The enlargement of organs and the respiratory problems can cause cardiovascular stress and can lead to heart disease later in life.

Patients with intermediate ASM activity tend to have more neurological problems than Type B but fewer problems than Type A. Because there is not a precise correlation between ASM activity and neurological involvement, it is not possible to accurately predict the severity of the disease by enzyme testing. There are approximately 1,200 cases worldwide, with the majority being Type B or an intermediate form.

Type C Niemann-Pick, although similar in name to Types A and B, is very different at the biochemical and genetic levels. Patients are not able to metabolize cholesterol and other lipids properly within the cell. Consequently, excessive amounts of cholesterol accumulate within the liver and spleen, and excessive amounts of other lipids accumulate in the brain. Type C causes a secondary reduction of ASM activity, which led all three types to be considered forms of the same disease.

There is considerable variation in when Type C symptoms first appear and in the progression of the disease. Symptoms may appear as early as in the first few months or as late as adulthood. Vertical supranuclear-gaze palsy (VSGP)—the inability to move the eyes up and down—enlarged liver, enlarged spleen, or jaundice in young children are strong indications that NPC should be considered. It is common for only one or two symptoms to appear in the early stages of the disease.

In most cases, neurological symptoms begin appearing between the ages of four and ten. Generally, the later neurological symptoms begin, the slower the progression of the disease.

About five hundred cases of Type C Niemann-Pick have been diagnosed worldwide. It is believed that the number of people affected is higher, but it is often difficult to make the correct diagnosis. Niemann-Pick Type C has been initially diagnosed as a learning disability, mild retardation, clumsiness, and delayed development of fine motor skills. It is not uncommon for a family to spend several years seeking a diagnosis before Type C is identified.

Type C is always fatal. The vast majority of children die before age twenty (and many die before the age of ten). Late onset of symptoms can lead to longer life spans, but it is extremely rare for any person to reach age forty. In the past, other types of Niemann-Pick were identified. The older forms include the following:

- Type D Niemann-Pick was described in the French Canadian population of Yarmouth County, Nova Scotia. Genealogical evidence indicates that Joseph Muise (c. 1679–1729) and Marie Amirault (1684–c. 1735) are common ancestors to all of the Nova Scotia cases. This is now recognized as a variation of Type C.
- Type E Niemann-Pick was described for cases of adult-onset. This is now considered a variation of Type C, where the metabolic processes are only partially dysfunctional, slowing the onset and progression of symptoms.
- Niemann-Pick affects all segments of the population, with cases reported from North America, South America, Europe, Africa, Asia, and Australia. However, a higher incidence has been found in certain populations:

  Ashkenazi Jewish population (Types A and B)
  French Canadian population of Nova Scotia (Type D)
  Maghreb region (Tunisia, Morocco, and Algeria) of North Africa (Type B)
  Spanish American population of southern New Mexico and Colorado (Type C)

Pick's disease is sometimes confused with Niemann-Pick, but Pick's is a different disease, involving the atrophy of the cerebral cortex.

What are the signs and symptoms of NPD?

Symptoms of all forms of Niemann-Pick are variable, so no single symptom should be used to include or exclude Niemann-Pick as a diagnosis. A person in the early stages of the disease may exhibit only a few of the symptoms. Even in the later stages of the disease, not all symptoms may be present.

Type A Niemann-Pick begins in the first few months of life. Symptoms may include the following:

- A large abdomen within three to six months
- Liver or spleen enlargement
- Cherry-red spot in the eye
- Feeding difficulties
- Progressive loss of early motor skills
- (Generally) a very rapid decline leading to death by two to three years of age

Type B is biochemically similar to Type A, but the symptoms are more variable. Neurological involvement, such as loss of motor skills, is slight-to-none. Common symptoms usually appear in infancy or childhood. Progression of Type B is generally much slower than with Type A, and many people live into adulthood. Symptoms are as follows:

- Liver or spleen enlargement
- Cherry-red spot in the eye
- Shortness of breath (may require oxygen)
- Repeated lung infections

Type C Niemann-Pick usually affects children of school age, but the disease may strike at any time from early infancy to adulthood. Symptoms may include these:

- Jaundice at (or shortly after) birth
- An enlarged spleen or liver, or both
- Difficulty with upward and downward eye movements (VSGP)
- Unsteadiness of gait, clumsiness, problems in walking (ataxia)
- Difficulty in posturing of limbs (dystonia)
- Slurred, irregular speech (dysarthria)
- Learning difficulties and progressive intellectual decline (dementia)
- Sudden loss of muscle tone, which may lead to falls (cataplexy)
- Tremors accompanying movement and, in some cases, seizures
- Psychiatric problems of unknown cause in teens and adults

Type C is the most variable form of the disease. Symptoms may appear and then disappear. Some symptoms may never appear. The rate at which the disease progresses is different from person to person. The rate of progress for an individual changes over time.

Type C is often incorrectly diagnosed, most commonly as attention deficit disorder (ADD), learning disability, retardation, or delayed development.

VSGP is highly suggestive of Type C. Parents often notice this when their child walks up and down stairs, watches TV while sitting on the floor, or is in similar situations. The child tilts his head to see instead of moving his eyes. Liver or spleen problems in the first few months after birth are also highly suggestive of Type C.

How is NPD diagnosed?

Type A and B Niemann-Pick are diagnosed by measuring the ASM activity in white blood cells. The test can be performed after taking a small blood sample from suspected individuals. Although this test identifies persons with Types A and B (two mutated genes), it is not very reliable for detecting persons who are carriers (only one mutated gene).

It is possible to diagnose Type A and B carriers by DNA testing because the gene containing the blueprint for ASM has been cloned and many of its mutations identified. The Mount Sinai Department of Human Genetics has identified certain populations (shown in the table) in which specific mutations account for a high percentage of cases. In other populations, the mutations must first be identified for the individual before DNA-carrier testing can be performed. The Mount Sinai School of Medicine, University of Pittsburgh, and UCSF-Stanford Lysosomal Disease Center can assist with DNA testing and diagnosis for Types A and B.

Type C Niemann-Pick is initially diagnosed by taking a small piece of skin (skin biopsy), growing the cells (fibroblasts) in the laboratory, and then studying their ability to transport and store cholesterol. The transport of cholesterol in the cells is studied by measuring conversion of the cholesterol from one form to another (esterification). The storage of cholesterol is assessed by staining the cells with a compound (filipin) that glows under ultraviolet light. It is important

Populations in Which Specific Genetic Mutations Are Known to Account for a Preponderance of Cases of Niemann-Pick

Population	Mutations	Percentage of Niemann-Pick Cases	Niemann-Pick Type
Ashkenazi Jewish	R496L, L302P	53	A
Saudi Arabian	H421Y, K576N	85	B
Turkish	L137P, fsP189, L549P	75	B
Portuguese or Brazilian	S379P, R441X, R474W, F480L	55	B
English or Scottish	A196P	42	B
Other	DeltaR608	12	B

SOURCES: O. Levran, R. J. Desnick, and E. H. Schuchman, "Identification and Expression of a Common Missense Mutation (L302P) in the Acid Sphingomyelinase Gene of Ashkenazi Jewish Type A Niemann-Pick Disease Patients," *Blood*, 1992, *80*, 2081–2087; C. M. Simonaro, R. J. Desnick, M. M. McGovern, M. P. Wasserstein, and E. H. Schuchman, "The Demographics and Distribution of Type B Niemann-Pick Disease: Novel Mutations Lead to New Genotype/Phenotype Correlations," *American Journal of Human Genetics*, 2002, *71*, 1413–1419.

that both the transport and storage tests be performed, as reliance on one or the other may lead to the diagnosis being missed in some cases.

Since 1997, over 120 genetic mutations related to Type C have been identified. The number of unique mutations precludes use of genetic testing as a general diagnostic tool. However, genetic testing can be performed to identify carriers in families where the mutation is known. The Mayo Clinic has done extensive DNA testing and counseling for patients and families with Niemann-Pick Type C. For additional information about options for genetic testing, contact Cate Walsh Vockley, the national Niemann-Pick disease coordinator.

Because Niemann-Pick Type C is rare and its symptoms are quite variable, it is not widely known, *even in the medical community*. Although education efforts by NNPDF have increased awareness of the disease, there are still instances of misdiagnosis and delayed diagnosis. If your child is exhibiting symptoms of Niemann-Pick, you may need to ask your doctor to consider the possibility that the disease may be present.

What treatment is available for NPD?

The news concerning treatments for all forms of Niemann-Pick is improving, but there is still much to do before definitive therapies are available. Just a few years ago, the cause of Niemann-Pick was unknown. Now the genetic sources of Niemann-Pick have been identified, and research is focusing on how the biochemical mechanisms work and how they can be corrected.

Potential treatments are described for informational purposes only. You should consult with your physician for medical advice about individual cases.

- *Types A and B:* Research into definitive therapies has progressed rapidly since the early 1990s. Mount Sinai School of Medicine is conducting research on bone marrow transplantation, enzyme replacement therapy, and gene therapy. These therapies have proven effective against Type B in the laboratory, but they have not been effective against the progressive neurological decline found in Type A.
- *Bone marrow transplantation* has proved effective in mouse models for many aspects of Type B when the transplant occurs early in life. Because bone marrow transplant is a complex medical procedure, it has only been done a few times on humans with Type B. The results of these transplants has been mixed. Patients who want more information can contact Dr. Edward Schuchman at (212) 241-9198; fax (212) 849-2447; e-mail: edward.schuchman@mssm.edu.
- *Enzyme replacement* has been tested on mice and shown to be effective for Type B. It has also been used successfully in other lysosomal storage diseases, such as Gaucher Type 1 and Fabray's. Genzyme Corp. is working with Mount Sinai Medical Center to develop outcome measures and tests necessary for a clinical trial of enzyme replacement therapy. Contact Dr. Robert Desnick to obtain more information on the clinical trial at (212) 241-6944; fax (212) 360-1809; e-mail: rjdesnick@vaxa.crc.mssm.edu.

- *Gene therapy* would allow the defective gene to be replaced by normal genes. Positive results have been obtained with individual cells, but testing on Niemann-Pick mice is just beginning.
- *Supportive treatment* can help manage the symptoms of Type B and improve the quality of life for Type A. Support may be needed from various specialists:

> Pulmonologist for respiratory problems
> Cardiologist for heart problems
> Liver and spleen specialist
> Nutritionist
> Physical therapist
> Learning specialist (if neurological difficulties are identified)
> Gastroenterologist

- *Type C*: There is no definitive therapy for Type C Niemann-Pick. Research is continuing to identify potential treatments that would either slow or stop the progression of the disease.

A clinical trial of Zavesca (or OGT-918) for Type C Niemann-Pick is under way in the United States and Europe. Zavesca slowed, but did not stop, the neurological decline when tested on NPC mice. Current information on this trial can be found on the NNPDF OGT-918 page.

A drug assay is being conducted by Laura Liscum, M.D. Nearly 50,000 compounds were tested by Bristol Meyers Squibb for potential effectiveness with Type C. Fifty compounds were identified as candidates for further testing, but none has proven suitable for human use. Work is continuing on related compounds.

Laboratory studies of neurosteroids have had encouraging results when tested on mice, but more work needs to be done before a clinical trial can be considered.

How is NPD transmitted?

All types of Niemann-Pick are autosomal recessive. This means that children with NPD have two copies of the abnormal gene. Each parent carries one copy of the abnormal gene without having any signs of the disease themselves. The parents are carriers, or heterozygotes. Siblings of the parents may also be carriers of the abnormal gene.

When both parents are carriers, chances are as follows:

- 1 in 4 that a child will have the disease
- 1 in 2 that a child will be a carrier
- 1 in 4 that a child will not have the disease and will not be a carrier

Carrier-detection testing for all families is not yet reliable.

The mutations for Types A and B have been extensively studied, particularly among the Ashkenazi Jewish population, and DNA tests for these forms of Niemann-Pick are available. Antenatal diagnosis (diagnosis in the fetus) of Niemann-Pick is available in a limited number of centers.

Wenda Greer, M.D., of Dalhousie University, has identified the genetic mutation related to Type D (now called the Nova Scotia variation of NPC). Carrier detection tests can be done for this mutation. Carrier detection is possible for other families only after their specific mutation is identified.

ᦉ *National Niemann-Pick Disease Foundation, Inc.*

Chapter 32

Tay-Sachs Disease

Tay-Sachs disease (TSD), in its classical form, is a fatal genetic disorder in children that causes progressive destruction of the central nervous system. Affected babies appear healthy at birth and seem to develop normally for the first few months of life. After this time, development slows and symptoms begin.

Babies with Tay-Sachs lack an enzyme called hexosaminidase A (hex A), which is necessary for breaking down fatty substances in brain and nerve cells. These substances build up and gradually destroy brain and nerve cells, until the central nervous system stops working. Symptoms of classical Tay-Sachs appear at four to six months of age, when an apparently healthy baby gradually stops smiling, turning over, grasping. Then the child becomes blind, paralyzed, and unaware of its surroundings. Death occurs by age five.

Cause: Tay-Sachs disease is inherited. A Tay-Sachs carrier, who leads a normal, healthy life, has one normal gene for hex A and one Tay-Sachs gene. When two carriers become parents, there is a 25 percent chance that any child they have will inherit a Tay-Sachs gene from each parent and have the disease, a 25 percent chance their child will be free of the disease and not a carrier, and a 50 percent chance that a child will be a carrier.

Treatment: There is no cure and no treatment for Tay-Sachs. Affected children can only be made as comfortable as possible.

Disease frequency: Tay-Sachs has been almost completely eradicated. In 2003, ten babies were born in North America with Tay-Sachs, but not a single one was Jewish. In 2004, no baby was born in North America with Tay-Sachs. Just one baby was born with Tay-Sachs in Israel in 2003, and no babies were born with Tay-Sachs in Israel in 2004.

Carrier frequency: Approximately 1 in every 27 Jews in the United States is a carrier of the TSD gene. There is also a noticeable incidence of TSD in non-Jewish French Canadians living near the St. Lawrence River and in the Cajun community of Louisiana. By contrast, the carrier rate in the general population, as well as in Jews of Sephardic origin, is about 1 in 250.

Diagnosis: A blood test can be used to diagnose Tay-Sachs.

Prenatal screening: A simple blood test can distinguish Tay-Sachs carriers from noncarriers. Prenatal tests, amniocentesis, and chorionic villus sampling (CVS) can diagnose Tay-Sachs before birth.

History: The disease is named for Warren Tay (1843–1927), a British ophthalmologist who, in 1881, described a patient with a cherry-red spot on the retina of the eye. It is also named for Bernard Sachs (1858–1944), a New York neurologist whose work several years later provided the first description of the cellular changes in Tay-Sachs disease. Sachs also noted that most babies with Tay-Sachs disease were of Eastern European, Jewish origin.

Future: The disease has apparently disappeared almost completely from the Jewish nation for two reasons. First, in Israel, at the expense of the state, the general public is advised to carry out genetic tests to diagnose the disease before the birth of the baby. If an unborn baby is diagnosed with Tay-Sachs, the pregnancy is usually terminated.

Second, the ultra-Orthodox association Dor Yesharim tests young couples to check whether they are genetically "suitable." If both the young man and young woman are Tay-Sachs carriers, the match is determined to be unsuitable, and the couple split up.

꧑ *Lisa Katz*

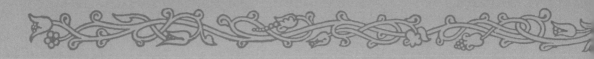

Chapter 33

Crohn's Disease

Crohn's disease is a chronic disorder that causes inflammation of the gastrointestinal (GI) tract. It most commonly affects the small intestine or colon, or both. Crohn's disease and ulcerative colitis are the two main diseases belonging to a group of illnesses called inflammatory bowel disease (IBD). Research has shown evidence of a genetic predisposition to IBD among Ashkenazi Jews.

The symptoms of Crohn's disease are as follows:

- Abdominal pain, often in the lower-right area
- Diarrhea
- Rectal bleeding, which may be serious and persistent, leading to anemia
- Weight loss
- Fever
- A greater risk of developing colorectal cancer
- Delayed development and stunted growth

Cause: Although environmental factors clearly contribute, there is strong evidence from studies of twins and affected families that IBD, especially Crohn's disease, has a genetic basis. Research has shown evidence of a genetic predisposition to chronic IBD among Jewish individuals of eastern European descent.

Treatment: There is no cure, thus the focus is on controlling the inflammation. Inflammation is controlled through powerful drugs such as corticosteroids. Surgery may be used to remove inflamed or damaged portions of the intestines. The doctor may recommend nutritional supplements, especially for children.

Disease frequency: It is estimated that as many as one million Americans have IBD, with that number evenly split between Crohn's disease and ulcerative colitis. American Jews of European descent are four to five times more likely to develop IBD than the general population.

Carrier frequency: The carrier frequency for Crohn's disease is unknown.

Diagnosis: Crohn's disease can be diagnosed through a thorough physical exam and a series of tests, which may include a blood test, stool sample, upper-GI series, colonoscopy, and X-rays.

Screening: No carrier or prenatal screening tests exist for Crohn's disease at this time.

History: In 1932, Dr. Burrill B. Crohn and two colleagues published a paper describing Crohn's disease.

Future: Although Crohn's is a serious, chronic disease with many complications, it is not a fatal illness. People with the disease may be hospitalized from time to time and need to take medications, but most people with the illness can lead productive lives. Even though there is no cure at this time, research and education programs are improving the health and quality of life of people with Crohn's disease.

Lisa Katz

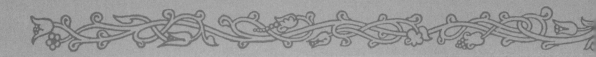

Chapter 34

Canavan's Disease

Canavan's disease (CD), which primarily affects children of Eastern and Central European Jewish (Ashkenazi) descent, is an inherited neurological disorder in which the brain deteriorates.

The signs of CD usually appear when the children are between three and six months of age. Symptoms include developmental delay (significant motor slowness), enlargement of the head, loss of muscle tone, poor head control, and severe feeding problems. As the disease progresses, seizures, shrinkage of the nerve to the eye and often blindness, heartburn (gastrointestinal reflux), and deterioration of swallowing develop. Most children with Canavan's disease die in the first decade of life.

Cause: CD is caused by a deficiency of an enzyme called aspartoacylase (ASPA). This deficiency leads to the buildup of N-acetylaspartic acid (NAA) in the brain. The accumulated NAA causes a chemical imbalance that destroys myelin. Myelin, commonly known as the "white matter" in the brain, protects nerves and allows messages to be sent to and from the brain. When the chemical imbalance makes this white matter spongy, the incapacitating symptoms of CD appear.

Treatment: No effective treatment is available yet.

Disease frequency: 1 in 5,000 Ashkenazi Jews is affected by CD.

Carrier frequency: 1 in 38 Ashkenazi Jews is a carrier of CD.

Diagnosis: The diagnosis of CD is made by detecting lack of the enzyme aspartoacylase in skin cells or by genetic testing of the gene for CD in blood.

Screening: DNA testing can tell with over 95 percent certainty whether someone is a carrier. Genetic counseling can assist at-risk couples in family planning. DNA-based prenatal testing, using samples obtained through CVS or amniocentesis, is available to couples who are both carriers.

History: The disorder was named for Myrtelle Canavan, the researcher who first described the disease in 1931.

Future: Because of the severity of CD, the lack of treatment for it, and its high incidence in the Ashkenazi Jewish population, population screening within the Jewish community is beginning to be offered using the model developed for population screening for Tay-Sachs disease.

Lisa Katz

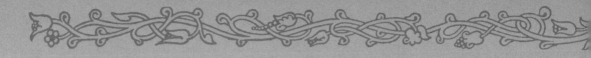

Chapter 35

Bloom's Syndrome

Bloom's syndrome—an inherited disorder carried by 1 in 100 Ashkenazi Jews—is characterized by photosensitivity and elevated dark red blotches on the skin, growth deficiency, reduced resistance to infectious diseases, and increased susceptibility to tumors.

The symptoms of Bloom's syndrome include the following:

- Short stature
- Narrow face with prominent nose
- Color changes in the face, which are more noticeable after sunlight exposure
- Butterfly-shaped facial rash, similar to rash caused by lupus erythematosis
- High-pitched voice
- Increased susceptibility to infections and respiratory illness
- Increased susceptibility to cancer and leukemia
- Possible fertility problems
- Possible mental retardation

The mean age of death is twenty-seven years and is usually related to cancer.

Cause: Bloom's syndrome is inherited in an autosomal-recessive pattern, which means two copies of the gene must be altered for a person to be affected by the disorder. The gene for Bloom's syndrome is located on chromosome 15; one particular mutation in the gene has been identified as the cause of Bloom's syndrome in the vast majority of Ashkenazi Jews.

186

Treatment: There is no treatment for the underlying cause of Bloom's syndrome. Preventive measures such as increased surveillance for cancer and decreased exposure to sunlight and X-rays should be taken. Bone marrow transplantation is a possibility.

Disease frequency: Since this syndrome was first described by New York dermatologist David Bloom in 1954, over 170 individuals have been recognized as being affected.

Carrier frequency: At least 1 in 100 Ashkenazi Jews is a carrier.

Diagnosis: The diagnosis of Bloom's syndrome can be confirmed or ruled out by a laboratory test known as a chromosome study.

Screening: A carrier screening requires a blood sample. Through the blood test, it is possible to detect the specific gene change that is seen in Ashkenazi Jews with Bloom's syndrome. The test is not as accurate for individuals who are from other ethnic backgrounds. CVS or amniocentesis, performed early in the pregnancy, can detect Bloom's syndrome in a fetus.

History: New York dermatologist David Bloom first described the disease in 1954.

Future: The gene for Bloom's syndrome, located on chromosome 15, was recently isolated. One particular mutation in the gene has been identified as the cause of Bloom's syndrome in the vast majority of Ashkenazi Jews. Screening for Bloom's syndrome is available now because of these recent findings, and perhaps a cure will also be found in the future.

Lisa Katz

Raising Our Children

Chapter 36

Infant and Child Care

The Hebrew word for infant is *tinok*, which means "suckling." The age span of the term corresponds to the period between birth and eighteen or twenty-four months of life. Modern psychologists note that the period of infancy is at its end when the baby utters a few phrases, whereas Talmudic scholars observed that the child begins to talk at about the time solid food is introduced (*Berachot* 38). Thus in Judaic literature, the word *tinok* is applied as long as the baby nurses (*Ketubot* 60a; *Iggerot Moshe* 2:6); according to Rabbi Eliezer, this is the first twenty-four months; according to Rabbi Joshua, up to five years of age (*Ketubot* 60a; *Yevamot* 43a).

Although the recognized period for nursing has diminished since biblical times, and most babies receive solid food, at the latest, by the age of fifteen months, the Hebrew word is still often applied to a child after that period of time to denote a sense of endearment. It thus symbolizes the Judaic philosophy of infant care and devotion to the newborn, based on love and tenderness. In accordance with halakhah (Jewish law), the word *tinok* is applied as long as the child still has the same status as a sick person not in mortal danger, allowing

---

From the Sources

The Jewish tradition of infant care is best summarized in the following statement: "A baby should be as well looked after as a king, a high priest, and a learned man."

A. Jellinek, *Beit Hamidrash* 11:96.

191

> ### *From the Sources*
>
> The physical needs of the infant are aptly summarized in the advice given to Abbaye by his competent and wise nanny: "The care and development of the infant requires first that he be bathed and anointed with oil; later, when he grows older, that he be given eggs and dairy products; and when he grows older still, that he be given the freedom to play with toys." These three principles of infant care are guidelines for healthy development: (1) personal hygiene, (2) proper nutrition, and (3) developmental play.
>
> Talmud, *Yoma* 78.

certain actions on the Sabbath, otherwise forbidden by rabbinical law, to fulfill his needs. Although the *Chazon Ish* defines this period as the first two or three years of life in normal cases and beyond that age if the child is still eating baby food (*Chazon Ish, Mo'ed*, 60, 59, sec. 4), we find that the limit is set at about ten years, depending on the child's state of development and health (*Minhat Yitzhak* 1:78).

PERSONAL CLEANLINESS AND HYGIENE

The emphasis on personal hygiene is better understood if we consider the Judaic viewpoint on the subject. We learn in the Talmud that "cleanliness leads to holiness" (*Sotah* 12:5; *Avoda Zarah* 20b). Personal hygiene is a spiritual duty, for it is only logical that proper hygiene should be applied at all stages of the child's development, as he or she is created in the image of God. The following are various aspects of hygiene related to children as noted in the Talmud. The laws and comments that follow offer sound advice on child care.

Bathing

Bathing the child is considered so essential that we find in the *Midrash Mei Hashiloach* the statement: "The existence of the world is maintained with six things and one of these is bathing."

Maimonides advised that one should bathe after dinner is digested and that anointment with oil should follow the bath (*Hilchot Deot* 4,15). This is excellent advice in the case of infant care and is recommended by many pediatricians. The benefit of such a schedule is pointed out by Rabbi Chanina, who attributed his vigor in old age to the baths and oil treatments he was given as a child (*Chullin* 20b). Bathing facilities are so important that a learned man "may not live in a town in which there is not, among other things, a public bath" (*Sanhedrin* 17b). Nevertheless, limits are recognized, for we find in the Talmud (*Avodah Zarah* 28) the warning that if a child has been bitten by a wasp or has a sting or a wound or a disease such as malaria, it is dangerous for him or her to be bathed. In all such cases, it is advisable to consult the doctor. Special regulations are stipulated in halakhah concerning bathing on Sabbath and holidays.

Washing the Hands and Personal Hygiene

Biblical law stipulates that the hands must be washed upon rising from the bed in the morning to protect against evil spirits (*Shabbat* 109a). It is forbidden to touch any part of the body before washing the hands according to the ritual. Washing the hands before meals is also required according to biblical law (*Chullin* 106a), and the Talmud states that the mouth must be rinsed after eating by drinking water

(*Shabbat* 41a). It is recommended that children be taught to wash their hands in accordance with these traditions. Even infants' hands are washed upon waking and before eating to assure maximum cleanliness, as their hands sometimes touch food even before they are able to feed themselves (*Shabbat* 109a).

The warning that an unwashed hand touching the ear may cause deafness exemplifies the harm done when hands remain unwashed (Chaim David Halevy, *Mekor Chaim* T. A. 1965, *1*(2), 7). On related matters of hygiene, the Talmud notes that coins should not be put in the mouth (Jerusalem Talmud, *Terumot* 7:4)—a very appropriate warning for infants and toddlers. In considering other elements of hygiene, the Talmud notes that one should not be kissed on the lips but rather on the back of the hand (to avoid spreading germs) (*Berachot* 8b), again, very appropriate in caring for children.

Outings

Jewish sages have always recognized that sunshine and fresh air are essential to health (*Ketubot* 110b; *Nedarim* 8b). Mothers and other caregivers should, however, keep in mind the commentary that damp air is harmful to the body (*Sotah* 47a) and schedule outings accordingly.

The sun does wonders with the sniffles and other ailments. It is, thus, advisable to expose a child with cold symptoms to the sun whenever possible, unless he or she is running a fever. Special regulations are imposed in Jewish law concerning the use of baby carriages on the Sabbath and holidays.

> ### *From the Sources*
>
> A regular outing during the day will do wonders to calm even the most fretful infant. The Talmud notes that "[w]hen the sun appears, the patient recovers."
>
> *Bava Batra* 16b.

Clothing

Parents and caregivers must make sure that children have adequate clothing for their needs and comfort. This is learned from the example set by the Almighty, who provided Adam and Eve with "clothing" so that they might be dressed properly (Genesis 3:21). Mothers who are encumbered with piles of washing-machine loads will be comforted to know that they are adhering to a biblical precept that clothes be washed frequently, for changes of clothes are indispensable to health (*Eruvin* 65a). The sages also point out that it is dangerous to wear damp clothing. All garments must be dried completely to avoid risk of skin disease (*Pesachim* 112b). Thus mothers must take care that the infant's clothes are kept clean and dry and meet their growing needs. In all cases, the law forbidding the mixture of linen and wool clothing must be obeyed (Leviticus 19:19). Special regulations are determined in halakhah concerning the care of diapers, rubber pants, and sheets on the Sabbath. To summarize the importance of hygiene, Rav Samuel said: "A dirty head causes blindness, dirty clothing brings on boredom, and dirtiness of the body brings on skin eruptions" (*Nedarim* 81).

Care of the Teeth

The Talmud notes that it is important to take good care of the teeth, for decayed teeth are a cause of malnutrition (*Niddah* 63a). According to a passage in *Berachot* 40a, it is advisable to drink water after eating and to gargle with aseptic and salt after meals. Thus infants may be given a bit of water to drink after meals to rinse out their mouth.

From the Sources

The Code of Jewish Law stipulates that the mouth is to be washed every day upon rising.

Orach Chayim 4:11.

According to a passage in *Shabbat* (123a), children's mouths were cleansed with *asube yanuke* (children's herbs)—a possible antecedent to children's toothpaste. Special guidelines are determined in halakhah for the care of the teeth on the Sabbath.

Care of the Nails

Nails should be trimmed periodically, and the parings should be disposed of in a manner to ensure that they are burnt (*Moed Katan* 18a; *Niddah* 17a). It is customary to cut the nails on Friday and not Thursday, so that good grooming becomes a part of the preparations for the Sabbath (*Kitzur Shnei Luchot Habrith* 61). The left-hand nails should be cut first, alternating the fingers rather than cutting in a row (*Orach Chayim* 260:1). The nails of the hands and feet should not be cut on the same day (*Zohar* III, 79a–b).

Care of the Hair

Hair should be routinely washed and combed. Not to comb one's hair is bad for the eyes, according to passages in *Shabbat* (41a) and *Nedarim* (81). According to the Talmud (*Shabbat* 41a), hair was washed with soda and soap and then anointed with oil. The hair of boys was not cut until they were at least three years old (so that they might grow the traditional side-curls). A feast was held (and is still celebrated today in many Hasidic circles) on the day of cutting the hair to symbolize the child's entry into the world of *mitzvot* (good deeds) (*Shaarei T'shuvah* 531:5; Leviticus 19:27). In Israel, the cutting ceremony (known as Halaka) is traditionally held at the tomb of Rabbenu bar Yochai in Meron.

Exercise

Biblical sages recognized that regular exercise is essential for mental health and stimulation of blood circulation, as well as an aid to sleep. Doing simple exercises with infants during diaper changes and whenever the baby is at ease serves the same purpose and helps to develop motor coordination.

> ### *From the Sources*
>
> The Bible mentions that children exercised with balls and weights according to the size of each individual child.
>
> Zacharia 12:4, commentary.

Sleep

The biblical perspective on child development recognizes that sleep is like food and medication for the body; the rest provided by sleep is life-giving (*Divrei Rabbi Eliezer* 12). Drowsiness is brought on by eating. A person (or infant) who has not eaten or has eaten little has difficulty in falling asleep, while one who has eaten well has a sweet sleep (*Tanchume Ki Tissa* 3; *Berachot* 61b). From the halakhah stipulated in the Mishna (*Shabbat* 2,5) that a light may be extinguished on the Sabbath to allow a sick person to sleep, we learn of the therapeutic importance attributed to sleep.

Cribs in biblical and talmudic times were made of wood (Genesis *Rabbah* 8:10) or glass (*Tosefata, Kelim*). They had short legs to ensure the baby's safety and prevent major injury if the child should fall out (*Oholot* 12:4). Bells were put on the cradle to help put the baby to sleep (*Shabbat* 58; *Berachot* 53). There were also swinging cradles that served the same purpose (Genesis *Rabbah* 8:10). A fan was used to keep flies away from the cradle, and rubber sheets were placed under the child to keep the bedclothes clean (*Chullin* 91b). Maimonides advised putting a baby to sleep on his or her side (a practice verified by recent studies carried out to prevent the tragic "cradle death" syndrome). Provisions for the infant's sleep in biblical times were essentially the same as those we make for infants today, with utmost consideration for baby's comfort. This attests to the importance attached to sleep for healthy development.

NURSING

The primary function that the mother fulfills upon the birth of her child is breast-feeding. According to halakhah, this is a task she carries out through her role as a wife (*Ketubot* 59b). By thus ensuring that each newborn is nursed, halakhah makes provision for the best possible nutrition for the child, as well as the opportunity for the mother to express her love for the infant. During the first three months of life, the infant functions mainly on the basis of reflex and stimulation. Physical contact is essential for the child's developing sense of self. As the mother cuddles and fondles the child during nursing, the infant learns the warmth of love and trust, which is the foundation for healthy mental development. Modern psychologists also stress the fact that love must be communicated physically, especially in the first few months of life (M. Jersil, *Emotional Development*. Hoboken, N.J.: Wiley, 1954).

If a woman does not have enough milk, this is considered a curse (*Ketubot* 59). The infant must not suffer on this account, however, and the mother may hire a wet nurse. The Hebrew word for wet nurse (*omenet*) is interchanged with the word *em* (mother), suggesting that the maternal role may be fulfilled by a woman who is not the natural mother, as long as she gives the child the love and warmth necessary for life (*Yoma* 78). Thus halakhah stipulates that a woman who is breast-feeding her child (or someone else's child) may not marry until the child is twenty-four months old (*Yevamot* 43; *Iggerot Moshe*, sec. 6; *Shulchan Aruch* 145:14). This law is very interesting, for beyond ensuring that the child will have the best source of nourishment in infancy, it shows a basic consideration for the emotional development of the child. As we now know, the first two years of life are crucial for the child's development of a sense of trust and a healthy mental state. The Bible makes sure that the child has all the technical opportunities to receive what is naturally due him or her— the care and attention of his mother (or mother substitute) for the first two years of life.

Natural Spacing

Another vital point inherent in this law is that it allows for natural spacing between children. Modern psychology has pointed out the importance of the first three years of life for the child's developing personality. Children who experience the birth of a baby brother or sister within that period of time are forced to share the attention they received until then with the new arrival. This causes a number of problems, including sibling rivalry, jealousy, and a deep sense of frustration at times when the child feels that he is receiving less attention. By setting the time span for breast-feeding at eighteen to twenty-four months, the rabbinical sages incorporated a built-in mechanism for spacing between children, for it is a law of nature that the lactating mother has slim chances of becoming pregnant (although this possibility is not entirely eliminated). In fact, nursing mothers are one of the three categories of women who may legally practice contraception in accordance with halakhah (*Yevamot* 12b, 35b; *Ketubot* 37). Nevertheless, the question of natural spacing is a complex one in Jewish law, and parents must discuss it with a competent rabbi before making a decision on the matter. In practice, the Talmud stipulates that the mother is required to suckle the infant only as long as he or she wants to nurse (*Ketubot* 60). If the infant recognizes his mother and wants to nurse only from her, she is compelled to nurse him, according to Rav, for three months; according to Rav Samuel, for thirty days at least; no set limit may be determined, for in each case it should be as long as the infant wants to nurse.

If the child is weak, breast-feeding is obligatory (*Ketubot* 59). The emotional and physical benefits of breast-feeding were known to be so important that a mother who refused or neglected to suckle her child was compared to an ostrich—a creature that has no feeling for her offspring (Job 39). A symbolic representation of such a mother is used by the prophet Jeremiah to represent cruelty (Lamentations 4:3–4). The mother's duty to breast-feed is upheld, even if she had vowed not to nurse. According to the school of Hillel, the husband may invalidate his wife's vow and compel her to breast-feed (*Ketubot* 59b). If the woman is divorced, the husband can compel her to nurse only if the child is over thirty days, in which case he must pay child

From the Sources

In modern responsa, we find the awareness that babies rarely want to nurse after fifteen months.

Iggerot Moshe, Even Haezer 72:6.

> ### *From the Sources*
>
> On the subject of demand feeding versus scheduled feedings, Judaism takes a clear stand: "The infant must nurse at any hour during the day or night."

support (*Ketubot* 59–60). Nursing is so basic a need for the infant that even if he nurses all day, no harm comes from it (*Tosefta, Sotah* 4:3) According to a *Midrash*, although mother's milk is of uniform quality, the baby finds in it various delectable tastes, so that he never tires of it.

There is no room for controversy when the infant's well-being is at stake. Until the infant settles into his own routine feeding schedule, he should be fed when hungry, even at midnight (Jerusalem Talmud, *Berachot* 9,3). A woman who is nursing a child must not do other work, as is exemplified by Hannah, who put aside all domestic duties in order to suckle her child (the book of Samuel). In this decision, she was wholeheartedly supported by her husband, Elkanah, who said to her, "Do what seems to be good, remain at home until the child is weaned" (1 Samuel 1:21–23). The same advice is offered today by pediatricians and by the La Leche League (the International Organization for Nursing Mothers), who recognize the importance of the mother's having a relaxed state of mind and freedom from tension if she is to nurse successfully. A woman must adhere to the laws of modesty during nursing; according to Rabbi Meir, a woman who nurses in the street may be divorced (*Gittin* 89a).

Wet Nurses

The mother's milk is always preferred to that of the wet nurse (*Avot de-Rabbi Natan* 31:1). However, if the mother is ill or if she has died, a wet nurse may be employed to provide the infant with natural mother's milk. The Talmud allows the wet nurse to take over the responsibility of nursing, even in cases where the mother's status prevents her from doing so (Exodus 2:7–9; *Ketubot* 60b). Halakhah thus makes allowances to ensure that each child has the possibility to nurse under all circumstances. Special allowances are made for nursing mothers on the Sabbath and holidays (Joshua Neubirt, *Shemirat Shabbat Kehilkhato*; J. Feldheim, 1965, chap. 23:25). Orphan babies were suckled by neighborhood women in turn or were fed milk and eggs, which were considered the second-best nutrition for infants (*Avot de-Rabbi Natan* 31:1). The wet nurse must not suckle more than one child if she is given a charge (*Yevamot* 42a). The wet nurse must be given abundant food (*Ketubot* 60b).

According to some rabbis, it is permitted for a gentile to suckle a Jewish infant if the infant is in mortal danger and must receive breast milk and if the gentile woman is the only person available (*Tanhuma*; Exodus 7:26; *Yurushalmi* 76). Others cite the case of Moses, who refused to nurse from a gentile woman and accepted nourishment only when given the breast of a Jewish woman (*Sotah* 12; Exodus *Rabbah*, *Tanhuma* 7). Contemporary rabbis have concluded that although it may be permissible in certain cases for a child to be nursed by a gentile, if this may be prevented, all the better (Responsa of Azriel, 10:80).

Diet of the Nursing Mother

The diet of a nursing mother is of importance for the well-being of the infant as well as the mother, for "all that the mother eats, the infant receives through nursing" (Song of Songs *Rabbah* 3). This has been confirmed by modern research pointing out the importance of a well-balanced, nutritious diet for the lactating mother. Thus rabbinical sages warned that a woman should not nurse if she must eat certain forbidden foods as a result of illness, for this will transmit a bad habit to the infant (Exodus 2:7). The following foods were considered bad for nursing women, according to Rav Kahana: green cucumbers or melons, young greens, small fish; Abbaye included the quince fruit. Rav Papa included palm leaves (which were eaten when soft) and unripe dates. Rav Ashi added sauces made from curdled milk and fish hash. All these foods have the effect of stopping the flow of breast milk or altering its composition (*Ketubot* 60b). Thus a lactating woman should make sure that she eats fresh dairy products to avoid upsetting her digestive system. It is beneficial for the nursing mother to drink a bit of wine (*Ketubot* 60–61), but no more than one cup was ever offered to a woman (*Ketubot* 65a). In considering the principle that the baby is nourished by whatever the lactating mother eats, the following food items are recommended for nursing women, for each has a beneficial effect on the child: old wine and meat will maintain the child's health, as well as the mother's; fish eaten during the nursing period will make the child graceful; adding eggs to the diet acts to produce large-eyed children; parsley is especially recommended to produce beautiful children; coriander acts to produce muscular children; and lemons serve to give children a pleasant odor (*Yoma* 78; *Ketubot* 60b). A nursing mother who finds that her milk flow has decreased or ceased is advised to eat eggs and milk (*Yevamot* 44). If a mother wishes to breast-feed successfully, she will do well to follow a well-balanced, nutritious diet in accordance with the recommendations of the pediatrician. This will help her bestow upon the child a great gift with which to begin life: "the blessing of the breast" (Genesis 49:25).

PLAY

In order to demonstrate the importance of play in a child's development, Rav Abbaye notes that Rabbah used to buy broken crocks at the market and bring them to his son so that he could play with them and break them if he wished to let off energy (*Yoma* 78b).

Throughout the Talmud, we find references to children's toys, such as a toy horse (*Tosefta, Shabbat* 10:3), the ball (*Zevachim* 88b), toy hats, and various fruits and vegetables used for play (Dr. N. Morris, *Toldot Ha-Chinnukh shel Am Yisrael*; T. A. Omanut, 1960, p. 297). It is customary among Orthodox circles not to give children toys with images of people or forbidden animals to play with.

It is evident that the principle of play as an important element in learning and motor development and as a pleasant pastime is recognized in Judaism. In light of the ever-increasing sophistication of children's toys, a number of guidelines have been established in the Code of Jewish Law and responsa so that parents may select the proper toys for use on the Sabbath by preschoolers.

> ### *From the Sources*
>
> The following anecdote, recited by the Sages, points out the importance of play for the infant. A man left a clause in his will stipulating that none of his belongings should be given to his son until the latter made a fool of himself. Rabbi Yose went to consult Rabbi Joshua ben Karcha about this case. When approaching his home, he saw the sage through the window as the latter was crawling on all fours with a piece of grass in his mouth, playing horses with his baby. Upon entering the house, he asked Rabbi Joshua about the case. Rabbi Joshua laughed and answered: "Why, the exact thing which you have asked me about has just occurred here. For when a man has children, he often makes himself look like a fool to amuse them."
>
> Genesis *Rabbah* 47.

SUMMARY

Biblical law determines the obligation of the father to feed and educate his children for a required number of years and the laws concerning the child's status in the family and society (*Kiddushin* 29a; *Ketubot* 65a, 49a; *Shulchan Aruch Yoreh Deah* 251d). The daily care of children, as discussed in this chapter, is a consequence of the parents' natural instincts. It is the motherly instinct to provide for her child's needs during the most vulnerable period of life. Nevertheless, this natural instinct is implicit in the very essence of Judaism, as we learn from the example set by the Almighty and imprinted as part of creation and human development. The fact that the Almighty created man after the universe was completed is attributed to the care he took to ensure in advance that all the necessities of life would be prepared for man's needs (*Eruvin* 18a). Likewise, the Talmud notes that in the creation of the universe, man was created last so that he would be able to eat and nourish himself immediately (*Sanhedrin* 38). The Almighty also provided man with clothing and all other needs for survival and development (*Gittin* 12). *Rashi* (man), who is created in the image of God, must learn from this example and provide for the needs of his offspring upon birth (E. F. Weinberger, *Yad Ephraim*, 1997), together with the additional element of the love and tenderness that are fundamental for healthy development.

The natural mother is the person most suited for this task. Her love for the child is natural. When the prophet Isaiah speaks of the comfort to be offered by the Almighty to the people of Israel, he uses the example of a mother comforting and caring for her child (Isaiah 66:13). The fact that each child is naturally considered fragile and unique by his mother makes her the one most suitable to fulfill his physical needs (Proverbs 4:3).

Attention to the spiritual and emotional needs of the child, by contrast, is a responsibility of both parents. The importance of providing for the emotional and spiritual needs of children should also be learned from the example set by the Almighty, who bestowed commandments for spiritual and emotional development to man immediately after his creation (Genesis 2:16; *Sanhedrin* 56b). This model dramatizes the view that man's most important task in life is to instruct his children in the way of the Lord, the way of life that ensures a healthy emotional development (Genesis 18:19).

The child's healthy physical development is a foundation and a prelude for his or her spiritual, emotional, and intellectual well-being, just as Israel's physical deliverance from Egypt was the prerequisite for its spiritual, emotional, and intellectual redemption at Mount Sinai.

If the parents are unable, for any reason, to fulfill their roles as caretakers and teachers, Judaism allows for substitutes to carry out the important tasks. Thus a governess may assume responsibility for the child's physical and emotional needs in infancy (2 Samuel 12; *Ketubot* 48,61). Sometimes, the grandmother assumed this role (2 Samuel 4). In other cases, the *bet din* (court) is responsible for appointing a parent-substitute or for making sure that the child's physical and spiritual needs are met in other ways (Rambam, *Hilkhot Nachalot* 11:10; *Sukkah* 2b).

Under no circumstances is any child to be neglected or denied his or her basic physical, emotional, spiritual, social, and intellectual needs. Provisions for fulfilling these needs are woven into the fabric of Judaism, as is evident from the references in the Bible to motherly love and the father's responsibilities to his children, as well as the numerous discussions in the Talmud concerning the child's needs, legal status, characteristics, and rights to a healthy life in accordance with the principles of biblical law. In this sense, one should recognize that the primary outline for the "universal rights of the child," including all the requirements for healthy physical, emotional, spiritual, and intellectual development, are inscribed in biblical law that preceded the United Nations document on the universal rights of the child by thousands of years.

✑ *Shoshana Matzner Bekerman*

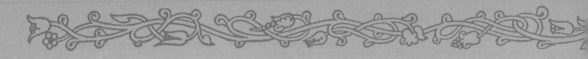

Chapter 37

Some Answers from a *Mohel*

Jewish babies are traditionally circumcised on the eighth day after their birth. Several types of practitioners are competent to perform a bris. Here are answers to some questions new parents of boy babies may have.

Why should I use a traditional rabbi or cantor mohel *instead of a doctor mohel?*

Because you want the most experienced religious practitioner of this ancient rite who will perform a proper bris gently and efficiently in accordance with all Jewish laws and customs. Take all of the following into consideration.

Experience. The traditional rabbi or cantor *mohel* is a super-specialist, an expert at his profession, who possesses more experience at performing brisses than doctor *mohels*. A traditional rabbi or cantor *mohel* may perform more brisses in a month than a doctor *mohel* will perform in an entire year.

Training. The training for a traditional *mohel* is an apprenticeship lasting one to two years covering all aspects of this ancient ritual. The training for a doctor is either a thirty-five-hour minicourse or a weekend seminar, often in violation of the Sabbath!

Availability. Doctors are usually involved full time in their medical practices. A doctor may be called away on medical emergencies and have to cancel participation in your child's bris unexpectedly. I have often been called in to perform brisses on behalf of doctors who had to cancel due to sudden medical emergencies. Also, a traditional *mohel* can perform a bris in any locale. Doctor *mohels* are limited to performing brisses in the state in which they are licensed, as they are

206

not permitted to practice medicine without a license in another state. A bris is a religious ceremony, not merely a medical procedure.

Knowledge of Jewish law and custom. Doctors are not proficient in the religious requirements of the *brit milah* ceremony. Dealing with the demands of their own busy practice, they will schedule brisses at religiously inappropriate times, such as before the eighth day or at night. A bris should be scheduled to take place during the daylight hours of the eighth day of life (which can be tricky to calculate at times, since the Jewish day begins at sunset) and never at night. The traditional *mohel* is an expert in the Jewish laws and customs of *brit milah* and will avoid such mistakes in scheduling, ensuring that your son's bris takes place at the religiously correct time.

Tradition. Brit milah is an ancient Jewish ritual, and practicing as a *mohel* has become a time-honored profession. If doctors continue to perform a *mohel*'s function, a spiritually rich and important Jewish tradition will be lost.

Technique. When a circumcision is performed by a doctor *mohel*, the baby is often strapped down to a cold, molded plastic body board or placed on a table, and the procedure can take up to half an hour or longer, depending on the ability of the individual doing the circumcision. The device that is used is called the Gomco circumcision clamp. It is very clinical and very difficult for the baby.

The technique that I (and other traditional *mohels*) use is very different. The baby is never strapped down. Instead, the baby rests on a double pillow, on the lap of the *sandak* (an honored guest, often the baby's grandfather), held by warm, loving hands. With this technique, the bris takes about twenty seconds. The device I use is called the Mogen circumcision clamp. My instruments are autoclaved (heat-steam sterilized), I wear gloves and follow the highest levels of sterilization and aseptic technique.

How much pain does the baby feel?

Simply put, we don't really know, but this is a controversial area. There is clearly some discomfort. Many studies have been done to try to ascertain how much pain the baby feels. These studies, however, reflect the clinical experience of hospital circumcisions, not traditional brisses that were performed by rabbi or cantor *mohels*. The baby will cry when his diaper comes off and he is exposed and when he is held down.

I believe the reason that this question is asked with such increasing frequency is because of the inexperience of doctor *mohels* and the nontraditional circumcision techniques they employ.

Is there any anesthetic that can be used?

This is related to the preceding question. If there were a topical anesthetic that was also safe and effective for use on newborns, I would be recommending it vigorously. There are a number of choices, but all of them have some drawbacks. Many of these are now available over the counter, but I strongly advise against their use due to the potential dangers and side effects.

EMLA cream is a topical anesthetic that needs to be applied about an hour before the circumcision. The problem with EMLA cream is that it can cause significant swelling of the tissue, which may prevent the bris from taking place. EMLA cream acts as a vasodilator and therefore causes more bleeding The package insert for EMLA cream contains a significant list of potential allergic and localized reactions. EMLA cream has been used so aggressively that it has caused a number of cardiac problems in newborns, and a death was reported due to toxicity. L.M.X. 4 is another type of topical anesthetic, but it is not recommended for use on children under the age of two.

Cetacaine or lidocaine in spray or ointment form may not work on this type of tissue. Also, although toxicity or the possibility that it may be absorbed by the baby is remote, it could cause seizures or cardiac arrest.

A penile block consists of multiple injections of lidocaine in and around the base of the penis. I never really understood why anyone would do this. I have observed the injections being administered, and it seemed to me that the pain of the injections was greater than that of the bris. Also, in my experience, the baby has never *not* cried after having been given a penile block. (Don't forget, he is exposed, and his legs are being restrained also.) And again, although the risk of toxicity or absorption is low, lidocaine could cause seizures or cardiac arrest.

Many parents have asked me about giving the baby infant acetaminophen (Tylenol). First, check with your pediatrician. The concern I have about giving the child acetaminophen is that it could mask a fever. I've seen it used, but it doesn't seem to do much for the baby.

Sugar water (a 25 percent solution) can be given to the baby to reduce his discomfort. In my experience, it is the least invasive and most effective substance to administer. The baby may suck on a gauze pad soaked in concentrated sugar water prior to and during the *brit milah* ceremony (*Harvard Health Letter,* June 1991). In my experience, it is the safest and best way to reduce the baby's discomfort. Kosher sweet wine can be given to the baby before the bris or following the bris during the naming portion of the ceremony. (It's the sugar content, not the alcohol content, that helps reduce discomfort.) Administration of wine and sugar water speeds the baby's recovery time significantly.

I performed a bris for one of the top pediatric anesthesiologists in the New York City area. He didn't use anything to blunt his child's sensations. When I asked him why, he said, "He'll have a bris, he'll cry a little, and he'll be fine."

I will suggest to parents (tongue in cheek) that the best anesthetic for the baby works as follows. Before the bris, they should take two glasses and fill them with wine. The mother drinks one and the father drinks the other. If they do that, I tell them, their baby will be fine.

My observations are experiential, not scientific. I have performed more than fifteen thousand brisses during my career as a *mohel.*

What do you do with the foreskin?

Traditionally, after the bris, the foreskin is buried—covered in dirt or sand. This custom may relate back to Adam, the first man, who, according to the Book of Genesis, was created from earth. Or, perhaps because, as it is written in the Book of Joshua, the Jewish people were about to enter the Land of Israel, and those who were not circumcised had to be circumcised before they could enter the land. The foreskins were buried in the desert sand.

Does jaundice prevent a bris from taking place?

Normal physiological jaundice is just that—normal. It does not prevent a bris from taking place. As long as the doctor agrees that it is normal physiological jaundice, the bris may be scheduled for the proper day. However, if the doctor determines that the baby may not have a bris for some health reason, the *mohel* may not proceed until the baby is declared fit and healthy by the doctor.

What if the baby is born prematurely?

The doctor will determine if the baby can have a bris. While there may be other health concerns, most parents want to know how much the baby should weigh before he can have a bris. Most doctors (and *mohels*) prefer that the baby's weight be at least five pounds. I have done brisses on babies slightly under five pounds, but it depends on the doctor and the comfort level of the parents.

When boy-girl twins are born prematurely, if the boy is healthy but the girl must remain in the hospital, the boy should have his bris on time, on the eighth day. If twin boys are born and one is healthy and one is not, the one who is healthy should have his bris on time and the other when he is healthy. Celebrate each bris separately. One should not delay the bris of the healthy twin until the other baby is healthy just so that both can be circumcised at the same time. Each child is special and unique and should be given the best possible start in life—spiritually and physically.

How do we explain to young children or the siblings of the new baby what a bris is?

My recommendation is to tell them it's a party for the new baby. I don't think very young children need to have the surgical aspects of a bris explained. In general, I recommend that children under the age of twelve not be permitted to watch the actual bris. I try to include the older siblings in the ceremony (before the actual bris takes place); you can tell them that part of the celebration is a big-brother or big-sister party.

If a Jewish child was circumcised in a hospital, does he still need a bris?

Yes. A circumcision is not a bris. If a baby was circumcised in the hospital on the first or second day, even if someone recited some prayers and blessings, that child still needs a *brit milah* on the eighth or proper day. A regular *brit milah* ceremony is held, but since the baby is already circumcised, a *hatafat dam brit* (symbolic circumcision) is performed.

The blessings are recited, a drop of blood is drawn from the penis with a pinprick, and the baby is named. This should be done as soon as possible, preferably before the baby is three years old.

If my son didn't have a bris, is he still considered Jewish, and can he still have a bar mitzvah?

If the mother of the baby is Jewish, then the child is Jewish whether or not he is able to have a bris. A circumcision before the eighth or proper day is not a bris, even if prayers and blessings are recited. One cannot have a bris without a circumcision. A ceremonial circumcision (removing only a small part of the foreskin) is not a bris either. The entire foreskin must be removed to uncover the glans completely.

One does not "have" a bar mitzvah; one *becomes* a bar mitzvah (literally, "son of the commandment"). It marks the point when one reaches the age of majority in Judaism. Traditionally, the girl becomes a bat mitzvah ("daughter of the commandment") when she reaches her twelfth Hebrew birthday and the boy becomes a bar mitzvah when he reaches his thirteenth Hebrew birthday. There is no ceremony, and nothing is required.

And if you don't do anything, it happens anyway!

Upon reaching the age of majority in Judaism, one's Jewish obligations begin, and they never end. Jewish education is ongoing, and Torah learning is a lifelong endeavor. Unfortunately, for many Jewish children, the bar or bat mitzvah marks the end of their Jewish education. If you never had a bar or bat mitzvah ceremony and you would like to celebrate your Jewishness in a meaningful way (no matter how old you are), I would recommend that you join a synagogue, take a Torah class, learn about Judaism, give *tzedakah* (charity), and try to redirect yourself and your family toward a Jewish way of life.

✎ *Cantor Philip L. Sherman*, Mohel

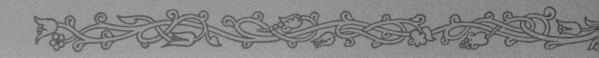

Chapter 38

Breast-Feeding

✎ Insights from the Torah and Sages

The American Academy of Pediatrics recommends breast-feeding for at least the first six months of life and encourages the mother to continue for up to one year. Numerous studies show that breast-feeding leads to healthier kids, but what about the spiritual side of breast-feeding?

LESSONS IN LOVE

King Solomon taught, "Listen my son to the advice of your father, and do not forsake the Torah of your Mother." What is the "Torah" of the mother? Rabbi Shimshon Raphael Hirsch answers that King Solomon is referring to "the nursing years." Rabbi Hirsch teaches in his book *Yesodot HaChinuch*:

> Mothers start worrying about the education of their children too late. . . . In my opinion, the most important period for education is that time when true *chinuch* (education) is most often ignored, a period of time when education is deemed not possible—the first years of the child's life—the nursing years.

Rabbi Hirsch does not mean for us to teach our newborns the story of Adam and Eve! Of course not! He is referring to lessons in love. When a baby is born, he is completely dependent upon others. Aside from physical needs, children also need to be loved. When people talk about children's physical needs, they tend to use the word

> ### From the Sources
>
> When nursing her newborn child for the first time, a mother should begin on the left side.
>
> *Tzava'at* Rabbi Yehudah HaChasid.

need, but when referring to their emotional needs, they use the word *want*. For example, "He needs to be fed," as opposed to, "He wants to be picked up." The truth is that babies need to be held, carried, and loved just as much as they need to eat and sleep.

When a mother nurses her child, she cares for her baby in the most special way possible. She is meeting his need for nourishment, and at the same time, she is providing physical affection. The mother is teaching her child how to love someone, and this is the essence of the Torah. As the sage Hillel explained to a potential convert, "Love your neighbor as yourself; all the rest is commentary."

LEARNING FROM OUR ANCESTORS: SARAH AND HANNAH

Sarah, the mother of all Jews, gave birth to Isaac at the age of ninety years. After God performed this amazing miracle, Sarah lactated and nursed her son until the age of two years. God does not perform "extra" miracles, so why was it necessary for God to allow Sarah to also nurse her newborn son? "Perhaps the fact that Sarah resumed lactating and nursed her child was not an additional miracle 'in vain' . . . ," writes Tehilla Abramov. "Nursing a baby is an intrinsic part of birth." In fact, the Hebrew word for "baby" is *yonek*, or "one who nurses" (*Straight from the Heart*, p. 36).

Hannah, who remained barren for many years, desired more than anything to have a child. She poured her heart out to God, begging for the opportunity to raise children. She prayed, "You have not created anything without a purpose. You have given me breasts, were they not intended to nurse a child? Give me a baby so I may use Your

> ### From the Sources
>
> . . . because the baby should have his first meal from the place that's closest to the seat of understanding—the heart.
>
> *Knesset Chachmei Yisrael* 914.

creation" (Talmud *Brachot* 31b). God answered her prayer, and she gave birth to the great prophet Samuel.

After the birth of her son, Hannah's husband, Elkanah, made a pilgrimage to the Temple to give thanks to God, but Hannah asked to stay behind, allowing her to take better care of her son and continue nursing. "And the woman sat and nursed her son until he was weaned" (1 Samuel 1:23). Traveling to the Temple in order to offer thanks to God is important, but Hannah knew that staying behind to nurse her child was more important.

A MYSTICAL INSIGHT INTO NURSING

The benefits of breast-feeding go beyond our understanding; perhaps nursing is as important to the Jewish soul as keeping kosher or observing the Sabbath. A story is told about a great rabbi, the Baal Shem Tov, which brings to light this mystical aspect to raising children. A married, childless couple came to the Baal Shem Tov in order to ask him for a blessing. They wanted to have children whom they could raise in the way of Torah. The Baal Shem Tov gave them a blessing, and so many months later, the woman became pregnant. She gave birth to a healthy baby boy. Two years later, after nursing and loving their gift from heaven, the child became deathly ill and passed away.

The couple returned to the Baal Shem Tov, and they questioned him, "What kind of blessing was that? So many tears have been shed throughout the years because we wanted nothing more than to have a child, and now, after a blessing from you, we are given a child, who is taken away from us. Why?"

The Baal Shem Tov explained that every *neshamah*, or soul, has a purpose, and every one of us must complete their mission, whatever it may be. He told them that this child possessed the soul of a righteous convert, and he deserved the highest place in heaven. There was only one problem—he never nursed from a Jewish mother. His sole purpose in coming back to this world was to nurse, and now, his soul would be able to rest in the heavens. "So," the Baal Shem Tov explained, "you have merited to nurse this special child."

Nursing a child is one of the most important decisions a mother, Jewish or not, will ever make. Unfortunately, some women and babies are unable to breast-feed for medical or emotional reasons, God forbid. Since God is in control of everything, there is a reason he placed both this mother and particular child together, and he knew that breast-feeding would not be an option. A mother who is unable to breast-feed can hold her baby close while bottle-feeding, stroke his head or arms, and make eye contact. At home, a mother can take her shirt off and bottle-feed her baby clad in just a diaper to nurture the need for close contact.

Breast-feeding affects our child's physical, emotional, and spiritual health. Their very essence—their *neshamah*—is affected in ways we cannot claim to understand. Isn't it worth giving it a try?

Rachel Gurevich

Chapter 39

Breast-Feeding Questions and Answers

Nishmat is a highly regarded woman's learning community, active in many areas of Jewish education for women. On the subject of breast-feeding, Nishmat states:

> Breast-feeding is halakhically encouraged, especially for the first two years of life. Up to the age of two, if a child has ceased nursing, he may resume breast-feeding even if he has only nursed for a few months or has never nursed. Above the age of two and until the child's fourth birthday (or if the child particularly needs it, the fifth birthday), nursing may be continued (but not initiated); however, anytime a healthy child above the age of two does not wish to nurse for 72 hours, breast-feeding may not be resumed. Expressed breast milk is kosher even for older children or adults.

On its Web site, Nishmat provides examples of answers to a wide range of questions related to women's health issues. Here are some of the questions regarding breast-feeding:

September 21, 2004

I am exclusively breast-feeding my son, who is five and a half months old. I have heard a full range of opinions on whether or not I must fast on Yom Kippur. From what I understand, the main question is whether I should drink or eat in *shiurim l'chatchilah* (small quantities spaced throughout the day), or if I should wait if/until I feel dehydrated and then drink, risking that I will have to drink more than a *shiur* at that point. I feed my son every three to four hours, and I am his only source of food.

Please let me know what to do.

Dear Questioner,

Thank you for your question.

The *Shulchan Aruch* clearly states that breast-feeding women should fast on Yom Kippur in the same manner as others (*Orach Chayim* 617:1). As in all areas of halakhah, if there is a medical risk, there is room for leniency in individual cases. A rabbi must be consulted in such situations.

Fasting by a breast-feeding woman raises questions as to the health of two people, the mother and the baby. Most breast-feeding women can fast without any risk to themselves. Many report, however, that fasting while breast-feeding is harder than it is at other times. They should make all efforts to drink a lot the day before the fast and to rest as much as possible during the fast. It is more important to fast than to attend *shul*. Couples with young children that need to be cared for during the fast should think about how to do this without overtaxing the breast-feeding, fasting mother—hiring a babysitter for example, or even having the husband remain home for part of the day to help. Women should *not* reduce the frequency of breast-feeding during the fast, as this is likely to lead to a breast infection.

As far as the effect on the nursing infant, there are almost no data on the effect of such a fast on human breast-milk. The only published article to date is by O. Shefi: "*Tzom Yom Hakippurim v'Hashpa'ato al Nashim Menikot,*" in *Assia* 14, *Elul* 5754. In her review article, the author found one human study that showed a slight difference in milk composition after an overnight fast. Studies in animals showed changes in composition and a small reversible decrease in milk supply the day following a twenty-four-hour fast. The author reported anecdotal data from women she interviewed of reduced milk on the day after the fast. However, no statistical data are provided. Based on my own experience as a pediatrician, lactation consultant, and breast-feeding mother, I feel that most babies can weather the fast with little more than slight fussiness. Mothers can help by being prepared with a bottle of expressed breast-milk from the day before that can be administered at the end of the day (either by bottle, syringe, cup, or spoon, depending on the age and nursing history of the baby). Mothers should arrange to have a quiet day the day after the fast when they can spend time with the baby and nurse more frequently to make up for any slight decrease in supply that might have resulted from fasting.

These are general guidelines. There are individual cases such as sick infants, difficult nursing situations, and past bad experiences where mothers should be told to drink in *shiurim* (small quantities). Any such case requires an individual medical assessment of the situation and an individual halakhic ruling.

February 1, 2005

I am breast-feeding my first child; he doesn't want to take my milk from a bottle at all, which makes me wonder what can I do if I need to breast-feed in public—a restaurant, metro car, or bus. Because of this I haven't left the house with him yet besides going to the doctor's office. What are the laws due to modesty?

I have also heard I should cover the *mezuzot* when breast-feeding. Is that true?

Thank you, sincerely,

Malka

Dear Questioner,

Thank you for your question.

As long as your breast is not exposed, there is no prohibition against nursing in public unless local feeling is clearly against it. The ability to nurse in public gives the mother much more freedom to pursue her normal lifestyle and thus should be encouraged.

Modesty is maintained by covering yourself with a blanket, your shirt, or a sweater that drapes over your shoulder while breast-feeding. You can even purchase a form of "bib" designed for this purpose; you may also be able to find clothing with an arrangement of slits and flaps to facilitate modest nursing. In a restaurant, you can often sit with your back to the other patrons. With practice, breast-feeding in public can be done discreetly so that only other knowledgeable nursing mothers will know what you are doing.

There is no need to cover the *mezuzot*.

This Internet service does not preclude, override, or replace the *psak* (halakhic decision) of any rabbinical authority. It is the responsibility of the questioner to inform us of any previous consultation or ruling. As even slight variation in circumstances may have halakhic consequences, views expressed concerning one case may not be applied to other, seemingly similar cases.

෨ *Nishmat*

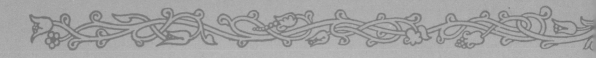

Chapter 40

Turning Your Kid into a Mensch

Turning your child into a mensch is a family affair. The first thing it takes is parents who are honestly willing to struggle with their own *Menschlichkeit* and who invite their children to join them in their quest.

Elie Wiesel tells the story of a Jewish boy who asks his rebbe, "What is a good Jew?" The rebbe then says, "Do you think you are a good Jew?" When the boy answers, "I don't know," the rebbe responds, "I think that good Jews are people, who when asked if they are good Jews, answer, 'We don't know.'"

Menschlichkeit starts with insecurity. Being a *mensch* takes insight and skill. To be a *mensch*, you have to get into MIT: you constantly have to be a *mensch in training.*

Begin your training by developing a list of *midot tovot*—good qualities by which a mensch is measured. Here are a few examples:

- *Shalom Bayit:* maintaining family peace
- *Talmud Torah:* emphasizing Jewish learning
- *Gemilut Hasadim:* performing acts of kindness to help others
- *Rodef Shalom:* being a pursuer of peace
- *Tzedakah:* contributing funds to others
- *Kibud Av va'Em:* honoring one's parents
- *K'vod ha-Briyot:* respecting and showing kindness to all creation
- *Bal Tashchit:* respecting the environment (not wasting)

- *Lashon Hara:* avoiding hurtful language or gossip
- *T'fillah:* making time for prayer and reflection

Participate in systematic acts of kindness. Although it is fashionable right now to encourage people to practice "random acts of kindness," consistent acts of kindness are the stuff *mensches* are made of. *Mensches* are people who are kind when they feel like it, and even when they don't.

Regular involvement in *tikkun olam*—actions that help repair and redeem the world—is a great foundation for families. Here are a few suggestions:

- Make a ritual out of giving *tzedakah* before lighting the Shabbat candles every week.
- Learn about the unique Jewish *tzedakah* practice for each Jewish holiday. For example, on Purim, it's *matanot l'evyonim*—gifts of food to the poor.
- Create a family *tikkun olam* ritual. It could be weekly, monthly, annually, but it should be something your family chooses to do. I know some families who skip dinner once a week and use the money to feed others. Other families spend Yom Kippur afternoon working in a soup kitchen.

Become an active member of a caring community. The more you are part of a circle of people who actively practice mutual care, the more *Menschlichkeit* will be actualized by you and your children. Such a community may not be readily available; you may have to take responsibility to create or transform it.

When I was a teacher at Akiva Schechter Day School in Chicago, the father of our beloved school secretary, Millie, died. Much to my surprise, Rabbi Harvey Well, the school principal, brought the entire fifth grade to her house. He said, "They have to learn how to show compassion." I asked him how they knew how to be compassionate. Harvey said, "We practiced before we went."

When children are part of a family who regularly make *shiva* calls, are part of a group who visit each other when one is sick or in the hospital, make calls of congratulations or concern, and take care of each other, they learn an important lesson. They learn that they are part of a wonderful network of people and that when something goes wrong or right, someone will be there.

Exercise empathy. Reading biblical tales with your children is a wonderful way of developing your family's skills in understanding other people's feelings and actions.

The Torah gives us the opportunity to embroider its stories with all kinds of personalizations. In the process of figuring out the story behind the biblical story, we practice our empathy skills. As you read the stories, ask your children, "What do you think the biblical character is feeling? What do you think this character will do next?"

Model times for saying "I'm sorry," and encourage children to feel safe admitting when they've just blown it, too.

Say the *Shema* with your child every night at bedtime—a great way to build self-esteem and inner security. It does so because of the special attention parents are giving each child. It does so because of the conversations it allows. And it does so because it makes God a living possibility in your child's life.

Make mensch-like responses when your children have done something wrong. Forget the notion of punishment. Replace it with ways that your kids get to make restitution and do *t'shuvah*—the Jewish concept of repentance.

Help your kids evolve into mensches. Remember that children are not born mensches. They are still human "becomings." Kids can be selfish, violent, heroic, thoughtless—and they can demonstrate moments of *Menschlichkeit.* They can manifest great hearts and wondrous acts of selflessness.

 Joel Lurie Grishaver

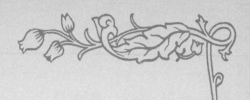

ℰ Special Focus

Infertility

Chapter 41

Infertility and the Jewish Couple

For many couples, teasing from friends and family about when they plan to start a family is inevitable. The ribbing and nudging often begin under the *chuppah* (wedding canopy), when the rabbi extols the virtues of being fruitful and multiplying.

But for some couples, each teasing remark is like salt in a fresh wound, as they struggle to bring a child of their own into the world. For many, the word *struggle* doesn't begin to cover the pain of infertility, which is felt on so many different levels.

Rabbi Michael Gold, in his book *And Hannah Wept: Infertility, Adoption, and the Jewish Couple*, suggests that based on his own observation, the number of couples experiencing infertility appears to be higher among Jews than among other groups.

"The reason is simple," writes Gold. "Jews tend to marry later and postpone having children longer than the general population." Studies have shown that fertility decreases with age.

 DID YOU KNOW?

Infertility is defined as the inability to become pregnant after one year of regular sexual relations without contraception. It also is defined as the inability to carry a baby to live birth. Between 15 and 20 percent of couples of child-bearing age in the United States are infertile.

HEALTH FACTS

In vitro fertilization (IVF) involves removing a woman's egg cells from her ovaries, fertilizing the eggs with sperm outside the woman's body, and implanting the resulting embryo or embryos back in the woman's uterus.

"Before anyone knew we were having problems, there was constant kidding and joking about starting a family," recalls Laurie L., who asked that her last name not be disclosed. "My father-in-law would end every phone conversation by saying, 'OK, go get off the phone and make me a grandchild."

"After we told everyone we were having problems, the family was supportive, but we still got a lot of 'just relax,' 'maybe you're trying too hard,' 'take a vacation.'" Laurie adds. "Most everyone experiencing infertility can tell similar stories."

"Unsolicited advice can be a real problem," explains Sherri Leisman, an infertility and adoption counselor with University Women's Health Care in Monroeville, Pennsylvania. "People say things and they mean well, but they can often be hurtful." Not only do remarks like "just relax" and "take a vacation" call into question the couple's own ability to choose well and wisely for themselves, they also ignore the fact that people sometimes have blocked fallopian tubes or bad sperm, Leisman points out.

"Infertility is a valid problem," echoes Laurie L. "It's not happening because we're not relaxing. It is a medical problem. I think a lot of people don't understand that and don't understand how devastating it is."

As time went on, Laurie's and her husband's families began to see that their infertility was a real, ongoing problem, and family members began to make offers of financial support. In just over two years, Laurie and her husband have been through numerous medical procedures and received a variety of fertility drugs administered orally and through daily shots, the effects of which are monitored by countless ultrasounds and blood draws.

The latest procedure was their first attempt at in vitro fertilization, bringing the tab to about $10,000, of which insurance covered nothing.

THE JEWISH VIEWPOINT

How does Judaism regard such medical interventions? As with most everything else, there is a range of Jewish opinions, says Rabbi Aaron Mackler, who is also a Pennsylvania college professor.

"In general, Judaism tends to be very open and supportive of medical intervention to combat infertility. The use of hormones and other medical intervention, on the whole, is supported," says Mackler.

Regarding IVF in particular, Mackler says some Orthodox thinkers would suggest that this form of reproduction upsets the natural order of things. And the question becomes more complicated when couples consider using donated sperm or eggs.

"It's more complicated because of the question of who is officially the parent in Jewish law. Some feel it's not appropriate to have other people's genetic material coming into a marriage," explains Mackler.

As reproductive technology continues to evolve, so does the body of literature exploring its relationship to Jewish law and ethics, but by-and-large, Rabbi Mackler asserts, Judaism is very much pro-children and generally in favor of medical intervention. In fact, to suggest that Judaism is pro-children is a bit of an understatement.

"Be fruitful and multiply" is the first commandment in the Torah. "And because of the focus on children in much of our religious and communal life," writes Rabbi Gold in his book, "infertility is particularly painful to Jews." Shabbat, Hanukkah, Passover, Sukkot—so many holidays involve special rituals for children that it's often difficult for couples experiencing infertility to participate in these and other life-cycle celebrations.

One veteran of infertility treatments, Naomi Z., recalls telling her best friend that she didn't know whether she and her husband would be able to attend the naming ceremony of her friend's second child.

"I told her it would depend on what kind of day we were having," explains Naomi. Her friend found that hard to understand, but they continued to talk about it. Ultimately, Naomi and her husband attended as the child's godparents.

Leisman tells clients to take care of themselves. "It may be difficult to attend a baby shower. You might feel guilty, but if you can't, you can't, and that's OK," she asserts.

SEARCH FOR MORAL SUPPORT

Although some Jewish rituals may prove difficult, Naomi found one to be especially helpful. As a teacher of *b'nai mitzvah* classes, she has always encouraged her students not to knock things until they try them. In that same spirit, she decided to try going to the *mikvah* (ritual bath) and found that it really meant something to her. When each month brought disappointment, she looked at going to the *mikvah* as a new beginning.

"OK, here's a rebirth, a fresh start; God cares about what's happening to me. Going to the *mikvah* was really important to me," Naomi explains. "When you're trying to become pregnant, your period really is a death. To go to the *mikvah* is to wash away a death and start working on a new life."

Naomi is expecting her first child any day. While she found comfort at the *mikvah*, her husband, Brian, struggled to make his own way. He resisted traditional sources of support, such as the counselor available to him through their doctor's practice and, he admits, "it was probably the wrong choice."

Part of the difficulty for men in dealing with this is that it's something men typically don't talk about. "Conversations are almost exclusively among women. Naomi had lots of people to talk to, but it's not something guys talk about," explains Brian. "I talked almost exclusively to Naomi, and it wasn't fair to her because she had her own issues to deal with." But that communication between the two of them, says Brian, is what enabled their marriage to survive the strain that infertility can cause.

"It's such a strain for so long, watching friends get pregnant," he says. "When you find someone who has gone through this or who you can talk to about it, it can be very important."

Indeed, people struggling with infertility speak a common language of pain and perseverance, of daily shots and so many blood draws each week that they begin to feel like human pin cushions, of tears shed and hormones run amok on the drug of the month, of time missed at work, and of the insensitive things blurted out by even the best-intentioned friends and family members. Less often heard are stories of what friends and family do right.

Naomi recalls that one of the best things someone did for her was a gesture by her rabbi. Naomi had gone to services on Shabbat at a particularly bad time and ended up in tears. The rabbi offered to call her at home, and when he called, he offered to bring chocolate.

"He came over with a huge grocery bag full of chocolate, ice cream, Pop-Tarts, all kinds of goodies. We shmoozed about nothing for two hours, and it was so important. We didn't even talk about [infertility]. It just made me feel really good," she says, "because he sent the message 'You're worth spending time with; you have value as a person in your own right.'"

SOLACE IN PRAYER

Some couples find solace in prayer or inward thought when conception is difficult. Naomi wrote the following prayer to say before going in the *mikvah* the night before she began the procedure that ultimately resulted in her pregnancy:

> Shechinah my God, God of all generations, I stand before you today as did my mothers, Sarah, Rebecca, Rachel, Leah, Hannah and Michal, to ask for your help in my quest for a child. As each of their journeys took a different path, so, too, I am mindful that my journey has many possible endings.
>
> I stand before you not to ask for a baby, but to ask for the strength to face all that lies before me with grace, dignity, and courage. Help me to remember that your covenant at Sinai bound those who were there with those who had not yet come to be, and to be mindful of the participation of both myself and the child I seek in that covenant relationship with you. Help me to accept the comfort and support of my family and friends as I walk this road, and keep alive in me the spirit of hope. Amen.

ॐ *Judy Wertheimer*

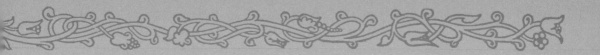

Chapter 42

Assisted Reproduction in Judaism

Be fruitful and multiply," Genesis 1:28 tell us; "fill the earth and subdue it." Nowadays most rabbis agree that the commandment to populate the world is so important that many modern technological developments for assisting infertile couples may be permitted by Jewish law. They say that in case natural reproduction does not succeed, it gives a tacit approval for assisted reproduction.

The implied flexibility of the Torah regarding assisted reproduction should not surprise us.

The narrative provides much of the human drama in the relationships between the matriarchs and their husbands, and between the matriarchs and God. The three matriarchs dealt in different ways with their tragic circumstances.

OUR MOTHERS

Sarah bitterly resigned herself to not having children and even laughed a cynical laugh when presented with the possibility of conception at an advanced age. Rebecca was more positive. She asked Isaac to intervene on her behalf, and Isaac's prayers were answered. Rachel used desperate measures. She declared to Jacob: "Give me children, otherwise I am dead." The commentator Rashi explains that this statement signifies that a childless person is accounted as dead.

Rachel's next act was even more desperate. Reuven, the first-born son of Leah, returned from the field with some plants called

HEALTH FACTS

Three out of four biblical matriarchs suffered from infertility. The Torah documents, in Genesis, the suffering of Sarah, Rebecca, and Rachel due to infertility.

dudaim (Genesis 30:14). The biblical commentator Nachmanides suggested that these plants were herbs that promoted conception. Reuven presented them to his mother for her use. Rachel observed this and begged her sister for the plants. Then she made a deal: in return for the *dudaim,* she would allow Leah to spend one night with Jacob. Ironically, Leah's fifth son was born as a result of this deal. And because of Rachel's desperation this "assisted reproduction" achieved its goal for her as well. Rachel was finally "remembered" by God, and she conceived and bore Joseph. She then states: "God has taken away my disgrace."

YESTERDAY AND TODAY

Infertility was not only a painful and tragic experience for the matriarchs, but it continues to afflict many Jewish couples. The biblical notion of infertility was that it was due to the female. Surprisingly, the cause of infertility among Orthodox Jewish couples today is predominantly due to male factors. Dr. Vincent Brandeis, who runs fertility centers in New York State, has estimated that in 60 percent of Orthodox patients, infertility is due to problems with sperm quality. This compares with close to 50 percent male-factor infertility in the general population. The reason for this difference may have to do with the low incidence of pelvic inflammatory disease among Orthodox women, who are generally sexually inactive before marriage. Pelvic inflammatory disease increases the rate of female infertility in the general population so that it slightly exceeds male infertility.

Talmudic ideas of reproduction in many ways reflect the notions of those times.

> Our Rabbis taught: There are three partners in man: The Holy One, blessed be he, the father and the mother. The father supplies the semen, the white substance, out of which are formed the child's bones, the sinews, the nails, the brain and the white of the eye. The mother supplies semen, the red substance, out of which are formed the skin, flesh, hair, blood and the black of the eye. God provides the spirit, the soul, the beauty of the features, eyesight, the power of hearing, ability to speak and walk, understanding and intelligence. (Talmud, Tractate *Nidda*, 30a)

Although the Talmud was unable to explain the scientific mechanisms of inheritance of traits, it was enlightened in assigning a role to the female "semen." Many scholars of that time believed that the female simply provided an incubator for the male seed to grow into a child. Even the Torah recognized the presence of a female seed with the passage: "If a woman emits a seed" (Leviticus 12:2).

MODERN CONCEPTS AND PRACTICE

Today, of course, we know of the genetic mechanisms of inheritance. There are many thousands of genes inherited by a child that control the child's physical attributes. For most traits, a child inherits two copies of each gene, one from the mother and one from the father. The individual copies of each gene can interact with each other. A copy from one parent may be dominant over the other and be preferentially

 DID YOU KNOW?

In IVF, conception takes place outside the body. This technique overcomes the problem of scarred, damaged, or blocked fallopian tubes (which prevent the sperm from reaching the eggs and the eggs from reaching the uterus). It also allows men with low sperm counts to conceive, as sperm samples can be concentrated and deposited adjacent to the ripe eggs. Only small numbers of viable sperm are needed for successful fertilization in a petri dish.

expressed in the child. Or the two copies may work together to produce a combination or blended trait.

Assisted reproductive technology that is available today enables many infertile couples to fulfill the biblical commandment to "be fruitful and multiply." Technological advances have led to the development of in vitro fertilization—when the sperm from the father and the egg from the mother are mixed together in a petri dish in the laboratory, and the sperm is allowed to fertilize the egg, producing a "test-tube baby." The fertilized egg is then returned to the biological mother's womb where it develops, and nine months later the baby is born.

A variation on this theme is intra-cytoplasmic sperm injection, or ICSI. With this technique a man who produces *no* sperm in his ejaculate can become a father. Pieces of tissue from the testicle can be used. Only a few sperm cells need to be isolated from the testis, and those cells can be mechanically injected, one by one, into individual eggs. Another variation involves a process called assisted hatching. In assisted hatching, a small opening is made in the clear zone, or "shell" around the egg. The process is done to allow the fertilized egg to emerge properly, as this can assist it to implant into the lining of the uterus.

FINDING IMPLICATIONS IN JEWISH LAW

How "kosher" are these techniques in terms of Jewish law (halakhah)? It is generally agreed by rabbinic authorities that IVF and related techniques are acceptable for Jewish couples when the husband's sperm and the wife's eggs are used. In husband-wife IVF, four problems, in particular, need to be addressed:

1. There is some controversy regarding how semen may be procured for the procedure. Because there is a biblical admonition regarding the "spilling of seed," some rabbis insist that the husband may not ejaculate to provide a specimen. However, since the intention of the procedure is specifically to enhance procreation, and the semen is not being wasted, ejaculation to produce the semen may indeed be permissible.

DID YOU KNOW?

It is generally agreed by rabbinic authorities that IVF and related techniques are acceptable for Jewish couples when the husband's sperm and the wife's eggs are used.

2. When more than one fertilized egg is implanted into the woman, this may result in a multiple pregnancy. When there are three or more fetuses growing in the womb, this results in a high-risk pregnancy; fetal reduction, or selectively eliminating one or more of the fetuses, may be recommended. Is this halakhically permissible? Ending the life of a fetus is not considered murder by halakhic definition, but it is not permissible either. This would only be permitted if the doctor has determined that some fetuses must be eliminated or they will all die. Even then, the decision is a very sensitive one and must be made by the doctor.

3. When IVF is performed the woman is stimulated by hormone treatment so her ovaries can produce up to twenty eggs per cycle. The eggs are harvested and fertilized, but only three or four can be used in that cycle. The rest can be preserved by freezing. How does Jewish law address the issue of extra embryos? The fate of extra embryos could include

- Use of them by the original couple to establish future pregnancies (rabbis affirm this use)
- Destruction of the extra embryos (permissible halakhically if this is done passively, by letting them thaw out and die on their own)
- Use of these extra embryos for research (because this is an active process and results, ultimately, in their destruction, this is not generally acceptable by Orthodox rabbis)
- Donation of the extra embryos to another infertile couple (not approved by many Orthodox rabbis because the "adopted" child may inadvertently marry his or her genetic sibling, resulting in incest)

4.   Although most IVF labs are reputable and try to be meticulous in keeping track of the sperm, eggs, and embryos of each couple, over the years some mistakes have been made. Even worse than inadvertent errors are the cases of deliberate tampering with sperm, eggs, and cmbryos that have been discovered in unscrupulous fertility labs. Because parentage is of vital concern, some Orthodox rabbis would like to see trained supervisors present during IVF of Jewish couples. One such arrangement has been made between the Star-K Kosher Certification and a New York clinic. The supervisors will reportedly be present during the entire procedure to ensure that halakhic protocol is followed and that meticulous attention to the accuracy in the process is maintained.

DONOR SPERM AND EGGS

The issues involved in using donor sperm or eggs can *create* halakhic problems. Artificial insemination has been performed for many years, and the question of the halakhic validity of this procedure has been discussed by many sources. It is clear that more rabbinical authorities approve of artificial insemination if the husband's sperm is used, as long as it is not wasted in the process; there are special devices recommended by rabbis for collecting the sperm in as natural a way as possible. However, the idea of using donor sperm has not been accepted by many rabbis. Although the use of donor sperm is not considered adultery per se, given that sexual relations are not involved, it is still considered an abomination by many and is strongly discouraged. Rabbinic sources generally agree that paternity is determined by who provides the sperm so that a baby conceived from donor sperm would not, halakhically, be considered the child of the infertile husband.

When an egg donor provides an egg for an infertile couple, the recipient, usually a sterile woman who cannot produce eggs, serves as the gestational and birth mother and she gives birth to and raises the baby as her own. In this case there are two categories of motherhood: a genetic mother and a gestational, or birth mother. These—now-separate—functions can be performed by two different people, who may or may not be related to each other and may or may not have any connection with each other (other than their individual contributions to producing and raising the child).

There are rabbinical authorities who reject outright the idea of using donor eggs. Others believe that a woman may receive donor eggs as long as her husband has consented. The question as to who is the mother is extremely complicated to answer. This is certainly a critical question, as it affects the status and identity of the baby. According to traditional Judaism, one is not a Jew unless one's mother is a Jew. When the genetic mother and the gestational mother are the same person, the issue is clear. But what happens when the genetic mother is a different person from the gestational mother? Which mother is considered the mother for the halakhic decision on religious status? If the genetic mother is not Jewish and the gestational mother is, what is the status of that infant? Rabbi Moshe Heinemann, rabbinic administrator of Star-K Kosher Certification, states unequivocally that if the egg is from a non-Jewish woman, the baby is not Jewish. In this very stringent ruling, when a donor egg is used, the birth mother is *not* considered the halakhic mother.

Other rabbinic authorities have addressed this question and have concluded that there is halakhic uncertainty regarding who the mother is. Rabbi Moshe Tendler writes that "the contributions of the gestational mother are quite consequential" (*Pardes Rimonim*, 1988). In fact, many halakhic authorities regard the birth mother,

---

 DID YOU KNOW?

The biblical commandment to have children is the first commandment given to Adam after he was created. A similar directive is given in Isaiah 45:18, which reads: "He did not create the world to be desolate, but rather inhabited." Because Adam was specifically charged to "be fruitful and multiply," that positive commandment has been interpreted as an obligation on the part of the man to reproduce. The quote from Isaiah, commentators have explained, pertains both to men and women: thus women are included in the obligation to fill the world.

rather than the egg donor, as having maternal status. The halakhah on many issues relies on what can be readily observed with the naked eye. For instance, microscopic or small amounts of nonkosher contaminants in kosher foods do not necessarily render the food nonkosher. Thus the decision on maternity may be based on which mother gives birth (an action that is incontrovertible and readily proved), rather than which mother provided the egg (a microscopic contribution, albeit a critical one). However, considering the important role *yichus* (inherited status) plays in some Jewish circles, genetic status could be of paramount importance, and perhaps the mother who provided the egg should determine Jewish status.

It is clear that the scriptures have directed Jews to procreate, and this directive is so critical that Torah scholars agree it could be accomplished by natural or artificial means. The challenge of assisted reproductive technologies will be to sort out the complex relationships created by artificial reproductive processes, and to determine where to draw the line in terms of what techniques are ethical and permissible, which advances are questionable, and which are unacceptable.

Miryam Z. Wahrman, Ph.D.

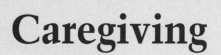

Caregiving

Chapter 43

The Physician's Daily Prayer

Almighty God—
You have created the human body with infinite wisdom.
In Your eternal providence,
You have chosen me
to watch over the life and health of Your creatures.

I am now about to apply myself to the duties of my
profession.
Support me in these great labors that they may benefit
humankind.
For without Your help, not even the least thing will
succeed.

Inspire me with love for my art and for Your creatures.
Do not allow thirst for profit, ambition for renown and
admiration
to interfere with my profession.
For these are the enemies of truth and can lead me astray
in the great task of attending to the welfare of Your
creatures.

Preserve the strength of my body and soul
that they may ever be ready to help
rich and poor, good and bad, enemy as well as friend.
In the sufferer let me see only the human being.

Enlighten my mind that it may recognize what presents
    itself
and that it may comprehend what is absent or hidden.
Let it not fail to see what is visible
but do not permit it to arrogate to itself
the power to see what cannot be seen
for delicate and indefinite are the bounds
of the great art of caring for the lives and health of Your
    creatures.

May no strange thoughts divert my attention at the
    bedside of the sick
or disturb my mind in its silent labors.
Grant that my patients may have confidence in me and
    in my art
and follow my directions and my counsel.
When those who are wiser than I wish to instruct me
let my soul gratefully follow their guidance
for vast is the extent of our art.

Imbue my soul with gentleness and calmness.
Let me be contented in everything
except the great science of my profession.
Never allow the thought to arise in me
that I have attained sufficient knowledge
but vouchsafe to give me the strength and the ambition
to extend my knowledge.
The art is great,
but the mind of a person is ever-expanding.
I now rise to my calling.

*Attributed to Maimonides; adapted by
Rabbi Simkha Y. Weintraub, C.S.W., for the
National Center for Jewish Healing*

From the Sources

Every town counted among its permanent officials a physician who supervised the circumcision of children and looked after the communal well-being. A scholar was forbidden to live in a city where there was no physician.

Sanhedrin 17b; *"Yad," De'ot,* iv. 23.

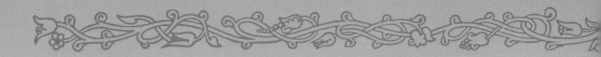

Chapter 44

The Many Worlds of Family Caregivers

Meet Marjorie, who could be your friend, neighbor, sibling, client, or you, yourself. (She is fictional, so she could also be Mark.) She has been worried about her mother's failing memory for some time; now Florence, her mother, has broken her hip after falling in the bathroom. Florence has had successful surgery and is coming home from the hospital. She needs considerable assistance with her exercises, with medications and special diets for her preexisting diabetes and heart disease, and with money management and household chores. Marjorie has already been helping out quite a lot, but her mother's level of need has increased dramatically. And it will go on increasing, because, after all, Florence is eighty-eight, and being in the hospital seems to have made her more anxious and fearful.

The home care agency that is providing a few weeks of post-surgical care considers Marjorie the "responsible party," meaning that she will have to take charge if the home-care aide does not show up or some other problem occurs. Researchers and policymakers consider Marjorie an "informal caregiver," because she is unpaid, although she is expected to perform the same tasks as a professional nurse and physical therapist. Secretaries and clerks at various offices and agencies involved in Florence's care consider Marjorie "the daughter," that is, her mother's agent in providing documentation, arranging payment, and making and keeping appointments.

The other people in Marjorie's life have also responded to her preoccupation with her mother. Marjorie's husband thinks she is spending too much time with her mother and too little with him and

242

their three children, one of whom is a teenager going through a bad patch. He doesn't like to bring it up, but Marjorie is also spending a lot of money for items that her mother needs but are not covered by Medicare. Marjorie's employer is sympathetic but is concerned because she takes so much time off from work and seems distracted even when she is on the job. Marjorie's friends tell her she is a "saint" but among themselves comment on how tired she looks and how she never seems to have time for lunch or a movie, or even a phone call. Marjorie and Florence belong to the same church, and the minister comes to pray with Florence. He tells her how blessed she is to have such a good daughter, but he never asks Marjorie how she is coping with all the added responsibilities.

And what of Marjorie herself? She hardly has time to think about it, but she wants to be everything to everyone—a dutiful daughter, a loving wife and mother, a valued employee, and a good friend. She also has her own private interests and projects. Yet the role she has taken on, with love but without realizing the consequences to herself or others, is not easily carried out with all her competing responsibilities.

Marjorie is a family caregiver—a person who provides essential, unpaid assistance to a relative or friend who is ill, elderly, or disabled. The two parts of the term are equally important. *Family* denotes a special personal relationship with the care recipient, one based on birth, adoption, marriage, or declared commitment. *Caregiver* is the job description, which may include providing personal care, carrying out medical procedures, managing a household, and interacting with the formal health care and social service systems on another's behalf. Caregivers are more than the sum of their responsibilities; they are real people with complex and often conflicted responses to the situations they face. In the past few years, family caregiving has moved onto the health policy and professional practice agendas in new and urgent ways.

FAMILY CAREGIVERS IN CONTEXT

Family caregivers may feel isolated, but they do not exist in isolation. Although typically considered part of the private realm of intimate relationships, family caregiving is greatly influenced by the cultural, political, and economic context of American society.

HEALTH FACTS

Since 1900, the percentage of Americans aged sixty-five and older has more than tripled, from 4.1 percent to 12.7 percent in 1998. In absolute terms, the number has increased from 3.1 million to 34.4 million. And the oldest of the old are increasing at an even higher rate; the number of people eighty-five and older was 33 times higher in 1998 than it was in 1900.

Currently, both families and health care are changing dramatically. While in earlier eras, some individuals lived to great old ages, the average life expectancy was decades less than it is now.

Although being old does not necessarily mean being frail or ill, there is an increase in diseases of aging, especially Alzheimer's disease, and the older one gets, the more likely one is to have illnesses or disabilities.

Because physicians had few effective treatments until the antibiotic age, most people who suffered severe trauma or serious illness either got better or died. Nature put a limit on caregiving. In the twentieth century, the advent of scientific medicine and the benefits of research, public health measures, better nutrition, and safer jobs have enhanced and extended lives. Moreover, some recent successes of acute care medicine (for example, in the care of newborns and trauma patients) have also created a population of individuals dependent, to unprecedented degrees, on technology and on other people for basic survival.

Although *family* is a basic organizing structure of all human societies, definitions of *family* have varied throughout history and by culture. American society today is made up of many different types of families—multigenerational, biracial, nuclear, blended, adoptive, immigrant, gay and lesbian, and others. Even in cultures where family is the primary unit of attachment, communities may supplement what families can provide or assume some caregiving roles, such as helping new mothers or caring for the dying. Religious institutions have a long history of providing care for the ill and dying; modern hospitals grew out of this tradition.

The shortcomings of care and abuses of human rights, as well as the economic costs of the past, are powerful deterrents to a return

HEALTH FACTS

Until the 1970s and 1980s, people in the United States with psychiatric problems, mental retardation, severe disabilities, and other conditions were routinely institutionalized.

to institutions for these populations. Still, it is interesting to note that even in our own time, rhetoric aside, families have not been expected to provide all necessary care.

Old assumptions and patterns of care do not fit present-day realities. Beyond the needs of an aging population and changes in family and household organization, these realities include prevalence of chronic rather than acute illness, women's increasing participation in the labor market, and, perhaps most decisively, the ongoing trend toward a health care delivery and financing system that uses hospitals and professional and public resources sparingly and patients' homes and family caregivers liberally.

The process of market-driven health care is still evolving, but trends are clear. Health care costs are being contained through reduced length of hospital stays; increased outpatient and community-based care; and reductions in home-care benefits available through insurance, managed care organizations, or public programs. A new industry has emerged that markets high-tech medical equipment for home use. Individuals and families are under increased pressures to pay more direct costs. Families are expected to provide more hands-on, often technologically complex, care; undertake greater burdens for longer periods of time; and forgo more educational, career, and social opportunities. Most families do not want and cannot afford to place their loved ones in long-term care facilities; only 4.2 percent of Americans over sixty-five are in nursing homes. Although alternatives such as assisted living have grown in the past decade, they are generally too expensive for most families. Nevertheless, the human and social costs of maintaining patients at home are very high.

Carol Levine

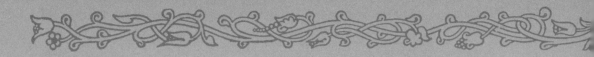

Chapter 45

Honoring the Elderly

My grandmother sold her home after my grandfather died and moved into an apartment. She was eighty-six years old. I remember that she was intent on renting one particular unit in the new building. When it came time to sign the lease, she was unhappily surprised to find that the apartment promised to her had been rented to someone else!

My grandma was literally a "little old lady," standing maybe 4 foot 10, yet she packed quite a punch when it came to standing up for her rights! She marched into the rental office and told the manager, "You're not pulling anything over on this old lady! I want *that* apartment!"

Needless to say, the young couple who had just begun unpacking was told to pack up and move to a different place!

Often those of us enjoying youth, young adulthood, and even middle age tend to forget that people who have reached retirement and beyond are people with feelings, sensibilities, intelligence, histories, and values. Yet the Torah teaches: "You shall rise before the aged and show deference to the old; you shall fear your God: I am the Lord" (Leviticus 19:32).

GROWING OLDER

Judaism, from its oldest teachings, places a premium on the *mitzvah* of *hiddur pnei zaken:* honoring the elderly. The *Midrash* says: "He who welcomes an old man is as if he welcomed the Shechinah (God's presence)."

God willing, we will all grow old. (As my mother-in-law is fond of saying, "It's better than the alternative!") The psalmist writes, "The span of our life is seventy years, or, given the strength, eighty years." For some, aging may mean losing physical, mental, and even financial resources. Aging can also mean growing in wisdom and experience, and in the ability to offer valuable insight as to how to live life.

As at every point along life's cycle, each person is unique, and each will age differently. Some people lead active lives in their own homes well into their eighties; some enter nursing homes with debilitating illnesses much younger; some suffer from Alzheimer's; and some complete their days in retirement homes or communities.

OBSERVING THE *MITZVAH*

Aside from the literal commandment of "rising up before a gray head," the Torah tells us little of what we can do, in practice. But there are so many ways to fulfill the *mitzvah* of *hiddur pnei zaken*.

First, begin at home by observing the commandment, "Honor thy father and thy mother." As grandparents live farther and farther from children and grandchildren, it is so important to keep those connections strong. Take the time to plan ahead to ensure that you celebrate holiday and life-cycle events together, including all the generations!

In addition, listen to the stories of parents and grandparents. Record them and write them down. Those histories are precious legacies for future generations; they remind those who are still young and healthy that, indeed, Bubbe or Zayde was once a child, a teenager, or a young parent!

REACHING OUT

Make telephone calls. It certainly can lift the spirit when a cheerful voice says, "Hi, Tante, how are you today?" Because so many elderly people are isolated—unable to drive or unable to leave their homes—a friendly voice is incredibly helpful in connecting.

There are also many ways to help not only family members but the aging in the community. Many synagogues have school and youth groups that visit nursing homes and geriatric centers, speaking with residents, performing, and celebrating holidays.

When I was a teenager in Toledo, Ohio, our youth group would go to the Jewish nursing homes to conduct the minyan (services) on Shabbat mornings. Following the short service, we would spend a little while with the residents. We learned not to fear holding the hand of an older person; we learned to appreciate who they were and to know their names.

In Philadelphia there is a program at the Neuman Senior Center called "Cook for a Friend." So many elderly are homebound and in need of food and groceries. Cooking and shopping for those who can't do so themselves are ways in which we show caring and respect.

Celebrating "Jewishly" is a wonderful way of enacting this *mitzvah*. I regularly visit a couple in their eighties. After greeting both husband and wife with a warm hug, we visit and listen to Yiddish music!

CELEBRATING LIFE

I remember that when my son was born we would bring him downtown to visit his great-grandparents every other week. It amazed me that my in-laws thought it was such a "big deal"! In reality, it was an honor. How wonderful it was to watch Grandmom hold her first great-grandchild! And how the Shechinah was present as the generations held onto each other and passed the past on to the future!

Life is precious, and Judaism puts the highest premium on life. May we all find ways to "rise before the aged and show deference to the old" among us.

ᐦ *Rabbi Sandra Rosenthal Berliner*

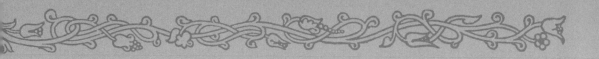

Chapter 46

Ten Guiding Principles of Long-Term Health Care Planning

It is important to be proactive, as opposed to reactive, when planning for health care.

   1. *Start long-term planning as early as possible.*

Plans are best made when you are not subject to the emotional stresses that result from the need for immediate decision making. If you start early enough, affordable long-term health care insurance (LTHC insurance) is available.

Effective long-term health care planning requires short-, mid-, and long-term considerations. To best accomplish this, the planning process should begin as early as possible. If you start before any major problems arise, affordable LTHC insurance is available. If you are able to get LTHC insurance, you should carefully review the policy before purchasing it. There is a virtual smorgasbord of policies available, and you should look for the one that best fulfills your needs and that is offered by a reputable company. However, very often we do not start the process of considering long-term health care planning until we are in the middle of a crisis. At such times, insurance will not be obtainable. In addition, because of the stresses and strains of the situation, we are often forced to have to make decisions under a great deal of pressure.

The planning process has many facets to it: financial, emotional, intra-family conflicts, location, dependency, and religion, to name a few. Because of all these and other factors, you must be proactive. You should start the planning process when minds are clear and before serious problems arise that will eliminate important planning options.

2. *Educate yourself about home health care, assisted living facilities, skilled nursing facilities, and continuing care retirement communities.*

In order to make the decision that is best for your family situation, you must know all the alternatives that are available in your community. New and innovative programs are being developed constantly, and they should be explored. Many communities have professional planners with whom you can consult.

Many options for long-term health care are available. For many, staying at home is the ideal situation. It allows the individual to maintain his or her habits and routines and to stay in touch with neighbors who provide companionship and support. For those who desire (and are able) to stay at home, many states have home health care programs. Most good LTHC insurance policies have home care provisions. In addition to private companies that provide nursing and custodial assistance, many religious communities have also responded to this need. If home health care is desired, you should choose the service carefully. While most providers are reliable, there are some who are not careful in the selection of caregivers. Remember that your loved one will spend most of his or her time with the caregiver and can grow dependant on that person. If the caregiver is not reliable or, worse, if that person is not properly skilled or trustworthy, much damage may result. It is also important that there be consistency in the relationship between the loved one and the caregiver. You do not want to have to switch caregivers too many times. You must also remember that the caregiver is not a substitute for family. It is important for you to maintain constant contact with both the caregiver and your family member.

If the conditions are such that remaining at home is not practical, then other alternatives exist. Assisted living facilities are now springing up everywhere. These facilities provide the opportunity for your family member to live somewhat independently, usually in an efficiency-type apartment. They meet the needs of older individuals who need some assistance in the activities of daily living but who do not require the skilled health care that is provided in a nursing home.

Generally, such facilities feature a community dining room, as well as kitchenettes in each living unit. They often have a medical staff and nurses on the premises. The staff makes sure that the family member's special needs are being met, including assistance with the taking of necessary medication and help in getting around, if necessary. Monthly fees are charged that include room and board; however, the cost of an assisted living facility is much less expensive than that of a nursing home. States can adopt "waiver" programs to provide government financial assistance for residents; however, many states have not yet made a serious attempt to provide financial assistance for assisted living.

For those individuals who do require skilled nursing care, nursing homes (also known as skilled nursing facilities) meet those people's needs. That is not to say that a person who needs only custodial care will not be admitted to a nursing home. However, if government assistance is sought, custodial care will not be covered. In the nursing home setting, the individual receives daily attention and assistance in the activities of daily living (ADLs). The ADLs include eating, dressing, bathing, transferring (getting in and out of bed or chair), toileting, and continence.

Nursing homes provide medical services and custodial care in one central location. Although very few individuals want to move into a nursing home, it sometimes becomes the only alternative available, especially when there is a need for medical supervision, and no family member is able to provide that level of care. Unlike residing in an assisted living facility, living in a nursing home, by definition, results in a loss of independence and privacy. Unlike residents in an assisted living facility who have their own units, residents in nursing homes generally share a room. Like assisted living facilities, nursing homes charge a monthly fee. Government assistance is available (in the form of Medicaid) for those who meet eligibility requirements. Nursing home costs vary throughout the country, but it is not unheard of to see costs as high as $6,000 to $7,000 per month. Remember that the quality of nursing homes varies greatly. Just because a nursing home charges more does not mean that its quality of care is better than a less expensive one. Before placing a loved one in a nursing home, you should check it out carefully.

Continuing care retirement communities (CCRCs) are facilities that combine all the methods described. They are very popular with middle- and upper-income individuals. Generally, if your loved ones are married, they move into the community together, as if it were a retirement community. There they can engage in recreational and social activities with members of their own age group. But what differentiates the CCRC from a retirement community is that the CCRC offers different living levels. If the need arises for your loved one to require assisted living, he or she moves into the assisted living part of the facility. If skilled nursing care is needed, the person moves into the nursing home section of the community (or, if there is no nursing home facility in the community, contracts for nursing home care are in place with local facilities). Generally, an admission fee is paid at the time of entry into a CCRC, and then a monthly fee is paid thereafter. The resident signs a contract with the CCRC that obligates the facility to provide housing, activities, and health care support. The admission fee varies from facility to facility, depending on the size of the living unit and the number of activities provided. Many contracts provide for partial refunds of the admission fee in the event of the "premature" death of a resident.

Also available in some areas are continuing care arrangements that allow the family member to remain at home until such time as skilled nursing care is needed. Under such plans, the provider will send home health aides to the family member's house, as needed. When a determination is made that skilled nursing care is required, the family member will be moved into a nursing home. An initial entry fee and monthly fees will cover all of the costs for such care.

3. *The entire family should participate in the planning.*

One person should not make the decision; all members of the family, including the person needing care, should participate in the long-term care planning process. Certainly, if the loved one is competent to give input, that input should be given great, if not total, weight. If all family members participate in the process, they then all have ownership of it. This certainly helps to avoid recriminations later on. It also helps family members deal with the inevitable guilt that sometimes arises. By having everyone participate, an understanding of the emotional and financial impact of the decisions can be shared by all. After the family agrees on the plan, certainly one person can be appointed to make the necessary arrangements. If that is the case, the designated person should keep all the other family members up-to-date on a regular basis. It is often a good idea to hold regular family meetings to discuss the process and to review how decisions may be affecting the loved one.

4. *Assemble the financial documents of the loved one and organize them as early as possible.*

Long-term health care is expensive. Generally, admissions offices request financial statements prior to a person's admission. It is important to assemble the financial information as early in the process as you can. Memories fade easily, and the location of financial records and even the existence of assets can be forgotten. Financial planning can be done to *lawfully* protect some of the assets of the loved one, but planners need accurate financial records. If an application for medical assistance such as Medicaid is going to be made, complete and accurate financial data will be needed. Often records dating back at least three years are requested. It is important that full disclosure is made both to the facility (if requested) and to the Medicaid officer taking the application.

5. *Assemble and review necessary legal documents.*

Regarding the issue of long-term health care planning, there are certain legal documents that must be prepared and executed by the family member while he or she is still legally competent to do so. Often routine documents such as the last will and powers of attorney should be specially prepared to take care of long-term health care planning. Powers of attorney should be drafted to deal with the issues of gifting (*if* the family member wishes to make gifts) and decision making. The powers should be checked to see if they meet with the state-of-residence requirements. They should also be checked to see if they are *durable.* This is especially important, because in many states, if the power is not durable, it will become invalid in the case of incompetence or incapacity.

If Medicaid will be needed, an attorney should also carefully check the wills. Proper drafting of the wills can minimize or avoid the loss of benefits of a Medicaid recipient if his or her spouse predeceases the patient.

Advance medical directives (AMDs) should also be discussed with the family members. Typically, there are two parts to an AMD. The first part is a *proxy* directive. This part appoints a person or persons to make medical decisions for the patient if he or she is incapable of making his or her own decisions. The second part is the *instructions* directive. This portion expresses the desires of the patient concerning end-of-life decision making. It is a *guide* for the holder of the health care proxy. It generally contains the wishes of the patient concerning the use of artificial means to keep him or her alive if death is imminent. Often hospitals and nursing homes request an AMD prior to admission. If the patient does not have one, these institutions generally provide prepared forms. In such cases, these documents are often executed under the stress of the situation and sometimes do not reflect the actual wishes of the patient. If your family member wants to execute an AMD, it is recommended that this be done well in advance of his or her admission to a facility and that it not be a boilerplate form but one that reflects the desires of the person.

If family members accompany their loved one to an attorney's office to have any or all of these documents reviewed or drafted, they must remember that the client is the loved one. The attorney should meet with the client alone to determine his or her wishes without any pressure from the family members. While family members can be present for a portion of the meeting, the attorney should excuse them when the actual details are being discussed, and they should not be upset or insulted when such a request is made.

6. *Choose a facility that allows for ease of visiting.*

When selecting the appropriate facility for your family member, pay careful attention to its location. While financial factors are important, the emotional need of the family member to spend time with family and friends cannot be overlooked. If placement in a facility is necessary, try to find a facility that is convenient to everyone, especially the spouse of the family member. While this advice seems so obvious, I have seen situations where the loved one is placed in a facility that is inconvenient for visits by the spouse who is living at home.

For many people, visiting a loved one in a nursing home is not easy. It can be depressing. The demand of visitation often conflicts with the family life of the children of a loved one who is in a facility. If distance becomes a factor, it can easily result in a reduced number of visits. For obvious reasons, one cannot overlook the importance of visitation to the institutionalized family member. For less obvious reasons, visitation by the children, grandchildren, and spouse is important to them as well. One cannot underestimate the guilt that is often felt by these individuals if they do not regularly visit their loved ones.

7. *Carefully scrutinize the facility.*

No matter what facility is chosen, due diligence is required. Check out its physical plant, staff, medical department, rooms, and dining facility. Often a good measure of the cleanliness and organization of a facility is the way the dining room is administered. Get and check references from other residents' families. Check with the local Department on Aging (or its equivalent) to see if any complaints against the facility have been lodged. If Medicaid is going to be required, make sure that the facility is certified. Make sure that you have the opportunity to carefully review the documents that are required to be signed for admission into the facility. If possible, have those documents reviewed by legal counsel with experience in the area of long-term care. In the case of CCRCs, it is especially important to check out its financial stability, in addition to the other factors mentioned, because CCRCs usually require a significant up-front investment in the form of an admission or entry fee. If the CCRC is not financially stable, that initial investment may be lost if the CCRC goes out of business. The Continuing Care Accreditation Commission certifies many CCRCs, although it must be remembered that such accreditation is expensive, and many fine CCRCs are not registered with them.

8. *Familiarize yourself with the federal, state, and foundation funding requirements.*

As you can see from the discussions so far, long-term health care is expensive. Depending on where you live, assisted living facilities can cost from $1,500 to $4,000 per month, or more. Skilled nursing facilities can cost from $3,000 to $7,000 per month. At some point, public or foundation assistance may become necessary. You should know in advance what programs are available and their requirements. Contrary to popular belief, Medicare pays for very little of nursing home care. Generally, Medicare will pay for the first twenty days, and then copay for the next eighty days (in 2000, the copay rate for the patient was $97 per day). *But* Medicare will only pay if skilled nursing home care is medically mandated, if it is for rehabilitative purposes, if rehabilitation is actually taking place, and if the admission to the nursing facility is from a hospital admission.

According to statistics, Medicaid pays for about half of all nursing home costs. Unlike Medicare, which is not a resource-based program, Medicaid determines eligibility on the basis of financial need. Both the resources and income of the applicant are reviewed to determine eligibility. The complexity of Medicaid (which is a federal-state cooperative program) is beyond the scope of this discussion. It is enough to say that the program is available for low-income and minimal-asset individuals who are blind, aged, or disabled. Advance financial planning can reduce the impact on individuals who will be seeking Medicaid. It is also important to know that while the federal government sets certain minimum financial standards, the states are free to establish less restrictive standards. Thus the Medicaid programs vary from state to state.

In addition to governmental programs, many private foundations, religious institutions, and charities provide assistance for long-term health care. Availability of these resources varies from community to community, and steps should be taken to determine whether such assistance exists in your community.

9. *Make a budget.*

Vital to sound financial planning is a well-thought-out budget. This is especially true when only one spouse is going into an assisted living facility or nursing home. Often inexperienced planners fail to take into consideration the ongoing costs of the "at home" spouse. If careful planning is not accomplished, especially when a person is in an assisted living facility where there is little in the way of government assistance, funds can be depleted during the lifetime of the individual. If that happens and the individual is not medically eligible for nursing home assistance, the financial burden of caring for the loved one will fall on the family members. This can cause a great deal of stress and, sometimes, resentment.

Since nobody has a crystal ball that will predict the future, a good financial plan will consider various scenarios. It is important that alternative funding sources are established in advance should funds be depleted during the lifetime of the family member, prior to Medicaid eligibility.

One must also be very careful about transferring of assets in order to speed up eligibility for Medicaid. While Medicaid does not now forbid such transfers, there are penalty (ineligibility) periods that can result from such transfers. If not done carefully, such transfers can result in Medicaid ineligibility periods that can extend beyond the available financial resources of the family member. And know this: nursing homes can legally require the removal of a resident for nonpayment of the nursing home bill.

10. *Most important of all, allow for the afflicted family member to retain his or her dignity at all times.*

The overriding factor in the planning process should be the dignity of the loved one. Family members should go into the planning process with the understanding that the loved one's quality of life should guide all the decisions being made. Financial factors such as the protection of assets, while important, should be secondary to the needs of the afflicted family member. Each of the planning items listed must be accomplished with full attention to the maintenance of the loved one's dignity. It is a terrible thing to lose control. It is even more so when control is taken away. When at all possible, explain what you are doing to your loved one and have him or her involved in the process.

∶ *Department of Jewish Family Concerns, Union for Reform Judaism*

Chapter 47

On the Quest for Resources

A Guide for Caregivers and Professionals

Among the difficult, frustrating, and tiresome tasks that caregivers must face, finding information, services, resources, and sources of support for care recipients and themselves is one of the most daunting. I spent close to a year on this task. However, even with the luxury of searching as part of my full-time job, without the urgency of being a hands-on caregiver, I was frustrated by the results. After spending countless hours on the Internet, sorting through dozens of books, and calling hundreds of organizations, I found that the information I was given was often limited, redundant, or out-of-date. There is an ocean of information out there, but it is often only an inch deep. While on my quest, however, I began to identify strategies that are likely to make the search faster, easier, and a little less frustrating.

- *Do not hesitate to give this job to someone else.*

Friends, family, or even acquaintances will often ask a caregiver if there is anything they can do to help. Looking for information and resources is an ideal task to pass on to someone else because it consumes excessive amounts of time and energy—two things that are most precious to a caregiver. What's more, the information can be easily conveyed to the caregiver when the work is done. High school or college students in the family may be able to take on this research project.

- *If you can, use the Internet.*

The Internet is an easy and quick way to obtain information for caregivers. Whether it is a Web site that specializes in providing moral support, a list of links to Web sites of disease-related organizations, a source of literature about medical conditions, or a means of ordering helpful books or supplies, the Internet offers an easy, convenient, and quick way to begin to find the help you need. If you do not have Internet access from your home, try your local library, schools, hospitals, or other community agencies, which may offer Internet access either for free or for a small fee. The time you spend looking for Internet access will pay off in the hours this helpful technology can save you.

The Web can be particularly useful when looking for books related to caregiving or home care. Even if a caregiver has the time to search in person, it is likely that many of the most helpful books for caregivers will not be on the shelf at local bookstores. A caregiver can order these books over the Web, making the search faster and easier.

One caveat: information on the Internet is variable and sometimes inaccurate. It is important, therefore, not to rely on one site alone. Also be sure to check out the sponsoring organization. Is it a reputable and reliable source of information? What is its financial stake, if any, in the information provided? When was the Web site last updated? If the site provides medical or scientific information, does it offer citations for the research or information provided?

- *Be sure to use* both *the Internet and the telephone to obtain information.*

Just as different agencies sometimes provide conflicting or contradictory information about the same topic, there are often discrepancies between the information an organization posts on its Web site and the information it sends through regular postal mail. That is why it is important to consult and compare all sources of information from an organization. Because the Internet provides an inexpensive and easy way to post a wide range of information, an organization's Web site usually has a more complete description of the types of services it offers than its printed pamphlets. However, a packet received in the mail is more likely to be tailored to your needs. A good practice is to look at an agency's Web site before calling to talk to one of its representatives.

Many agencies will send you information that overlaps or repeats information you have already received from other organizations. Many organizations refer their callers to the same national or specialized organizations. Therefore, if you obtain a good list of places to call for help, do not waste your time looking for other lists until you have exhausted your current one.

- *Before you call an agency, write down specific questions to ask the agency representative, and be as concrete and detailed as possible.*

When you call an agency or organization for information, rarely will you get the opportunity to speak to someone in person the first time you call. Even if you do, chances are the person on the other end of the line will give you the most general and brief overview, take down your name and address, and then end the conversation as quickly as possible. That is why you need to be ready. By looking on the Internet first, you can obtain the background you need to identify specific questions and needs.

If you are at the very beginning of your search for resources or have just recently become a caregiver, identifying your needs and questions may be particularly difficult. Spending time to assess your situation and your concerns, however, will save a lot of time in the long run. Take advantage of the fact that there is actually someone on the line to talk to you. If you find this person to be helpful, take down his or her name and ask to speak with this person if you need to call again. Many times, even after I asked specific questions, I received only general information that was not helpful and had to call back to clarify my needs. Knowing whom to speak with and what to ask for enabled me to get what I needed much more quickly. Keep in mind that this process can take months, so save time and have your questions ready.

- *Be aware: there will be a delay in receiving information you have requested.*

Many organizations have a heavy workload, which delays their sending the information to you right away. Make sure you let the agency know that you need the information as soon as possible, and ask for information over the phone to tide you over until you receive materials in the mail. If you have not received materials within two weeks, chances are you never will. Do not hesitate to call back and request them again. Usually, a second request receives prompt attention.

- *When calling an organization, if you have to leave a message, be sure to call again.*

Many agencies that help caregivers are too small to have someone available to answer the phone more than a few days a week. If this is the case, you will probably reach a voicemail system or answering machine. Leave a message, but be sure to call again if you have not heard back in a few days. Sometimes it took organizations several weeks to return my call. At times, depending on the agency and the services it provides, it may not be worth the effort to call again. Following up, however, even several times, always produces the best results.

- *Consider major disease-specific organizations for general information.*

Some large disease-specific organizations, such as the American Heart Association and the American Cancer Society, have an extensive amount of general information about caregiving and potentially helpful referrals that are useful and relevant to most caregivers, even if their loved one does not stuffer from heart disease or cancer. Call and ask for their general information packets. You may find helpful resources.

- *Be creative.*

Many of the services offered by even the largest agencies do not serve everybody. Even caregivers who live in a large metropolitan area and are more likely to have resources available to them than those living in rural areas or outside city limits are often ineligible for services for myriad inconsistent and dumbfounding reasons. It is in these most frustrating times that being creative in finding resources can work best. This means creating your own personal resource network. This could include contacting community-based agencies to find out what kinds of support services are available in your area. It could involve contacting your local grocery or drug store to create special arrangements for home delivery of food, medications, or other items. You might consider contacting local businesses, boys and girls

Community Resources

Administration on Aging: (202) 619-0724; http://www.aoa.gov

Alzheimer's Association: (800) 272-3900; http://www.alz.org

American Cancer Society: (800) 227-2345; http://www.cancer.org

American Diabetes Association: (800) 232-3472; http://www.diabetes.org

American Heart Association: (800) AHA-USA1; http://www.americanheart.org

American Psychiatric Association: (888) 357-7924; http://www.psych.org

Arthritis Foundation: (800) 283-7800; http://www.arthritis.org

Cancer Care: (800) 813-HOPE; http://www.cancercare.org

Children of Aging Parents (CAPS): (800) 227-7294; http://www.caps4caregivers.org

Medic Alert Foundation: (888) 633-4298; http://www.medicalert.org

Medicare Rights Center: (888) 466-9050; http://www.medicarerights.org

National Association of Professional Geriatric Care Managers: (520) 881-8008; http://www.caremanager.org

National Center for Jewish Healing: (212) 399-2320

National Hospice and Palliative Care Organization: (800) 658-8898; http://www.hospiceinfo.org

Parkinson's Disease Foundation: (800) 457-6676; http://www.pdf.org

Visiting Nurse Association of America: (888) 866-8773; http://www.vnaa.org

Well Spouse Association: (800) 838-0879; http://www.wellspouse.org

clubs, or schools to find out if they have special volunteer programs that might be of assistance. Being creative could also include speaking with government representatives for help, support, and referrals to services. Some places may seem unorthodox but may also be able to provide valuable assistance. It never hurts to ask for what you want, and when you do, people can usually find a way to accommodate you and your needs.

- *Be persistent.*

No matter how much you may want to, do not give up. You may have to go through several series of phone calls, letters, agencies, programs, and institutions to get what you need. The saying "the squeaky wheel gets the oil" is unfortunately true. People out there can help you. It just might take a lot of time and energy to get their attention.

Alexis Kuerbis, C.S.W., with Andrea Y. Hart

Chapter 48

A Crisis of Caregiving, a Crisis of Faith

On April 10, 1986, at 11:05 in the evening, my wife collapsed in our home from the rupture of two brain aneurysms. That began a phantasmagoria of events that has since determined the structure of our lives. In a traumatic second, she went from being an articulate public speaker, college administrator, teacher, and extraordinary wife and mother to a severely damaged woman. In the past twenty years, she has defied almost every statistic. Few people survive the level of cerebral damage she sustained. If, by some miracle, they do survive, the extent of brain damage that usually accompanies the rupture of a brain aneurysm, let alone two bleeding centers, results in severe cognitive disruption.

The attending physicians predicted that Elaine's death was certain and imminent. But after weeks in a coma she awoke, only to face overwhelming challenges. She was diagnosed with severe expressive Broca's aphasia. She had the typical symptoms of this form of aphasia, which for years impaired her ability to speak except for occasional utterances of a nonsense syllable. Though cognitively sound, able to understand spoken language, and physically whole, her inability to transmit her thoughts into words, spoken or written, frustrated her constantly. A remarkable and determined woman, she has battled valiantly to adjust to this brutal, daily challenge.

If this catastrophe struck her, it happened to our family as well. We are the parents of four sons, each of whom has made a major mark in his field. We were living a wonderful life of public service and commitment to our own careers. Everything seemed to be unfolding according to a well-designed plan when the facade collapsed. We were a public family, living in the spotlight of congregational and community activity, and our agony was not to be a private affair.

MANAGING THE IMMEDIATE CRISIS

In the beginning, loyal friends and concerned supporters rallied to my side, flooding the hospital. Eventually, hospital staff members asked me to restrict the number of visitors, as there was not enough room for all of them. Day and night, people would visit and ask, "What can we do for you, Rabbi?"

Through it all I was truly indefatigable. My adrenaline flowed as I conferred with physicians, comforted family members, and made important medical decisions on Elaine's behalf. In no way do I wish to make light of the situation, because it was horrible, but it was an incredible drama. I listened to the flood of medical advice from physicians in my congregation. We have over two thousand members in our synagogue, and a sizable number of them are doctors. They provided invaluable help in managing Elaine's clinical condition and helped me with referrals to the best available specialists. That outpouring of support remains one bright note in a period of intense stress and despair.

Then I began to hear disturbing advice. Over and over my congregants would tell me, "Rabbi, be strong. God will be good." I said to myself, "If God were so good, why did this happen in the first place? What did Elaine do to deserve this?" I discovered that I was relying on the great philosopher, Woody Allen, who once said that God is an underachiever.

"Rabbi, you give us strength," they would say. All the while I was screaming inside for someone to help me. So it was not only a crisis of practical response, it was a crisis of faith at a time when everyone expected me to be the symbol of unwavering faith. I was the rabbi, and I was supposed to set the example for the best possible way to handle this trial.

CAREGIVING WITHOUT TRAINING

I am still amazed that I was able to watch myself, almost from a detached perspective, as I tried to make sense of the unfolding horror. It should have come as no surprise, because I supposedly had all the proper credentials to be a caregiver. As a rabbi I have counseled many people. I have been on the faculty of three medical schools and have a specialty in medical sociology and bioethics. I had spent years on ethical review boards that dealt with research and clinical protocols. I had lectured extensively on the relationship of the health care community to patients and family members. Therefore, I assumed that I was somewhat sophisticated and knowledgeable about the health care delivery system. Who else would be so well prepared to be a caregiver? It was a disaster.

I found that I was bewildered and under total emotional siege. Even though I had, in my classroom, inveighed against the passivity of patients and caregivers, I found myself accepting, all too readily, the comfort of leaving the decisions to the doctors. It was so much easier to be lulled by the authority of the health care professional. I had to constantly battle to maintain my sense of perspective and a modicum of control. This became more of an issue as my wife's acute condition settled into a chronic state over months and years. An emotional fatigue gripped me and required that I call for more outside help and advice. At the same time, though, I realized that the basic decisions were mine. As much as I wanted relief from the constant onslaught of responsibilities, it was my mandate to be in charge.

In retrospect, I realize that I had been thrust into the role of caregiver without any preparation. None of the health care professionals caring for my wife, nor any of the doctors in my congregation, ever told me how to manage the transition from acute emergency to chronic illness, from being a husband to also being a caregiver. Acute illness has a clear definition of time and clinical activity. Chronic illness is more of a response to a daily regimen that has no time parameters. This transition is still happening twenty years later.

When the immediate crisis subsided, the people who we considered among our closest friends disappeared. They were unwilling to adjust to the sudden change in our lives.

That phenomenon seems to be common for people who experience dramatic shifts: those who become widowed, couples who divorce or separate, and those who become chronically ill or disabled. When a serious injury or illness renders an individual unrecognizable, many friends are unwilling to make the emotional adjustment necessary to continue the relationship. These losses can lead one to feel disillusioned, betrayed, and lonely. We were no exception.

With all of my experience and supposed sophistication, I realized I had to learn a new vocabulary. Before my wife's collapse I had never heard of aphasia. As I was introduced to clinical therapies for my wife's condition, which were almost primitive in 1986, I learned the technique of tonal intonation. A therapist had discovered that the brain processes speech and music in different areas. Although aphasics' abilities to put their thoughts into words are damaged, the therapist found that they might eventually be able to regain speech ability by reciting words as recitative. Since the portion of Elaine's brain that processes music was not damaged, I used the technique to reintroduce language to her. The technique helped her think about words in song and, eventually, to express herself, albeit in a limited fashion. I became an expert in responding to aphasia, not by study alone but by the trial of a beloved.

How devastating it was in those early years to talk and listen to someone who had been so articulate yet whose speech was now limited to a nonsense syllable. In the first two years after she became ill, she was able to articulate only one word I could understand: "prison." She was in a prison of verbal isolation. In many ways I was also in that prison, a prison of existential horror that was not of my choosing—the prison of caregiving. We had been companions in so many ways. We had a loving marriage of giving and sharing.

We had a relationship of care, admiration, and concern. We depended on each other's talents for mutual support and growth. Now I was required to be the decision-maker. At a time when I needed her strength and sagacity as never before, she was in the midst of her own battle against an indescribable isolation that required all of her energy and resilience.

There were other issues, which I can talk about only now, more than twenty years after that chilling moment. I wasn't prepared for the role reversal—a man caregiving for a woman. On one particularly upsetting occasion I found myself screaming at my wife's gynecologist on the phone, "What do I do?" I had been married to her for over thirty years, and I had no idea how her body functioned. A woman's gynecological needs, daily and monthly, are handled by her in discreet privacy and not before her husband. Now it was my responsibility.

SEEKING SUPPORT

In the midst of all of these imponderables, one of my sons said to me, "Dad, you have it so much easier than we do." I was taken aback. "What are you talking about?" I asked. "You only have to worry about Mother," he said. "We're worried about both of you." My sons insisted that I see a therapist. I did and realized that, after about a half-hour, he was telling me his problems. After all, I was a rabbi and it is my function to listen to problems. I told him, "I don't have to pay you $125 an hour to hear your problems. I listen to problems all day long." That was my first cautious step into therapy. The second—a more challenging one as it had a certain philosophical impact—occurred when a psychiatrist said to me, "Rabbi, let me ask you a question. If someone came to you with this problem, what would you say to them?" That was a shattering, cold moment. I knew that he was saying to me, "You know the answer as well as I do." I did not realize at the time that what I really needed was just to let loose. I just needed to be able to cry, to be able to scream.

In 1991, I discovered a helpful source of support—the Well Spouse Foundation. Its motto explains its mission: "When one person is ill, two need help." That group was vital, not only for mutual support with fellow caregivers but also for helping me develop a vocabulary to understand what I was experiencing. Before I encountered Well Spouse, I had never heard of the term *caregiver*. I realized that the group had already begun to articulate the existential issues with which I was grappling but had not formulated into words. I learned that I was part of a defined category of people and, at the same time, I was struggling as an individual to make some sense and purpose out of a dramatic life change. Well Spouse helped me identify that I was on a separate, but parallel, path from Elaine, which had its own distinct challenges. Caregivers are a group that has always existed but had just begun the process of self-identification and self-definition.

TAKING A TOLL

Recently, I realized that, for years, I had turned emotionally inward in an attempt to maintain control. I banked many of my emotions in the name of efficiency. I internalized my own sorrow, anger, frustration, and fear for the sake of my wife, who was battling her own inner struggles. It took its toll. Twelve years ago I had a heart attack.

The health conditions of caregivers are rarely discussed. We become ill as a result of the stress we experience. Caregivers provide an average of 17.9 hours of care per week and many provide forty hours or more, meaning they are in an almost constant state of caregiving.[1] Their clinical status is even starker: caregivers are more likely to experience health problems due to caregiving, and some face the risk of serious illness, including cardiac problems.[2] I am part of that statistic. Most disturbing of all, caregivers who experience emotional or mental strain are at a greater risk of dying.[3]

As I lay in the intensive care ward and listened to the pronouncements of the cardiac surgeon, I was beset with a familiar bifurcation of emotions. Of course, I was worried about myself. This was an attack on my mortality. I was to undergo emergency bypass surgery. My life was in danger and I was frightened. At the same time, Elaine was on my mind. Who would take care of her? Our sons and their wives are extraordinarily attentive, but they have their own lives. No one would take care of her as I had throughout these years. At that moment of ultimate personal challenge, I did not even have the time to luxuriate in my own health crisis. Elaine sat by my bed and held my hand. I could see the fear in her eyes; she was worried about me. She later told me that she could see the fear in my eyes. I was worried about her and me.

FINDING COMMONALITY

As former First Lady Rosalynn Carter said, there are only four kinds of people in the world: those who have been caregivers, those who are currently caregivers, those who will be caregivers, and those who will need caregivers. This makes caregiving a universal problem.

If this is true, then how can we better prepare caregivers to enter this role? I have heard the suggestion that caregivers should make their needs better known. Most caregivers struggle with this advice because it takes time for them to recognize that they are care-givers. In addition, caregiving consumes so much of the day that caregivers rarely have the time to seek help from outside sources.

If caregivers did seek assistance, where would they begin? With health care professionals? God help them if they do, because health care professionals work in institutional settings and generally provide little assistance to help people make the transition to the role of caregiver.

For most of the health care community, the emphasis is on the patient, and the family caregiver is visible only as a surrogate for the ill family member. Caregivers' needs are rarely on health care professionals' agendas, but the fact is that they need support as much as do patients.

Should they seek help from social service organizations? The social service community is just becoming aware of caregivers' cir-cumstances, and has yet to respond with adequate support services. Any programs these organizations create must have the flexibility to meet the varied needs of caregivers as patients move through differ-ent stages of illness. More important, services must be developed to support caregivers through the long periods when their ill or disabled loved ones remain in a steady, chronic state.

How about the clergy? There are no rituals for caregiving. There are traditional and modern rituals and liturgies for dying, but not for caregiving. And what are you going to pray for? Traditional pastoral care has tended to view the caregiver only in relationship to the ill family member. Religious leaders and secular counselors pos-sess little understanding of caregivers' needs.

In 1998, I completed the text for a book called *Mrs. Job: Caregiver in the Shadows.* Has anyone ever thought about Mrs. Job? The Book of Job tells the story of a good man who suffers the onslaught of disease and the loss of everything he values, including his children. Mrs. Job watches her husband suffer and lives through these losses, but no one comes to comfort her. Only one statement is attributed to her in the book. She says to her husband, "Curse God and die!" Throughout the years, commentators have condemned her statement as the ultimate blasphemy. But I understand what she's saying: "Let me out of here. I want an end to it." It is the cry of desperation.

The emotional drain on caregivers can indeed be intense. There is an unrelenting progression of exhaustion, anger, isolation, and resentment, mixed with the guilt that one should not have these feelings about someone you love but whose condition has nevertheless bound you in a daily emotional prison. Day after day, caregiving also involves financial management, and chronic illness creates horrendous financial hemorrhaging. Philosophy, theology, and even skill in complex home care fade in significance before the dismaying onslaught of financial strain. Perhaps the most frightening part of all is watching life's accumulated treasures disappear.

ENJOYING SMALL VICTORIES

The years since Elaine became ill have featured daily challenges, with the constant strain of her needs and the mourning of the end of previous expectations. But Elaine has made some remarkable progress. Intensive therapy helped her regain some language skills. She can speak in short phrases, achieved by a tremendous amount of effort. Her writing hand is immobile, but she can write with her other hand, however illegibly. She can read a newspaper or a detective novel, although her concentration is limited. She has a specially outfitted automobile, which allows her precious individual mobility. As with all aphasics, life is tremendously frustrating. While cognitively acute, she still struggles with self-expression.

Amid the trials of the last twenty years, there have also been the marriage of our sons, the birth of grandchildren, and public recognition for professional achievement. Elaine, with her verve and talent, founded a unique aphasia center at a rehabilitation hospital in Philadelphia, which has become a prototype for other needed centers. My own work with health care and bioethics has been a salve for the emotional battering that has characterized these years. Our greatest collective success has been in the ability to help identify caregivers as worthy of attention of the health care, religious, political, and media communities. It is no longer the lonely battle it once was to expand awareness and to effect response.

On my desk I have a picture of my wife holding her first grandchild for the first time. Ariel is looking at her grandmother, who is as much a miracle as is she. I keep it before me as a reminder that success is multileveled. Some questions were answered; some are still shrouded in silence and have yet to be voiced. The fact that there are still questions to be asked and answered is the greatest hope of all.

℘ *Rabbi Gerald I. Wolpe, M.A., M.H.L., D.D.*

Notes

1. National Alliance for Caregiving and AARP. *Family Caregiving in the U.S.: Findings from a National Survey.* Publication no. D16474. Washington, D.C.: AARP, 1997.

2. B. S. Rabin, *Stress, Immune Function, and Health: The Connection,* Hoboken, N.J.: Wiley, 1999; A. H. Glassman and P. A. Shapiro, "Depression and the Course of Coronary Artery Disease," *American Journal of Psychiatry,* 1998, *155,* 4–11; J. Keicolt-Glaser, R. Glaser, S. Gravenstein, W. Malarkey, and J. Sheridan, "Chronic Stress Alters the Immune Response to the Influenza Virus Vaccine in Older Adults," *Proceedings of the National Academy of Sciences USA,* 1996, *93,* 3043–3047; W. S. Shaw and others, "Longitudinal Analysis of Multiple Indicators of Health Decline Among Spousal Caregivers," *Annals of Behavioral Medicine,* 1997, *19,* 101–109.

3. R. Schulz and S. R. Beach, "Caregiving as a Risk Factor for Mortality: The Caregiver Health Effects Study," *Journal of the American Medical Association,* 1999, *282,* 2215–2219.

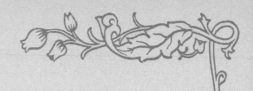

ℰ Special Focus

Hospice Care

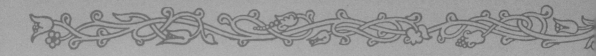

Chapter 49

What Is Hospice?

Hospice is a special concept of care designed to provide comfort and support to patients and their families when a life-limiting illness no longer responds to cure-oriented treatments.

Hospice care neither prolongs life nor hastens death. Hospice staff and volunteers offer a specialized knowledge of medical care, including pain management. The goal of hospice care is to improve the quality of a patient's last days by offering comfort and dignity.

- Hospice care is provided by a team-oriented group of specially trained professionals, volunteers, and family members.
- Hospice addresses all symptoms of a disease, with a special emphasis on controlling a patient's pain and discomfort.
- Hospice deals with the emotional, social, and spiritual impact of the disease on the patient and the patient's family and friends.
- Hospice offers a variety of bereavement and counseling services to families before and after a patient's death.

 DID YOU KNOW?

Hospice is not a place but a concept of care. Eighty percent of hospice care is provided in the patient's home, family member's home, and in nursing homes. Inpatient hospice facilities are sometimes available to assist with caregiving.

274

The Origins of Hospice Care

The word *hospice* stems from the Latin word *hospitium*, meaning "guesthouse." It was originally used to describe a place of shelter for weary and sick travelers returning from religious pilgrimages. During the 1960s, Dr. Cicely Saunders, a British physician, began the modern hospice movement by establishing St. Christopher's Hospice near London. St. Christopher's organized a team approach to professional caregiving and was the first program to use modern pain-management techniques to compassionately care for the dying. The first hospice in the United States was established in New Haven, Connecticut, in 1974.

Hospice care is a philosophy—an approach to caring for terminally ill patients—rather than a place. It provides aggressive comfort care when curative efforts are no longer effective.

A hospice team of physicians, nurses, social workers, rabbis, physical therapists, counselors, and volunteers provides expert medical care, pain management, and emotional and spiritual support for patients and families expressly tailored to the patient's wishes. Hospice staff provide telephone access twenty-four hours a day to answer questions, discuss concerns, or assist in solving problems.

The goals of hospice programs are to enhance the quality of life by keeping the patient as comfortable as possible, by relieving pain and other symptoms, and by supporting and reassuring both patient and family, thereby helping them understand and cope. Hospice care may be provided at home, in a nursing home, or in a home-like setting operated by a hospice program. Inpatient care is provided for crisis care and brief respite.

In summary, hospice care neither hastens nor postpones death. Rather, it affirms life and regards dying as a normal process. It offers support to help the patient live as actively as possible until death.

Hospice Foundation of America

Chapter 50

Frequently Asked Questions About Hospice Care

Who is eligible for hospice care?

A patient diagnosed by a licensed physician as having a terminal illness with a life expectancy of six months or less. Medicare, Medicaid, and many private insurers cover hospice care.

Can my own doctor continue to care for me if I become a hospice patient?

Yes, the patient's doctor can continue to supervise care; however, the hospice medical director can make home visits if needed.

Is hospice care covered by insurance?

Medicare and Medicaid cover hospice care. Other private or managed care insurance plans may also cover hospice care.

Should Jews use hospice care?

Hospice care can be very helpful to Jewish families. Most hospice programs are very respectful of their patients' religious needs.

Does hospice care shorten patients' lives?

Hospice care neither hastens nor postpones death. Rather, it affirms life and regards dying as a normal process. Its goal is to offer support to help the patient live as actively as possible for as long as possible.

Is hospice care only for cancer patients?

Hospice care serves any terminally ill patient. In addition to cancer, frequent diagnoses include heart disease, AIDS, lung disease, and neurological diseases such as Alzheimer's and ALS.

Must my physician make the initial referral for hospice care?

The patient or family may make the decision to enter a hospice program and may contact the hospice provider. A physician, however, must certify that the patient has been diagnosed with a terminal illness and has a limited life expectancy—generally six months or less. However, because it is impossible to predict death, the physician need only certify that it is *likely* that life expectancy is six months or less. There are situations when a patient's life is prolonged because of the quality of hospice care.

Must the patient be bedridden to be eligible for hospice care?

Hospice care is appropriate at the time of the terminal prognosis, regardless of the patient's physical condition. Many patients served by hospice continue to lead productive and rewarding lives.

ᴇᴏ *Hospice Foundation of America*

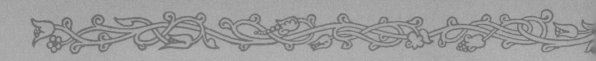

Chapter 51

Hadassah Hospital Kay Hospice for the Terminally Ill

We meet our patients and families at the most difficult times in their lives, when there is nothing false or artificial, but only the truth. It is a point of many mixed feelings, where both love and hate may be felt, where we worry, where the phrase "quality of life" is more than just words. It is meant to be a "window for hope" where compassion and professional excellence combine in an effort to control or prevent our patient's suffering, and where pain no longer has any right to exist.

Eleven years ago, Sara's sister died peacefully in our hospice; we were successful in helping her sister and their family, but our success is also your success. From the very first minute we opened our gates in 1986, Hadassah members have always provided us with the support that enables us to apply what we know and to always give our best.

When Sara's sister died, we were still young, not unlike a young child who is only four years old. We were young and without much experience, but we had many dreams and hopes for a better future. We wanted to mature quickly, but, alas, that doesn't happen so fast. Growing takes time, and that's how it should be. Growing means making mistakes and learning from them; it means learning as a result of doing; it means exploding myths and breaking taboos within the professional community by introducing new ideas and new ways of thinking.

In the beginning, we had certain criteria for admitting patients. After a number of years, we came to understand that those criteria were for the young and that we no longer needed them. We now have enough confidence in ourselves to admit and care for almost any patient who needs us. After all, who are we to judge if this patient really needs us, or if this patient does not? We now admit confused patients, even unconscious patients, as we believe that everyone has the right to benefit from our expertise. In addition, after much deliberation, we also decided to admit patients suffering from ALS (amyotrophic lateral sclerosis)—a very different category of patient, and as a result we have become pioneers in this field.

Indeed, over the past few years, we have reached new horizons in medical care. For example, by using certain well-known medications in an innovative way, we have been able to dramatically reduce the usage of certain drainage tubes in some of our patients, thus improving the quality of their life. We have introduced art therapy to our unit, and through pictures, we are able to better understand our patients and their families. We know that black clouds symbolize serious concerns, and a house without windows is a reflection of emotional problems. But a house with smoke coming from the chimney symbolizes life. The child who drew this picture was about to lose the aunt with whom he had a special relationship. Through his painting, he allowed us to enter his private world.

Over the last few years, the Hadassah hospice has become a clinical training ground for many professions. Nursing students, medical students, and students of social work spend valuable time in our unit and learn the significance of what it means to really care for patients and their families. It means learning to listen, learning to care with compassion and sensitivity, and learning that what really matters is not the procedures, laboratory tests, or statistics but the individuals who need our help during this critical phase of their lives.

We are always seeking new horizons. Recently, we joined a combined American Israeli mission to Riga, Latvia. Working together, our goal is to upgrade and improve the only Jewish hospital that exists in Latvia. After the initial fact-finding trip, one of our staff nurses traveled to Riga as part of a professional delegation to work toward improving the standard of care in their hospice.

Another new horizon opened for us when we received an unusual request from Japan. Mr. Abe asked if he could come to Israel to visit our hospice. He was actively involved in the development of a new hospice in Japan and had heard about us from one of his Israeli friends. His connection with us continues, since he has chosen our hospice as a model of excellence in palliative care. He told me, "Ruthie, in the United States, I saw how the system works; in England I came to understand the theory behind the system. It was only in your hospice that I saw how you combined the theory with the system and modified it to suit your culture." So now, Hadassah has a base in faraway Japan, where our hospice is loved and respected, even though our cultures are so different from each other.

We are continually involved in conducting research studies in our hospice with the clear goal of disseminating the findings in order to improve the quality of life of all terminally ill patients and their families. We have walked this beautiful and complicated path together, as a multiprofessional team. Teamwork is not just a token phrase in our hospice; it is our reality; it is a combination of all of our hearts, our minds, and our souls, and I believe that this is perhaps the key to our success.

Ruth Gassner

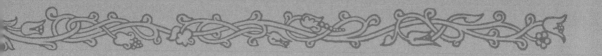

Chapter 52

Myths and Facts About Hospice, Pain, and Dying

MYTHS AND FACTS ABOUT HOSPICE

Myth: Hospice is where you go when there is "nothing else to be done."

Reality: Hospice is the "something more" that can be done for the patient and the family when the illness cannot be cured. It is a concept based on comfort-oriented care. Referral into hospice is a movement into another mode of therapy, which may be more appropriate for terminal care.

Myth: Families should be isolated from a dying patient.

Reality: Hospice staff believe that when family members (including children) experience the dying process in a caring environment, it helps counteract the fear of their own mortality and the mortality of their loved one.

Myth: Hospice care is more expensive.

Reality: Studies have shown hospice care to be no more costly. Frequently, it is less expensive than conventional care during the last six months of life. Less high-cost technology is used, and family, friends, and volunteers provide 90 percent of the day-to-day patient care at home.

Myth: You can't keep your own doctor if you enter hospice.

Reality: Hospice physicians work closely with your doctor of choice to determine a plan of care.

MYTHS AND FACTS ABOUT PAIN

Myth: Dying is always painful.

Reality: Many people die without experiencing pain. If pain does occur, it can be relieved safely and rapidly.

Myth: Some kinds of pain can't be relieved.

Reality: Some types of pain require "multimodality" (combined approaches) pain relief. Recent advances in analgesia ensure that all pain can be relieved by using commonly available medications or a combination of approaches that may include chemotherapy, radiation therapy, nerve block, physical therapies, and whatever else is appropriate.

Myth: Pain medications always cause heavy sedation.

Reality: Most people with severe, chronic pain have been unable to sleep because of their pain. The opioid analgesics (morphine, codeine, and the like) produce initial sedation (usually about twenty-four hours) that allows patients to catch up on their lost sleep. With continuing doses of medication, they are able to carry on normal mental activities. Sedation often occurs because of other drugs, such as antianxiety agents and tranquilizers that have been prescribed for other reasons.

Myth: It is best to save the stronger pain relievers until the very end.

Reality: If pain is not relieved by the lesser-strength analgesics (aspirin, NSAIDs, codeine, hydrocodone, and the like), then it is best to change to a stronger analgesic to bring the pain under continuing (twenty-four-hour) control. Pain that is only partially or occasionally controlled tends to increase in severity. This leads to two mistaken assumptions: the patient mistakenly fears that the pain is so severe that it can never be controlled; the doctor mistakenly believes that the patient is becoming addicted or is developing tolerance to the analgesic medication. In most cases, an adequate dose of a stronger analgesic such as morphine, prescribed on a regular basis, usually brings the pain under control.

Myth: Patients often develop tolerance to pain medications like morphine.

Reality: When morphine and other opioid analgesics are prescribed for the management of pain, the dose is sometimes raised to be sure that pain is well-controlled twenty-four hours a day, seven days a week. Opioids given to relieve pain generally do not lead to the development of tolerance. As a disease like cancer progresses, more opioid may be needed to control the pain on a continuing basis.

Myth: Once you start pain medicines, you always have to increase the dose.

Reality: In fact, the converse is true. Once pain is under control and the dose of opioid held at a steady level for several days, the dose of opioid analgesic can be lowered without the pain recurring. Levels of opioid can be raised safely as needed to control increasing pain. Also the dose can be lowered gradually if pain has been controlled on the same dose for several days. This change in dose to meet patient needs is known as "titration." The fact that the dose of opioid can be lowered once pain is controlled is one of the paradoxes of treating severe, chronic pain.

Myth: To get good pain relief, you have to take injections.

Reality: Until the mid-1970s it was believed that morphine was not an effective analgesic when administered by mouth, so it was universally administered by injection. We now know that morphine is effective when given by mouth or by suppository. Patients generally do not like injections, as they are painful in themselves. There are several excellent long-acting opioid analgesic preparations. Morphine and related opioids are available that control pain for twelve hours when used on a regular basis twice daily.

MYTHS AND FACTS ABOUT DYING

Many pervasive cultural misconceptions about dying exist that can interfere with people receiving the best possible care at the end of life. Debunking these myths and understanding the realities can allow caregivers to better support dying persons and their loved ones.

Myth: Death is too frightening to talk about. It's not normal to talk about death.

Reality: Death has been remote, hidden away in the back rooms of hospitals. There is a taboo about talking of death, even though death is a normal part of life. Everything that lives, dies. Death can be a positive experience, not only for the dying person but also for family and friends. In order to be a positive experience we must recognize the needs of dying persons as well as the needs of their caregivers. The family must be aware that dying persons have special needs that can be met.

Myth: People die as they have lived.

Reality: This is generally true, yet it is also possible for people to change. If people receive excellent care during their last illness, there can be great opportunity for reminiscence, for forgiveness of past difficulties, and for spiritual growth. This is only possible if there is good communication and openness among patient, caregivers, and family.

Myth: Dying is always painful.

Reality: This is one of the most common misconceptions about dying. Pain can be relieved safely without any danger of death or addiction. Hospice caregivers and most doctors are familiar with the proper use of analgesic drugs. When given in the correct dose at the right time, pain can be relieved without sedating the patient. When pain is relieved, patients can experience a good quality of life until the time that death occurs. Good pain management does not shorten the course of life. On the contrary, patients who receive excellent pain management tend to live longer than expected.

Myth: While dying, people see a white light, a tunnel, or something like that.

Reality: In general, this is not true. As people die there are physical and chemical changes in the brain that result in a gradual loss of consciousness. Some people experience what are known as delusions, illusions, or hallucinations, similar to dreaming while still awake. Some persons relate seeing relatives who have previously died. In almost all instances, these last visions are pleasant and offer comfort to the dying person, especially regarding the prospect of reuniting with deceased loved ones.

Hospice Foundation of America

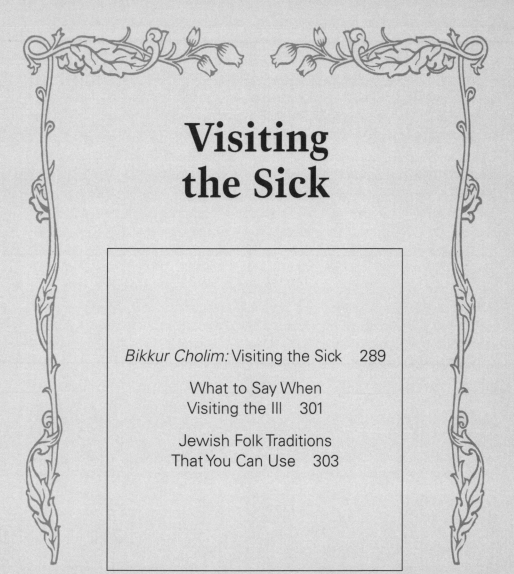

Visiting the Sick

Chapter 53

Bikkur Cholim:
Visiting the Sick

Hope is the gift we bring when we visit the sick. By sitting with a bedridden friend, we let that person know that he or she is not forgotten, that the outside world still cares. We offer hope by discussing plans for the future, by sharing the latest news from work, the latest adventures of a mutual friend, or the most recent cultural event. By bringing information from beyond the four walls of the sick room, we expand the horizons of the sick person, allowing him or her to enjoy a renewed fullness of vision and a sense of belonging. Of course, the most precious gift we can offer is our concerned attention. We can listen to the individual who is suffering from an illness.

Anyone who has ever been sick remembers how important such visits were. Each of us carries memories of the time someone touched us, of a gift that brought a sense of expectancy and a promise for the future, of a phone call at precisely that moment when we were feeling lowest. To be able to lift someone's spirits by such

From the Sources

The Holy Blessed One visited the sick, as it is written, "Adonai appeared to him by the terebinths of Mamre," and so you must also visit the sick.

Babylonian Talmud, *Sotah* 4a.

a simple gesture as sending a card or visiting for a few minutes is to make ourselves truly *shutafei haKadosh Barukh Hu* (partners with God).

Yet even as we recognize the importance of *bikkur cholim* (visiting the sick), even as we feel grateful to those brave and loving people who came to visit us in our sickness, we still feel hesitant, awkward, and fearful when it comes to visiting the sick ourselves. Resistance to visiting the sick is quite common and emerges from several different concerns, among them the following:

• *We are afraid of illness and death.* Watching someone wrestle with a serious illness is terrifying. It conjures the thought, "that will be me some day." Most of us apportion our time as though we will live forever. Visiting someone who is sick or dying forces us to confront our own mortality and the recognition that our time is finite—a limitation most of us would rather ignore.

• *We fear a loss of control.* When visiting the sick, we are forced to confront the terrifying reality that life does not tailor itself to our desires or our demands. We are forced to acknowledge that many aspects of life are beyond human control, that health and fitness—and life itself—are gifts. We may be able to affect them positively, but ultimately they remain beyond our manipulation.

• *We are uncomfortable in one another's presence.* We rarely reveal our personal concerns, hopes, and fears to other people. Rarely do we share the issues and goals that motivate one another's lives. Instead, we seek ways to be distracted together. We watch movies, television shows, or plays in silence. We find activities that fill our moments with other people—in sports or culture or eating. Visiting someone who is sick precludes all of these escapes from direct, personal interaction. At a sickbed, there is no alternative but to speak with one another, and doing this often forces one to delve into fundamental concerns and questions. At a hospital, the distraction of activities cannot provide an escape from the discomfort we feel in the presence of another human being.

For all these reasons and for countless personal ones, a chasm separates the discomfort we feel in the presence of illness from our recognition of the importance of *bikkur cholim.* This chapter is a bridge across that chasm. Confronting our fears and our frailty can bring us an acceptance of reality. It can help us appreciate every day of life as a gift and a blessing, and it can bring about a deeper involvement with our families and communities. The sense of concern and hope that a sick person receives from *bikkur cholim* is impossible to provide in any other way. Only the visit and attention of a friend, relative, or member of the community can inspire the sick with the knowledge that they are not alone, that they are not abandoned.

The steps that follow are a means to begin providing that care.

• *Upon discovering that someone is sick, send a brief card or a note.* It may be impossible to phone or visit the person for a few days. Rather than allowing a silence to isolate the sick, send a note to provide a sense of contact. Don't provide false cheer or lie about the sick person's prognosis. A note as brief as "I'm thinking of you" or "I want you to know that we love you" can be a great boost to someone who is ill. In addition to ensuring that the sick person hears from you (in case the phone is busy or it's impossible to visit right away), the card also provides a tangible symbol of love. Almost every hospital room I've visited has the cards taped proudly to a wall, in a place where the sick person can see them; they are a constant reminder that people do care.

• *Alert the sick person's rabbi.* Call the synagogue to say that there is someone who might benefit from a rabbi's visit. A rabbi is able to represent the Jewish community in ways that no one else can. Although a visit from a rabbi is often of great comfort, many people forget to notify the synagogue when someone is ill. As a result, the synagogue or local rabbi doesn't reach out, and the sick person often feels neglected. It is certainly preferable that a synagogue office get too many notices of someone's illness than that it not find out until the sick person is offended. Before notifying the synagogue, be sure to consider whether the patient will be upset by having his or her illness made public. If the patient is not Jewish (and the Talmud affirms that it is a *mitzvah* to visit the sick, whether or not they are Jews), try to notify his or her church, mosque, or temple.

• *Plan to visit the sick.* There is no substitute for the physical presence of caring people. They can banish loneliness and provide tangible evidence of a concerned community. A close friend or family member should visit immediately. If the hospitalization will be protracted, acquaintances and business associates should wait a day or two (the Talmud suggests waiting three days) before actually visiting. Many hospitalizations are for less than three days. For such short stays, it is certainly appropriate to visit sooner.

• *Don't plan a long visit.* Hospital patients have a busy schedule, and sick people often tire easily. It is better to visit briefly but repeatedly than to visit once for a long time. Be sensitive to the condition of the person and his or her stamina. When the patient tires, leave courteously with a promise to return another time. I remember one visit early in my rabbinate. We were in the middle of a stimulating conversation, or so I thought, when the patient blurted out, "Thank you for coming, rabbi." Unaware of her exhaustion and insensitive to her need for rest, I had put this sick woman in the position of having first to tolerate, and finally to dismiss, her rabbi.

• *Schedule your visit appropriately.* The Talmud counsels not to visit the sick early in the morning or late at night. Most hospitals have visiting hours in order to enable doctors and nurses to perform tasks unencumbered. Be sure to respect such restrictions. Early in the morning is often the only time a patient is able to sleep, and late at night may be a time of fatigue. Similarly, don't plan to visit on the day of an operation unless the patient or the patient's family specifically requests your presence.

• *Before visiting the patient, phone ahead to let him or her know you are coming.* This simple gesture creates the anticipation of a visit, giving the sick person that much more pleasure. Calling in advance provides a second advantage as well: it puts the patient in control. Being sick, whether at home or in a hospital, often results in a forced passivity. Doctors, nurses, and family members make and impose a range of decisions that a person normally would be able to make for himself or herself. When you phone and ask if it is all right to visit, the patient is able to exercise some control. If the patient declines the visit, don't insist or argue. Express the hope for a speedy

From the Sources

One who visits the sick causes them to live.

Babylonian Talmud, *Nedarim* 40a.

recovery, invite the patient to call you in the future, and politely end the call. Never visit someone who doesn't want to be visited.

   • *Prepare for a visit carefully and thoughtfully.* You can take certain steps that will lessen the sick person's discomfort and demonstrate your concern:

> *Don't wear perfume or after-shave lotion.* Illness often makes people more sensitive to smell, and artificial odors can be disturbing to the person who is sick.
>
> *Don't bring bad news.* No patient need hear of an additional tragedy. Disasters in the news, a personal crisis, even the illness of a mutual friend or relative, are all inappropriate topics to initiate. A significant part of *bikkur cholim* involves just listening— letting the sick person discuss whatever he or she desires. Try to restrict topics to those that will make the patient feel good. Focus on interests, loved ones, or hobbies.
>
> *Select one or two topics for discussion: perhaps an issue from the day's newspaper, a sports event, the weekly Torah portion, a movie or book that people are talking about.* The choice of topic should reflect the interests of the person who is ill. Preparing yourself with a few possible subjects for discussion can help you feel ready to sit and talk.
>
> *Bring the patient a small, practical gift.* A newspaper or magazine can reinforce a sense of connection to the outside world and leaves tangible evidence of the visit. Consider bringing a picture or poster and hanging it on the wall to enliven the room. One of the gifts I cherished most as a hospital patient was a bonsai tree. That little tree linked me to the outdoors and allowed me to feel less trapped by my hospital room.

   • *Before entering the patient's room, be sure to knock and ask for permission to enter.* This is another way to allow the patient to feel in control. Many people (doctors, nurses, therapists, and social workers) walk into sickrooms, often from necessity, without announcing themselves or asking permission. By simply knocking and asking if you may come in, you will help restore to the patient some sense of control.

   • *If there are already many visitors, wait outside until a few people leave.* Trying to juggle a room full of friends can be exhausting, and another visitor may simply be a strain. If there is time, wait. If not, then say, "I see that you are well cared for now. I wanted you to know I'll be thinking of you, and I'll come back when there are fewer people." It's important, when making this or any other promise, to fulfill the commitment. A promise creates an expectation where none had existed previously; to fail to visit again will transform that expectation into disappointment and heighten the patient's sense of isolation. Let the patient know when to expect the next visit, and then be sure to visit again.

• *When visiting, help with concrete tasks.* One of the crucial aspects of *bikkur cholim* is the kind of caring that can be demonstrated only in person. Help by making the bed, watering plants, straightening up the room, or any other chore that helps the sick person and makes the surroundings look well attended. Of course, it is important to get the consent of the sick person before tampering with the room. Anything that can increase his or her sense of control and dignity is an added gift.

• *Try to be with the patient during a meal.* Eating is a social act, and the presence of company during a meal can communicate additional closeness and caring because it suggests forethought. Be sure to ask whether the patient would like you to stay during the meal; many people are embarrassed to eat in another's presence.

• *Don't feel you have nothing to talk about.* At the heart of our discomfort with visiting the sick is a sense that we won't have anything to say. The following specific guidelines might help:

Be alert to objects in the room that might prompt a pleasant discussion. Photographs of people can lead you to ask who they are and to a discussion of their activities, interests, and relationships. A book lying by the bed can lead to a discussion about the book, its author, or the topic.

Don't criticize the hospital, the doctors, the food, or the medical procedures. Criticizing a patient's medical care may diminish his or her confidence in it. If the patient is frustrated, then listen sympathetically without committing yourself to agreeing. If the complaint is specific and reasonable, consider sharing it with a close relative of the sick person. If the patient is a member of your immediate family, then find out whether there is a possible solution to the particular problem.

Don't evaluate a procedure or the veracity of a medical progno-sis. A visitor's purpose is not to provide medical opinions. Disagreeing with the procedures selected by the sick person's pro-fessional caretakers undermines his or her confidence in the doc-tor's ability to provide the best possible care. Again, if there are reasonable doubts about the medical staff's performance, then inform a close relative of the patient. If the patient is a family member, then it might be worthwhile to call another doctor for a second opinion. At the same time, don't deny a poor prognosis. The patient may want someone who will listen openly and not brush aside the patient's feelings of hopelessness or despair. *Don't defend God, religion, or nature.* None of those needs defense. Being sick is a legitimate cause for anger, and expressing that anger or rage is the quickest way to be able to move beyond it. We can best help by listening sympathetically and by saying, "It must be very difficult to go through what you are going through. It really isn't fair. I'd be angry too if I were you." *Don't talk about someone who died of the same disease.* The last thing someone sick needs to deal with is the inexorable conclu-sion of a terminal illness.

- *Don't be afraid to sit in silence.* As with any situation where we are trying to bring comfort and friendship to someone who is suf-fering (whether from emotional or financial loss, or physical disabil-ity), the primary statement we can make is not through any words we speak but through our presence. Simply being with someone in a time of need is an articulate assertion of love and caring.

- *Listen.* Besides demonstrating our involvement by offering our physical presence, we can do so by allowing the sick to speak of their concerns. In fact, this is the main service we can offer. If people who are sick want to speak about their illness, then listen. If they want to talk about their families, then listen. All of us have a need to be heard, most of all when we feel strained or ill. By providing a receptive ear, we allow the sick person to validate his or her inner feelings, fears, and needs.

- *Offer your hand.* As a corollary to providing a loving pres-ence and a listening ear, don't hesitate to touch the person. There is no more immediate way to demonstrate that you will not abandon a person to illness than by reaching out and placing your hand on the patient's shoulder or by taking the person's hand in your own. The calm, love, and stability that a touch provides are without equal.

Touching may be especially difficult between men, with whom the social taboos are still strong. Yet illness is a time of particular vulnerability, a time when the need for connection is most intense. Actions not ordinarily performed can affirm a link that transcends words. Every time I have held a man who was suffering, he has burst into tears, even though we both hesitated before I reached out to him. I know that being a rabbi makes me an exception to the societal prohibition preventing men from holding one another, but the comfort and warmth transmitted are so real that this prohibition is worth being ignored by everyone.

- *Offer to pray with the patient. Bikkur cholim* is more than just visiting the sick. It is also the performance of a *mitzvah.* Of all the events in a person's life, illness is one that calls for the assurance of holiness and connectedness that Jewish tradition can provide so well. A willingness to observe Shabbat or other holiday and, more especially, a willingness to pray together can establish a living link to the Jewish community and to God. The rabbis of the Talmud often made a point of praying in the presence of the sick, some even claiming that a visit that did not include a prayer did not constitute *bikkur cholim.*

> *Prayer can be informal.* A simple wish of *refu'ah sh'leimah* (complete healing) or "God be with you" can bring a level of comfort that ordinary conversation cannot. Jewish tradition offers a brief prayer linking the experience of the individual to the broader community: "May God show compassion to you, together with all the other sick of the people Israel."
>
> *If possible, visit before Shabbat or a holiday, and bring some item that will allow the patient to celebrate that holiday.* On a Friday, consider bringing two small challah rolls and a little wine or grape juice (depending on what the patient is allowed to drink). Before Purim, bring some hamantaschen; provide honey and apples before Rosh Hashanah or matzah and a Haggadah for Passover. Linking your visits to the Jewish holidays is an effective way to combat the disorienting quality of being sick and reconnect the suffering individual to what other Jews are experiencing beyond the walls of the sickroom.

Read a psalm together. This simple gesture can add tremendous depth to your visit. Psalm 23 ("Adonai is my shepherd") can be a source of great comfort. Another possibility is Psalm 121 ("I lift my eyes to the hills") or Psalm 130 ("Out of the depths I call to You"). These readings link the present moment and the individual's pain to a continuity that stretches back in time to include the great figures of our biblical and rabbinic heritage. By using their words, we affirm a community of belonging that transcends illness, sorrow, and pain.

- *Offer to make two specifically Jewish gestures:*

Offer to attend a synagogue worship service and to have a Mi Sheberach *(literally "may the One who blessed") recited after the Torah reading.* The *Mi Sheberach* is a prayer for the sick. Be sure to find out the patient's Jewish name, as well as the Jewish names for his or her parents, because in the Jewish tradition a person is known as So-and-so, son or daughter of So-and-so and So-and-so. By asking the rabbi to recite a *Mi Sheberach,* you ensure that the community is informed of the illness, that more people will pray for that individual, and that the sick person has the comfort of knowing that a congregation of Jews cares.

Make a contribution to a synagogue or a charitable cause in honor of the sick person. In Jewish tradition, *tzedakah* (literally, "righteousness," a monetary contribution) is a highly cherished form of demonstrating respect and concern. Giving money in someone's name gives the person credit for an additional good deed and further links him or her to the values and activities of the larger community.

- *Reestablish the ancient Jewish tradition of* va'ad bikkur cholim. The mitzvah of bikkur cholim is an obligation that falls on all members of a caring community. Rather than relying on our own personal network of people who will "take care of their own," it is time to reestablish the ancient Jewish tradition of *va'ad bikkur cholim* ("committee to visit the sick").

Contact a nearby synagogue, and offer to work with the rabbi or executive director to organize such a project. All you need is a few volunteers and a willingness to put in some time. The visits of a *va'ad*

> ### *From the Sources*
>
> The Talmud tells a story about a disciple of Rabbi Akiba who became ill. When Rabbi Akiba discovered that no one was attending to the student, he himself went to the student's home, ordering his other students to sweep and clean the house for the sick student. Because of their care, the student recovered more rapidly. In gratitude, the student said to Rabbi Akiba, "My master, you have revived me." Immediately, Rabbi Akiba taught that "a person who does not visit the sick is comparable to one who sheds the blood of another."

bikkur cholim do not replace the efforts of the rabbi or the cantor. By providing regular hospital and sickbed visits by congregants, however, the *va'ad bikkur cholim* demonstrates that Judaism is not just for paid professionals and that the community, as a community, takes care of its members.

• *Visit nursing home residents, longtime hospital patients, and elderly shut-ins.* Many people suffer from chronic illnesses, suffering for such a long time that we often stop remembering that they need our care. The rules of *bikkur cholim* apply to these people, too.

Life is full of disappointments, mysteries, and pain. Although we cannot eliminate suffering completely, we do have the power to diminish its sting. By holding out our hands to one another, by providing company and comfort, we may not be able to make our world a paradise, but we shall surely make of our community a haven, a hope, and a home.

The *mitzvah* of *bikkur cholim* enables us to be fully human and fully alive to that which one human being can give to another. The time to begin giving is now.

ꙮ *Rabbi Bradley Shavit Artson*

How Friends Can Help

There are so many ways that we want to be of assistance to our family and friends when they are in a fragile and vulnerable state. Advocacy comes in many forms that you can perform on behalf of others. Each person has her own unique abilities. Each task is not for everyone, but as with everything in life, you should do what you enjoy and what you do best. We have itemized a few suggestions. We are certain that you will add to the list.

- *Some medical-based needs are as follows:*
  Offer to take your friend to the doctor for treatments or visits. Ask if she wants you to be present when the doctor or nurse discusses her illness, treatment, or medication schedule.
  Offer assistance through the maze of social service and health care providers and resources.
  Offer assistance in filling out forms and health care paperwork.
- *Household activities provide numerous opportunities for assistance:*
  Offer to make phone calls, organize dinners, feed and walk the dog, do the weekly shopping, fill the car with gas.
  Offer to go to the pharmacy, dry cleaners, post office, or the library.
  Offer to help organize a corps of volunteers for ongoing household needs.
- *There are times when your friend needs your company and friendship:*
  Read a book; play board or card games; listen to music; watch a favorite video, movie, or TV show together. Prepare snacks that the person is able to enjoy.
  Offer to take her to the wig maker or beauty parlor or one of many support groups that help recovering patients renew their self-esteem and enhance their personal appearance.
  Offer to take her shopping for clothes, or shoes, or whatever she might want. Offer to take her out to lunch, or to a movie.
  Offer to help her celebrate holidays in her home with her family: buy a challah each week, organize Shabbat dinner

through your network of friends and family. During the year, bring (when appropriate) Hanukkah candles, *lulav* and *etrog* (ritual items for Sukkot), books, cards, or special holiday foods and flowers for Shabbat.

Help her organize her day so that she builds in sufficient time for rest and recuperation.

Be a friend and take the time to listen.

Rabbi Hillel said, "If I am not for myself, who will be for me? If I am only for myself, what am I? If not now, when?" We are not expected to complete the full task, but we certainly are expected to do our share in helping others and in making a difference if only in one person's life.

From the Hadassah publication *Take My Hand.*

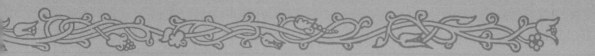

Chapter 54

What to Say When Visiting the Ill

"I am about to visit a friend who has just been diagnosed with a very serious illness. What do I say?"

Visiting someone who is seriously ill can be anxiety-provoking. To be with a person who is ill can stir up many strange feelings: our own fears of sickness and death, sadness we suffered when a loved one died, or discomfort with what is unfamiliar. Often we feel at a loss for words when we see this person in such great distress. Or we may feel nervous that we will say something that will make the situation worse. For all these reasons, it is understandable that one would want guidance in saying the right thing.

The truth is, however, that there is no "right" thing to say. Nothing you can say will shrink the tumor, remove the fear, or make things the way they used to be. What you can do is be present with this person wherever he or she happens to be; this is the spiritual gift you bring when you fulfill the *mitzvah* of *bikkur cholim*.

Being present is what *bikkur cholim* is all about. By visiting, we hope that the one who is sick feels less isolated, more loved, and more truly in the company of God; our presence should be a vehicle for magnifying the person's feeling that God is near. In the laws of *bikkur cholim* we learn that God's presence (the Shechinah) dwells at the head of a sick person's bed and that therefore we are not to sit there. I understand this *halakhah* (Jewish law) as a metaphorical teaching: whatever we say or do when we visit, we should make sure that we are not an obstacle to the Shechinah! We should not be focused on our own agenda or desire to find the "right" words that we fail to be present with our loved one.

To be lovingly present with another person, we must learn how to quiet our own internal dialogue ("He looks awful." "Why isn't she angry about what's happening? She must be in denial." "I wish I hadn't just said that." "Why is he talking about the football game?"). We must learn to be aware of those times when our own agenda, judgments, or preoccupations interfere with our ability to stay present with the thoughts and feelings of the person we are visiting.

To establish connection and be present with our friend, relative, or neighbor, not only is it helpful to quiet our own internal dialogue but also to follow the person's lead in conversation, to be able to listen, to be comfortable with silence, to be willing to communicate nonverbally, to be willing to show love, and to be oneself. In the course of visiting, we might say, "I love you," "I'm sorry that this is happening to you," "I'm here for you," or "I'll pray for you; you'll be in my thoughts." Such comments can express true love, care, and respect.

Although there is nothing magical to say to someone who is seriously ill, it is usually *not* helpful to say such things as the following:

"Cheer up!"
"Don't feel upset (or angry or depressed or sad)."
"It could be worse" or "Count your blessings."
"It's God's will" or "God gave you this for a reason."
"It's going to be OK" (you usually do not know this).

Remember that what you say is less important than who you are. Your presence really says it all.

Rabbi Nancy Flam, for the National Center for Jewish Healing

Chapter 55

Jewish Folk Traditions That You Can Use

A number of Jewish folk traditions, rituals, and ceremonies can be shared with an ill friend.

FOLK TRADITIONS

Many of the following rituals can be done alone or with a group of friends or family members.

Making Amulets

An *amulet* is an object with potential healing powers; it may be used to ward off evil and sickness. Consider bringing your friend one that you have made or purchased. In Israel, healing amulets have become extremely popular in the last few years. Judy Siegel wrote in the *Jerusalem Post* of May 17, 2000, "The use of amulets to speed the recovery of hospital patients, especially children, is increasing," and amulets may "express the families' need for emotional and psychological support in a crisis." Siegel observed that many different objects constitute healing amulets, for example, holy books, notes written by rabbis, pictures of rabbis, bottles of holy water, and bottles of holy oil. Researchers studying the use of amulets told Siegel that hospital staff members should "understand, help, and encourage families who use amulets as an extra treatment."

The *hamsa* is the most popular Jewish amulet. It is a picture or figurine of a hand, and the word *hamsa* derives from the Hebrew word *hamesh,* meaning "five." *Hamsa*s are used throughout the Middle East as a protection against the evil eye (a symbol of ill fortune). Some Jews call them the *hamsa* of Miriam. The *hamsa* may be made of metal, wood, or glazed clay. It can be worn as a necklace or placed on the wall as a plaque. Frequently, a wall plaque *hamsa* is decorated with prayers or blessings. A *hamsa* may also be decorated with an eye (to symbolically ward off the evil eye) or with blue or red stones. Both red and blue are considered colors that have apotropaic (protection from evil) powers. *Hamsa*s are sold at many Judaica stores, and they are also fun to make. Children can easily make a *hamsa* by tracing their own hand on paper and then coloring and decorating. When hospitals prohibit children from visiting loved ones, encourage children to make a *hamsa* and promise to display it near the sick person's bed. In this way, the patient will feel the love that the child is sending.

Tying Red Ribbons

Some of our mothers, grandmothers, or great-grandmothers protected us by *tying red ribbons* around us or by sticking a piece of red thread in our clothes or shoes. They sometimes followed this with three spits and the sounds, "tfu, tfu, tfu"—or in my family, "pooh, pooh, pooh!" You might create a healing ritual today by joining with others to encircle your friend with a red ribbon. Conclude by snipping off pieces of the ribbon for each person, so that all can share in the memory of a circle of loving friends united in prayer.

Making a Wall Plaque

Consider making a *mizrah* wall plaque. The Hebrew word *mizrah* means "east." The word also refers to a work of art that hangs on the eastern wall in both homes and synagogues to indicate the direction of Jerusalem. By facing the *mizrah,* we can direct our prayers to the east, to the site where the Holy Temple stood. Consider posting a *mizrah* that you have made or purchased in your friend's room.

SACRED SPACES

Transform your friend's room into a more healing place. Help to display cards, letters, or photographs in your friend's room in the hospital or skilled care facility or in your friend's sickroom at home. If too many flowers have accumulated, offer to distribute them to those who need cheering. If your hospitalized friend is ambulatory or can get around in a wheelchair, she might enjoy helping you distribute the extra flowers. By brightening up the lives of others, she may be able to feel that she can make a difference in the world, even now, when she herself is in the hospital. At holiday times, help your friend display the ritual objects and decorations that will establish a link to sacred Jewish time. Encourage others within the Jewish community to reach out to your friend at holidays as well.

- *Rosh Hashanah and Yom Kippur:* Arrange for someone to come in and blow a shofar. Bring white flowers, small round *challahs,* and apples and honey.
- *Sukkot:* Give your friend a *lulav* and *etrog* to keep by the bedside. The *etrog's* special fragrance is a wonderful bonus. Create an *"ushpizot* ritual"—a ritual in which you symbolically invite great Jewish women from history and from your own lives to join you now and to share their gifts and their blessings.
- *Simhat Torah:* Read the last chapter of Deuteronomy and the first chapter of Genesis to your friend.
- *Hanukkah:* If possible, provide a Hanukkah menorah and light Hanukkah candles with your friend. If lighting candles is impossible, provide an electric Hanukkah menorah, a dreidl, and enough gold-foil-covered chocolate coins for your friend to distribute to all who care for her. Alternatively, line up pillar-style candles as a symbol of the holiday.
- *Passover:* Prepare a Seder plate. Offer to create and hold a brief version of the Seder that covers the highlights of the ceremony.
- *Shavuot:* Decorate the room with the branches of just-flowering trees. Read the story of Ruth together.
- *Shabbat:* On Friday afternoon, bring a tape recorder and cassette of Shabbat music for your friend to play. Pack candles and candlesticks, too. If your visit will take place in a space where no candle lighting is allowed, electric Shabbat candles or a pair of night lights can serve as substitutes. Bring along a small challah, a little bottle of grape juice, a decorative plate and napkin, and also some spices for *havdalah.* Even if your friend feels too sick to "make Shabbat," her family may feel elevated by the opportunity you create to do so.

BLESSINGS FOR YOUR FRIEND

Alone or with a group of friends, hold a healing ceremony. If your sick friend likes the idea, hold the ceremony in her presence; if not, hold the ceremony at your home or the home of another friend. Create a ceremony as formal or as informal as you and your group wish and as Jewish, in language and in rituals, as you and your group feel comfortable with. There is no right way to proceed! Do, however, decide on a general outline beforehand, so that you and your group know what to expect. If friends can prepare special readings or bring special objects, they will feel more involved. A healing service held for a particular individual might include songs, psalms, shared wishes, and the *Mi Sheberach* prayer, either the standard version (found in a *Siddur*) or the lovely rendition by singer Debbie Friedman. Your group might also collaborate in creating a healing amulet for your friend, one that will express your love and shared concern for her.

THE TRIED AND TRUE

Bring your friend a kettle of chicken soup. Either the delicious soup will be healing in itself, or your friend's laughter will do the trick. In a pinch, bring a can of chicken soup to display as an amulet.

Some of the most learned rabbis of our age have suggested that, in times of crisis, the best thing a friend can do is bring ice cream or rich chocolate cake. According to sages, truly noble friends bring an extra spoon or fork, and offer to stick around and share.

ℰ *Vanessa L. Ochs*

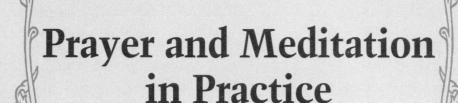

Prayer and Meditation in Practice

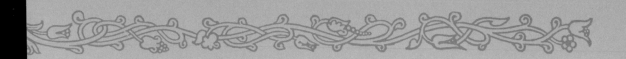

Chapter 56

Eight Possible Ways in Which Prayer May "Work"

1. Prayer may work in that one may have asked God for something that indeed came about.
2. Prayer may work by invoking a greater sense of God's presence.
3. Prayer may work by way of distraction, momentarily pulling the person out of his or her pain and suffering into a place of beauty or transcendence. (This is comparable to the Lamaze technique used in preparation for childbirth.)
4. Prayer may work by focusing more deeply on the pain or discomfort in the suffering person's life; in this way, prayer can be deeply grounding and clarifying. (This is comparable to the Bradley method of childbirth preparation, which helps women enter the pain more deeply and wholly.)
5. Prayer may work by quieting or centering the self.
6. Prayer may work by significantly connecting the one praying or being prayed for with Jewish community and tradition.
7. Prayer may work by helping the one praying or being prayed for connect to a deep level of the self that is already healed and whole, reminding the person of his or her essential wholeness. Music, for instance, often has the capacity to put us in touch with that deep place of essential wholeness.
8. Prayer may work by focusing the praying person on the blessings in his or her life, thereby enhancing the person's sense of gratitude.

Rabbi Amy Eilberg for The National Center for Jewish Healing

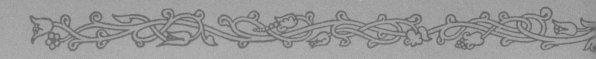

Chapter 57

Healing at Bedtime

ᐤ *The Traditional* Kriat Sh'ma

For people dealing with illness, bedtime can be a time of heightened vulnerability, anxiety, and stress, as well as a special opportunity for openness, intimacy, comfort, and reassurance.

Jewish tradition offers a bedtime ritual with some very beautiful and sensitive prayers that can be particularly moving, meaningful, and supportive for those who are ill, their loved ones, and caregivers. Without denying the very real fears and tensions, they can facilitate an ambience of hope, trust, and confidence.

Reproduced here are some elements from the traditional Jewish bedtime ritual, *Kriat Sh'ma Al HaMitah* (the "Bedtime Shema"), accompanied by an original translation. These prayers, of course, provide a time-hallowed framework for the expression of deep sentiments and profound beliefs, and one should feel free to integrate original, individual prayers alongside them. For many people, simple breathing exercises; repeated chanting of syllables, words, and phrases; and other relaxation or meditation techniques might also prove useful and evocative.

Following are excerpts from the traditional ritual Shema said at bedtime.

> *Who Closes My Eyes: A Blessing at Bedtime*
> Praised are You,
> Adonai, our God,
> Ruler of the universe,
> who closes my eyes in sleep,
> my eyelids in slumber.

310

May it be Your will,
Adonai,
My God and the God of my ancestors,
to lie me down in peace
and then to raise me up in peace.
Let no disturbing thoughts upset me,
no evil dreams nor troubling fantasies.
May my bed be complete and whole
in Your sight.
Grant me light
so that I do not sleep the sleep of death,
for it is You who illumines and enlightens.
Praised are You,
Adonai,
whose majesty gives light to the universe.

Here are excerpts from the Shema itself (Deuteronomy 6:4–9):

God Is a Faithful Ruler
Hear, O Israel, Adonai, our God, Adonai, is One.
Blessed be the name of His glorious majesty forever and
ever.

> You shall love Adonai your God with all your heart,
> with all your soul, and with all your might. And these
> words which I command you today shall be in your
> heart. You shall teach them diligently to your chil-
> dren, and you shall speak of them when you are sit-
> ting at home and when you go on a journey, when you
> lie down and when you rise up. You shall bind them
> as a sign on your hand, and they shall be frontlets
> between your eyes. You shall inscribe them on the
> doorposts of your house and on your gates.

Hashkivenu: "Lie Us Down"
Lie us down,
Adonai our God,
in peace;
and raise us up again,
our Ruler,
in life.
Spread over us Your Sukkah of peace,
direct us with Your good counsel,
and save us for Your own Name's sake.
Shield us;
remove from us
every enemy, pestilence, sword, famine, and sorrow.
Remove all adversaries
from before us and from behind us,
and shelter us in the shadow of Your wings.
For You are our
guarding and saving God,
yes, a gracious and compassionate God and King.
Guard our going out
and our coming in
for life and peace,
now and always!

A Prayer for Protection at Night
In the name of Adonai
the God of Israel:
May the angel Michael be at my right,
and the angel Gabriel be at my left,
and in front of me the angel Uriel,
and behind me the angel Raphael.
and above my head
the Shechinah (Divine Presence).

Rabbi Simkha Y. Weintraub, C.S.W., for The National Center for Jewish Healing

Chapter 58

The Lubavitcher Rebbe on Health and Healing

ATTITUDES AND HEALING

Here are some of the Lubavitcher Rebbe's ideas concerning attitudes and healing.

The Healing Effect of Positive Attitudes

The Rebbe always stressed the importance of positive words and attitudes concerning healing. Our words in a very real way create our reality. Positive words create a positive world for us to live in. We live in a world of words. People relate to us based on what we say, and we relate to ourselves according to the way we think and speak. There is a teaching in the Kabbalah that says our souls are made of words—words engraved in the soul. Choose them carefully. There is even a discussion in the medical fields of what would happen if there were no word for disease or death. Would people get sick? Would they die? That there is even such a discussion illustrates the power of words. Not all cultures get sick in the same way. Illness is very much a cultural phenomenon. Two people may have the same disease and receive the same treatment. Yet one is optimistic and positive and the other is gloomy and negative. Guess which one fares better?

Not Dwelling on One's Disease

In keeping with the advice of the Rebbe in keeping a positive attitude, he also instructed people not to research their diseases and not to know too much about them (for example, knowing how a given disease progresses and what symptoms will develop). A person should put his mind to positive healing such as *bitachon* (faith) in *Hashem* and how he is the healer of all flesh. It is best, the Rebbe said, to choose a trusted doctor and allow him to do his work. Remember that it is not man who heals; it is *Hashem*. As long as we do our share, *Hashem* has no shortage of means of sending a cure. This freedom from worry and anxiety frees up a person's mind to allow the healing to take place. When a person dwells on disease it creates anxiety and worry, blocking up a person's energy and mind and creating a very negative attitude, not conducive to healing.

Meditation: Good for the Mind

In the 1970s, the Rebbe instructed people to develop a simple Jewish meditation that could be taught to Jews. There are many great health benefits to be derived from meditation, including peace of mind and freedom from anxiety.

It is now known that many diseases are started and worsened by stress and anxiety. Meditation offers a simple, effective remedy to alleviate suffering. Many people are drawn to meditation and end up practicing Eastern disciplines that are, in fact, thinly veiled idol worship. It may seem odd that the Rebbe would need to make a call for Jewish meditation when the entire edifice of Chabad philosophy rests on the daily practice of intense meditation. I think the answer is that the Rebbe is requesting a different type of meditation—one in which the goal is pure relaxation and mastery of the mind over the body. Most meditative disciplines come packaged with teachings. Yet with Jewish meditation, when a student wants to learn more, there will be a rich, kosher heritage from which to draw. The Rebbe teaches that true relaxation only comes from the study of Torah. The only way to quench the burning beast within is by the cool waters of Torah, which is aptly called *mayim chaim* (waters of life).

The Immune System of the Soul

There are two general approaches to healing; one is attacking a pathogen that has invaded the body, and the other is to strengthen the body's own immune system so that it can fight off pathogens that have invaded the body. There are times when a disease is not caused by any pathogen but by a weakness of the body. In this case there is no other treatment but to strengthen the immune system. There are other times when the body has been suffering from weakness for a long time and then develops a pathogen. Usually in such times, drugs that would be used to cure the condition are too strong for the person, and they require nurturing, either beforehand to make the body strong enough to handle the medication or the nurturing is administered concurrently with the treatment to mollify the unwanted side effects. Commonly, nurturing is administered afterward also to help the body recover.

The same is true for the soul. One answer is to scour out negative aspects residing in the soul and to "fix what's broken" in the soul. The other answer is to strengthen and nurture what is good and healthy in the soul. Being that it is a singular unit, by strengthening one aspect of the soul, the whole soul becomes healed. The Rebbe took the later approach and emphasized the good. In fact, it says in Proverbs that "the Torah's ways are pleasant, and all its paths are peace." Torah is the blood of life. It is the blueprint of creation and our daily sustenance. The Torah places greater emphasis on the positive, nurturing role.

The Moderating Effects of Opposites

In practice it may not be as simple. There is a concept in the teachings of the Hassidic rabbis of *achlifu duchtaihu* (the reversal of mediums), whereby opposites are moderated by each other. Kindness is moderated with severity, and severity is moderated with kindness. For example, if one were to show pure love to another, it would smother the one being loved. So a person moderates his love by holding back a little

---

From the Sources

A doctor's healing is allowed, and is not considered interfering in the Divine plan.

Talmud, *Berachot* 60a.

(*gevurah*). Furthermore, if a person were to chastise another person in a manner of pure severity, it could be devastating. Therefore, a person chastises with compassion and love. We see this principle also in medicine. In Chinese medicine there is rarely a time when we prescribe a pure tonic formula. These formulas are always formulated with an aspect of rectification, or cleansing, if only mildly so. So too with cleansing formulas. They are always modified with a tonification aspect to protect the body. Not all medical systems practice like this. Western allopathic medicine takes a one-sided approach to treatment. All of its treatments are of the *gevurah* aspect. This kind of treatment usually leads to bodily imbalances and thus side effects.

TREATMENT

The Rebbe speaks on treatment as well.

Rapei Yirapei

The Rebbe teaches that the *possuk Rapei yirapei* ("Heal, he shall heal") comes to tell us that doctors have the right to heal and that the word of a doctor, in essence, is the word of God. It is the will of God that healing comes through natural means. After the Rebbe would give a *bracha* (blessing) and advice, he would regularly tell people to go to a doctor. We should not, however, disassociate the human act of healing from the divine. By doing so we are neglecting our responsibility of being partners with *Hashem* and doing our part in purifying the world.

The world was created without any disease or death. It was man who brought these things upon us. By healing through natural means, we are also healing our world. What constitutes natural means? The Alter Rebbe once gave a person some *shmura* matzah and water to drink as a cure. This seems to be the minimum requirement of natural means of healing.

Scientific Discoveries

The Rebbe in a letter writes, "The Torah bestows upon science—in certain areas at least—a validity much greater than contemporary science itself claims. The Halakha (Jewish law) accepts scientific findings, in many instances, not as possible or probable, but as certain and true."

There is a discrepancy between science and medicine, with science generally being a few years ahead of medicine. Many times patients are offered a medical treatment from their doctors, yet they find scientific research that challenges the treatment and offers new possibilities. This scientific research carries halakhic weight and should be taken into consideration. The ramifications of many recent scientific discoveries have yet to be fully understood. In fact, modern science validates many alternative and traditional therapies. Although these therapies may not be fully integrated into our cultural medical system, they are still useful and helpful.

The Rebbe gave many *brachas* to alternative therapists to heal, and when patients consulted the Rebbe concerning alternative medicine, he didn't discount it based on it being "alternative."

Instructions to Doctors

The Rebbe instructed doctors that due to their station in life they have even a greater obligation to promote the teaching of "knowing Him in all your ways." He furthermore implored doctors to refute the materialistic school of thought, inasmuch as the soul is primary in healing. Doctors were instructed to maintain a happy, positive attitude during their treatments, being that this attitude was infectious and extremely beneficial for the patients' well-being. He even told doctors to encourage their patients in the manner of *mitzvot* and Torah study.

Predicting the Future

Doctors cannot predict the future. They do not create health and healing; they only create the *how* of healing. Doctors are the vessels in which healing flows forth. When we do our share and do what is within our means to bring *refuah* (healing), then there is no lack of means of *Hashem* bringing *refuah*.

Going to a Specialist

The Rebbe always stressed the importance of going to a specialist. A person with a heart condition should be under the care of a cardiologist. It would be folly to go to a podiatrist for a respiratory problem.

Part of the *hishtadlut* (spiritual exertion) that a person is required to make in healing is to search out and find a doctor who is most proficient in a given field. Even this may not be enough. If there is a specialist within a given field who has more clinical experience in a particular disorder, seek him out. It is important to maximize our chances of success.

Second and Third Opinions

The Rebbe advised people to get second opinions concerning medical procedures. If the two opinions differ, get a third or consult with a Rav before making a decision. There were times, if the condition was serious, that the Rebbe advised getting three opinions from the beginning.

Heisenberg's Uncertainty Principle

Where is there room for God in a treatment? A doctor does A and the effect is B. This is a basic law of nature—or is it? Perhaps this kind of thinking was dominant in the nineteenth century, but since then, science has proved that it cannot "prove" anything. The most it can do is give the probable odds that a certain cause will produce a given effect. This is called the Heisenberg Uncertainty Principle. In fact, there is plenty of room between, for example, the striking of a match and the match igniting—an infinite amount of time, if you let it. God is everywhere and in all that we do. Anything less would be denying the six constant *mitzvot* to have God before us at all times. This has profound implications for us in treatment. It may seem that the doctor is healing, but in reality it is the kindness of *Hashem*.

There's a story in the Gemara of a Tanna (sage) whose daughter accidentally filled the *Shabbos* candelabra with vinegar instead of oil. By the time the mistake was realized, it was too late to change it. The Tanna said, "Light the wicks. He who makes oil burn can make vinegar burn." And it did.

Ya'akov Gerlitz

Chapter 59

Meditation

Judaism has many important facets that work together synergistically for our wellness, happiness, and evolution:

- Holy days to make us aware of our joys and foibles
- Life-cycle events to surround us with community for the celebration of transitions
- Torah study to focus our attention on how we treat one another
- Prayer to enhance our sense of blessings and to find the prayer of our heart

Jewish meditation offers a way to infuse each of these facets of Judaism with deeper meaning, greater connection to the Source of Life, and more meaningful human interactions. It is not an end in itself but a beginning.

Can meditation be an authentically Jewish experience?

Yes. Jewish mystics of all generations have used meditation practices as spiritual tools for expanding awareness, happiness, and holiness. The ancient Kabbalist, Eleazar Azikri, distinguishes study as the practice for the intellect and describes a Jewish meditation practice known as *hitbodedut* ("seclusion") as sevenfold more helpful to the soul.

In the Talmud our sages are described as meditating for an hour before and after services. In the Torah we are told of Jacob, who went out into the field to meditate. Rabbi Akiva is described as spinning in circles and deflecting off the corners of his room while praying. (This meditation practice is reminiscent of the Sufi whirling dervishes.) Even yoga-like sensibilities are depicted in the Talmud, such as the recommendation that when bowing in prayer one should "hyper-extend the spine until one can read the words on a coin set in front of your feet on the ground."

Although the practices of mindfulness or movement-based meditations, like yoga, are delightful to do in a Jewish setting, these are not the ancient arts of Jewish meditation. Some of these ancient forms are described further on in this chapter.

What is the purpose of Jewish meditation?

Just as healthy foods nourish us through the bloodstream, so Jewish meditation nourishes our "soul stream." Meditation can transform Judaism from the purely intellectual process most of us grew up with into a spiritual practice that links us to Judaism in the most profound way. Meditation gets under our intellectual defenses and helps us to feel at one with creation and to experience an expanded life that is rich in conscious awe and joy.

Each holy day and cycle of life has its own rhythm, nuance, taste, and character. Jewish meditation can help us shift into these holiday cycles, deepening our connection to them.

Should meditation be done in a group or alone?

Both. Recent biomedical studies in the field of psychoneuroimmunology indicate that group meditation enhances the benefits of solitary meditation. When a minyan of Jews meditates together, there is a reciprocity of caring, support, and spiritual energy.

Meditating alone has its advantages, too. Solitary meditators can experience a wonderful closeness to God, the flow of what Kabbalists call "the river of light" (which may, in fact, correlate with what scientists have identified as the electromagnetic fields of the body) which can add energy and delight to your day.

Are there different kinds of Jewish meditation?

Yes! An exciting variety of approaches exists. Depending on your emotional makeup and the circumstances and the effect you desire to create, one might suit you better than another. But whatever technique you choose, the benefits of a regular program of Jewish meditation will intensify with daily practice, and delicious nuances of experience and awareness will emerge over time.

Most types of Jewish meditation are simple to learn under the auspices of a good teacher. Some are more complex and require careful preparation and guidance. It is important to experiment and find the technique and teacher that work best for you.

Is Jewish meditation for everyone?

No. For those with borderline personality or schizophrenia, meditation of any kind can be unsettling, even dangerous. Meditation may also be problematic for those with addictive tendencies. Further, some forms of meditation will not work for everyone. Research shows that perhaps as many as 10 percent of humans do not have the "hard wiring" to benefit from guided visualizations.

Can Jewish meditation be practiced as a substitute for the rest of Judaism?

No. In small, sweet doses Jewish meditation can deeply enhance one's experience of Judaism. However, I do not recommend an extensive practice of meditation alone without Torah study, prayer, and the celebration of holy days and life-cycle events. The goal of Judaism is to give us a variety of tools for living the fullest expression of life possible, including the grounding, inspiration, and moral strength to work on making the world a better place. Meditation without the natural balances inherent in Judaism can lead us out of the joys of physical and communal life and decrease our ability to make the most of living in the here and now.

How do I find a good teacher?

Look for courses taught by the following Jewish master teachers of meditation. Not all those who call themselves teachers of Kabbalah and meditation are legitimate. I have attended sessions offered at major centers by so-called Jewish meditation teachers who seemed to be making it up as they went along.

Major methods of Jewish meditation include

- Chanting of verses from psalms, Torah, and prayers
- Focusing on a *shviti*—a special Jewish graphic that helps induce a mystical state of consciousness
- Meditating on the names of God or on the letters of God's name

- Visualizing, with guidance
- Walking, dancing, and meditating through movement
- Focusing on the levels of an external or inner flame
- Working with the "Tree of Life" (*sefirot*) (a model based on personality characteristic polarities, which correlate in some ways with the *chakra meridian* system and are designed as a holographic paradigm)
- Attaining a state of Eyin—the "no state"—which is all (often through attention to breath and silence)
- Sounding of vowels or letters, with guidance
- Studying ancient sacred Jewish texts, specially designed to induce mystical encounter
- Becoming attuned to the power of special blessings in connecting us to what mystics experience as "the river of light"

Rabbi Goldie Milgram, D.Min., M.S.W.

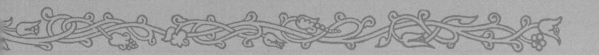

Chapter 60

What Is Reiki, and Is It "Jewish"?

Reiki is a hands-on modality of healing that was introduced by Mikao Usui in Japan during the 1920s. According to Western sources he was a seminary student who dropped out of his studies to search for the healing techniques of Jesus. The Eastern sources, however, seem to substantiate that he was a Buddhist monk, who at the culmination of a twenty-one-day meditative fast had an epiphany about energy and healing, which he then began to teach.

The understanding that spirit affects the body is pivotal to understanding Reiki. When there is disease in the spirit, it eventually manifests as disease in the body. Reiki works by channeling energy through the practitioner to the recipient. The practitioner may work by placing their hands on twelve different locations on the body. As important as the actual technique is the intention held by the Reiki practitioner. At its best, the one giving Reiki should be working from a place of love and respect for the recipient. They should also remember that they are just a conduit and maintain a *kayn yehi ratzon* ("may it be your will") attitude. A session usually lasts for about one hour. For those recipients who have experienced sexual abuse or other trauma, the practitioner may work several inches away from the body. The experience for most Reiki recipients is one of deep relaxation. Many may also experience a sense of electrical current or have dreamlike visions.

Although the lineage of Reiki is Japanese, the concepts behind it are deeply compatible with Jewish spirituality. If you read the prayer for healing, the *Mi Sheberach* in the original Hebrew, we pray first for *refuat ha nefesh* (healing of the soul) and then for *refuat haguf* (healing of the body). As Jews we understand that healing occurs first in spirit before moving to the body. We also understand that at some point there will not be a healing of the body but that a *tikkun* can still be made for our soul.

Channeling healing energy is also ancient Jewish knowledge that was practiced daily by the *cohanim* (priests) when the temple was still standing. This practice, now known as *duchening* is still practiced in Orthodox shuls during the three pilgrimage festivals. The *cohanim* stand before the congregation with *tallit*s over their heads and hands raised in the position that many of us know as the sign of "live long and prosper," made famous by the *cohain* Leonard Nimoy in his role as Mr. Spock. Before they recite the blessing, they recite a line saying they are to bless the people with love. Like Reiki, the *kavanah* (intention) of love is absolutely imperative to the proper performance of this *mitzvah*. They then recite the beautiful three-line blessing:

> May the Lord bless you and guard you.
> May the Lord show you favor and be gracious to you.
> May the Lord show you kindness and grant you peace.
> (Numbers 6:24–26)

The ceremony concludes with the line, "You will put my name on *bnei yisrael* and *I* will bless them." Note that it is not the *cohain* that is blessing the people but is serving as a pipeline for divine blessing that comes directly from God. The *cohain* is not the source of the blessing, but the conduit. Jewish parents serve the same function as a conduit when they bless their children every Friday night.

As a Reiki master and committed Jew, I feel a deep compatibility between the teachings of Reiki and the spiritual knowledge of the Jewish tradition. The Torah asks us to become a nation of priests. Perhaps Reiki is an avenue to open the door of blessing to all Jews.

Bonnie Cramer

Keeping Healthy in a Changing World

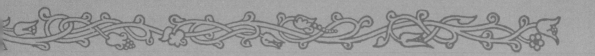

Chapter 61

The Challenges of Maintaining a Healthy Lifestyle in Today's Society

Although medical discoveries, state-of-the-art research, and increased awareness are enabling people to live healthier lives than ever before, the modern world also sets up a surprising number of obstacles to that goal. Here are some examples:

• *The nightly news.* Daily headlines and sound bites confuse women about what they should believe and do about taking charge of their health and wellness. Research studies seem to contradict each other. Is hormone replacement therapy recommended or not? Calcium supplements? Which is better, a diet rich in soy or dairy products? Should you have a Pap smear every year? At what age should you start having mammograms? Can low-dose aspirin prevent heart attack? Should we eat broccoli to prevent colorectal cancer? Sorting through all the latest information is a job in itself. You don't know what to believe.

• *Myths from Madison Avenue.* Ask most women what the leading killer of women is, and they will tell you it's breast cancer. But the truth is that, for women and men, heart disease is the leading cause of death. The emphasis on breast cancer has made women aware of its importance and encouraged millions of women to have an annual mammogram. This is wonderful news, but women also need to focus on heart disease and diabetes and on how to control their risk factors.

- *Stress.* Women over age forty face many daily challenges, including their jobs, taking care of aging parents, and raising their families. One way the body responds is to release stress hormones. Combine these hormones with the metabolic slowdown that comes with menopause, and you get fat around your middle—the worst place for it.

- *Taking care of others, not themselves.* Women are the care- givers in the family. For many, it has been ingrained in them to take care of their husbands, children, and parents. They are not used to taking care of themselves. Women need to retrain themselves. They need to learn how to make time for exercise and relaxation and to get the health screenings they need. Most women know their husband's cholesterol test results but have never had one of their own.

- *The shape of our neighborhoods.* Moderate daily exercise like walking can lower the risk of heart disease, stroke, diabetes, and colorectal cancer. But too many of us live in places where walking is a challenge. Suburban neighborhoods without sidewalks and unsafe and overcrowded city streets make it much easier to take the car or stick close to home. We end up having to pay to walk by joining a gym or buying a treadmill.

- *A world of abundance.* It's hard to stick to a healthful diet in a world where high-fat, high-calorie food is available everywhere. Practically every gas station, for example, has a mini-mart stocked with candy bars and chips. Restaurants specialize in huge portions. Food like red meat and rich dessert that was once saved for special occasions is now available every day.

- *Social isolation.* Many women, especially older women, live alone. It turns out that women who do not have a close friend and confidant have the same health risks as someone who is obese or a heavy smoker. Finding ways to be independent and involved is a health challenge.

Education is the key to meeting all these challenges. The more women know about their general health and wellness, as well as about specific conditions, the better prepared they are to be their own health advocates. Today's health care professionals look to patients as part- ners in maintaining health, as well as curing disease. Hadassah can help you to be better prepared so that you can effectively partner with your doctor. Women's Health has a wonderful booklet: *Questions to Ask Your Primary Care Physician About Breast Cancer* (R716 in the *Hadassah Resource Catalogue*).

The best prescription—healthy diet, regular exercise, and routine health screenings—is also the hardest to fill. It is also the one with the highest return on the investment.

⊘ Elizabeth A. Battaglino, R.N.

Chapter 62

Alternative Versus Complementary

What's the Difference?

W e've all heard of so-called miracle herbs and alternative therapies that alleviate pain and aid in healing. We've read about
antioxidants and the purported benefit of soy consumption. Now
Dr. Andrew Vickers, assistant attending research methodologist at
Memorial Sloan-Kettering Cancer Center in New York City, takes
Hadassah's *Health Memo* inside the world of complementary medicine, as Hadassah questions Dr. Vickers.

*Could you explain the difference between complementary medicine
and alternative medicine? Is integrative medicine a new term?*

Alternative medicine refers to therapies used instead of conventional care. *Complementary medicine,* which includes acupuncture,
massage, botanical (herbal) medicines, hypnosis, music, and meditation, is administered alongside conventional care. Memorial Sloan-
Kettering Cancer Center describes such techniques as "integrative
medicine," to emphasize that they should be an integrated part of a
patient's care, not separate from or as a substitute for conventional
medicine. The field in general is often referred to as CAM (complementary and alternative medicine).

*Can or should any complementary methods be used without med-
ical supervision?*

In general, you can use a CAM therapy without seeing your doctor if
your problem wouldn't usually require a doctor visit. But cancer is a

330

life-or-death situation. So with cancer patients, we are very strong on the distinction between complementary medicine, used alongside conventional care to treat symptoms such as pain, and alternative medicine, which means rejecting treatments such as surgery, chemotherapy, and radiotherapy. We treat cancer-related symptoms, not the cancer itself, with these therapies. We also research anti-cancer herbal medicines, but we don't treat patients with these medicines yet, simply because they haven't been shown to work.

What complementary methods have you found effective? Do certain patients or illnesses respond better to one treatment over another?

Some advocates might have you believe that all complementary therapies are effective for all symptoms. This is not the case. Similarly, skeptics' claims that no complementary therapy is effective for anything also seem to be misplaced. The truth is somewhere in between: some complementary therapies are effective for some conditions.

The best evidence comes from randomized controlled trials in which patients who receive a complementary therapy are compared with a randomly chosen group who do not. Such trials have shown that acupuncture helps pain and nausea. Randomized trials have also shown that massage reduces levels of anxiety in cancer patients and in general. Hypnosis and other relaxation techniques (like yoga and systematic relaxation) can help with nausea and pain. Hypnosis and relaxation can also help general anxiety or anxiety directly associated with an operation or other medical procedure. Music therapy, which has been shown to enhance your mood, can also be used to effect a medical change.

As far as which therapy to use for which condition, there is some evidence that how well someone does after receiving a complementary therapy depends on how much they thought it was going to help.

When you spoke at the National Breast Cancer Coalition meetings, you distinguished between "proven" methods and possibly harmful therapies. How would you define proven, and could you give an example of a potentially dangerous therapy?

As a general rule, most complementary therapies we provide are proven to control symptoms. But alternative therapies have often been disproved and can be harmful. I define *proven* in terms of evidence from randomized trials. I define *harmful* in general terms: a therapy can be harmful, not just because it directly causes a health problem but because it prevents patients from receiving effective care or because it involves undue time, travel, or expense. A patient with late-stage cancer who travels to Mexico, spending thousands of dollars on an unusual alternative cancer cure, may be harmed, not only by the unavailability of good palliative care, which is so important to treat pain, depression, and a host of other symptoms common in late-stage patients, but by having wasted valuable time away from friends and family.

Are there risks to herbal medicines?

Many herbs known to effectively treat symptoms such as depression can actually interfere with cancer treatment. A good example is Saint John's wort. In simple terms, it makes the liver work harder to break down the drug and excrete it more quickly, so the drug is in your system for a shorter period of time. In cancer, this means that chemotherapy has less opportunity to kill cancer cells.

Is there scientific evidence that any of the popular strategies (for example, the consumption of foods containing soy or antioxidants) are worthwhile?

There is a difference between prevention and cure. The American Cancer Society advocates a diet high in fruit and vegetables to help prevent cancer. One theory is that antioxidants in fruit and vegetables mop up chemicals called free radicals that can cause cells to mutate and become cancerous. But once a cell has mutated into cancer, there's no reason to believe that eating a certain diet is going to stop its growth. There is no strong evidence right now that taking antioxidants in supplement form will help reduce risk of cancer, and in some cases it could actually increase the risk of cancer.

The data on soy are difficult to interpret. Some researchers believe that soy consumption during puberty is protective but that the sudden use of large amounts of soy in a person's mid-thirties or forties isn't, and it might actually increase the risk of cancer.

We have heard that garlic has properties shown to fight cancer in a laboratory. Can we extrapolate that garlic might be beneficial to humans with cancer?

Advocates of alternative therapies will wave mouse trials or test-tube experiments as "proof." But the short answer is no. If everything that worked in the lab worked in people, there would be no cancer. Laboratory studies are just a model—a pointer that something else might be of interest in the future. The bottom line is that we need large clinical trials in humans to determine whether an herb such as garlic might help fight cancer.

Esther D. Kustanowitz

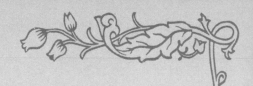

✑ Special Focus

Medical Research

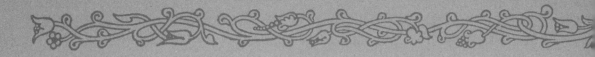

Chapter 63

Clinical Trials

✍ *The Way We Make Progress Against Cancer*

New discoveries in cancer research are occurring rapidly. As scientific advances bring us ever closer to answering unsolved questions, each new approach requires testing in people in order to determine its safety and efficacy. These tests are called *clinical trials. Cancer clinical trials* are research studies conducted with people who volunteer to participate in order to evaluate new ways to prevent, detect, diagnose, and treat cancer. Today's treatments are the direct result of knowledge gained from past clinical trials, and the future of care will be determined by current studies.

There are different types of cancer clinical trials:

• *Prevention trials* test new approaches, such as medicines, vitamins, minerals, or other supplements, which doctors believe may lower the risk of certain types of cancer. Behavioral approaches are also studied, such as the modification of lifestyle factors, including improved diet, increased exercise, and smoking cessation. An example is the National Cancer Institute (NCI), which is sponsoring a national breast cancer prevention trial called STAR (Study of Tamoxifen and Raloxifene). This study compares two drugs that may reduce the occurrence of breast cancer in women who are at increased risk for the disease.

• *Screening trials* test the best way to find cancer, especially in its early stages. The goal is to develop screening tools, such as imaging or laboratory tests, which will find the cancer earlier. This is extremely important, because for many types of cancer, detecting and treating the disease at an early stage can result in an improved outcome—a better chance to shrink the cancer, minimize its effects, or cause it to go away completely.

The NCI is currently evaluating the results of a national trial to determine whether screening tests for prostate, lung, colorectal, and ovarian cancers (called the PLCO trial) will reduce the number of deaths from these cancers.

• *Cancer diagnosis studies* seek to develop better tools to aid doctors in the diagnosis and clinical management of cancer patients. These trials may be aimed at finding new cancers or at better determining the spread or extent of previously diagnosed cancers. One example is an NCI-sponsored diagnostic trial evaluating whether a breast MRI improves the ability to detect a suspected breast cancer more accurately than current methods.

• *Treatment trials* test untried cancer treatments such as new cancer drugs, new approaches to surgery or radiation therapy, new combinations of treatments, or new methods such as vaccine or gene transfer therapy.

• *Quality-of-life trials*, also called *supportive care studies*, examine approaches that help to improve the quality of life for patients fighting cancer, for their families, and for cancer survivors. These trials seek better therapies or psychosocial interventions for patients experiencing nutrition problems, infection, pain, nausea and vomiting, sleep disorders, depression, infertility, and other effects of cancer or cancer treatment. Some supportive care trials target families and caregivers to help them cope with the patient's and their own needs during the illness.

Cancer researchers are learning more each day about how cancer arises from a cell that behaves abnormally, which eventually leads to the development of a tumor. Discoveries in cancer biology and the human genome are enabling researchers to design therapies that target the machinery of the cancer cell. With progress, future treatments may prove to be more effective and less toxic for patients than current approaches by being able to target and kill cancerous cells without harming normal cells. This can only be accomplished through clinical trials.

Fewer than 5 percent of adults with cancer participate in clinical trials, but as more people participate, the answers needed to cure cancer will be found more quickly. The knowledge gained through this careful, investigative, clinical trial process will be translated into improvements in health care, which ultimately benefits society as a whole.

To learn more, use these free resources from the National Cancer Institute (NCI): (800) 4-CANCER (422-6237); TTY: (800) 332-8615; http://cancer.gov. NCI's Cancer Information Service is a national information and education network for patients, the public, and health professionals. NCI's comprehensive Web site contains the latest in-depth information about clinical trials, cancer prevention, screening, treatment, genetics, supportive care, and complementary and alternative medicine, as well as a registry of over eighteen hundred cancer clinical trials and how to find them.

Andrea M. Denicoff, R.N., M.S., C.A.N.P.

Chapter 64

Judaism and Stem Cell Research

With one spectacular development tumbling over the next in ever more rapid succession, our generation is witnessing the compression of history in the scientific and medical realm just as much as in the geopolitical realm. Indeed, it may well be that in the long term, the direction of humanity and its history ultimately will be affected more profoundly by these scientific and medical developments than even by the current unprecedented global political upheavals.

Medical ethics concentrates largely on the opposite ends of life. For example, the beginning-of-life questions relate principally to abortion, contraception, and conception issues, even before birth. At the other end of life, inquiries relate to the management of dying, the moment of death, autopsies, and organ harvesting—even before death.

I outline here the essential medical facts pertaining to stem cell research and therapy, and summarize the principal approaches in Jewish law that have been proposed thus far. Clearly, given the novelty of these innovations, the medical and scientific questions, as well as the Jewish legal answers, are in flux and must be tentative.

WHAT ARE STEM CELLS?

Every discussion of medical ethics must be governed by the axiom: good ethics (and good Jewish law) require good facts.

HEALTH FACTS

All the various parts of a plant or tree—the trunk, branches, leaves, and fruits—develop from the stem. Similarly, all the cells of a living organism develop from precursor cells, known as stem cells.

Mammalian development begins with the union of a male's sperm cell with a female's egg. The resultant cell has the inherent potential to develop into the entire gamut of cells forming the organism. This prime cell divides, within several hours of fertilization, into two identical duplicate cells, each of which retains this broad potential. After several more divisions (by about the fourth day), these cells begin to specialize, forming a hollow sphere called a blastocyte, which is composed of an outer and inner layer of cells. Cells of the outer layer are destined to form the placenta and other supporting tissues of pregnancy. The inner-layer cells go on to develop into all the organs and tissues of the developing fetus.

These cells are now somewhat more limited in their potential. They can give rise to many but not all the types of cells necessary for fetal development. As stem cells "mature," their potential to develop into any kind of human tissue decreases. Soon after, these stem cells undergo further specialization (called differentiation), becoming cells committed to developing into a given line of cells.

Ultimately, stem cells develop into "master cells," designed to multiply into specific tissue types. For example, blood stem cells will develop into the various types of blood cells; skin stem cells into the various types of skin cells. Once they reach this level of specialization, they're committed to developing specific tissues.

The cells related to developing the blood are the best-understood stem cells. They reside in the bone marrow of all children and adults, and are, in fact, usually present in very small numbers in the circulating bloodstream as well. Because red and white cells in the peripheral blood have limited life spans, the stem cells are crucial to maintaining an adequate blood supply in the healthy person.

DID YOU KNOW?

At present there are several sources of stem cells:

- *Early human embryos.* In general, these embryos are developed as a result of couples using in vitro fertilization to conceive a child. The union of sperm and eggs in a petri dish produces many embryos. Implanting them all into the mother's uterus would present a grave danger to her in the event that all the fetuses become viable, obligating her to carry them all to term. Therefore, only a few are implanted; the remaining are leftover. These unimplanted embryos are a widely used source of stem cells.
- *Tissue obtained from aborted fetuses.*
- *Cells obtained from the umbilical cord of newborns.*
- *Cells obtained from blastocytes.* Using somatic cell nuclear transfer (SCNT), an adult cell's gene-containing nucleus can be combined with an egg from which the nucleus has been removed. Using special techniques, the resultant cell can be induced to divide and develop as an early stem cell to form a blastocyte from which very potent cells can be obtained. This is the basis of cloning.

IMPLICATIONS FOR THE FUTURE

Why isolate and develop pluripotent stem cells, that is, stem cells that have the ability to become any human tissue? At the most fundamental level, stem cell research will help enormously in understanding the complex events of early mammalian development. Second, such research could dramatically change the way drugs are developed and tested. Specific healthy and diseased cell lines could be exposed to specific drugs, largely obviating the need for much more dangerous and expensive human testing.

The most far-reaching applications would come in the area of cell therapies. Thousands of people are on waiting lists for organ transplants. Because the supply of donors is much smaller than the number of waiting patients, many patients will die of their illnesses before suitable donors can be found. Ultimately, it is hoped that stem cells could be stimulated to develop into a source of replacement cells to create banks of transplantable human tissue. There is already reason to believe that this will be possible in replenishing the diseased or absent brain cells caused by Parkinson's or Alzheimer's diseases, strokes, spinal cord injuries, various heart diseases, diabetes, and arthritis.

JEWISH LEGAL CONSIDERATIONS

We begin the outline of the Jewish legal approach to stem cell research by stressing some general, overarching principles. In contrast with other religions, Judaism has no problem with "playing God," provided we do so according to God's rules, as expressed by authentic Jewish legal mandate. Far from being shunned, "playing God" in the Jewish tradition is, in fact, a religious imperative: the concept of emulating God is implicit in the mandate to heal and provide effective medical relief wherever possible. Of note, the only two "professions" ascribed to God are those of teaching and healing. By teaching or healing, or both, we fulfill the obligation to play God.

There's no reason that microscopic manipulation of a faulty genetic blueprint should be any different from the surgical manipulation of a defective macroscopic—that is, visible to the unaided eye—tissue or organ. Normative Jewish law sanctions—indeed, encourages—medical intervention to correct both congenital and acquired defects and makes no distinction between stem and somatic (body) cell tissues.

The crucial distinction here is between the permissible act of correcting a defect and the forbidden act of attempting to improve on God's creations (generally proscribed by the laws of cross-breeding). For example, it would be permitted, were it possible, to correct the genetic defect that leads to Down syndrome, but manipulating genes to produce a "perfect-bodied" six-footer with blue eyes would be prohibited.

There would, therefore, be no Jewish legal problem with using stem cells derived from adult tissue. Similarly, it would appear that using cells from umbilical cord tissue would be permissible. A rather minor concern here might be the following: May one have umbilical tissue collected and frozen so that the cells will be available in case one requires stem cell therapy sometime in the future? Is this degree of effort, in trying to ensure one's health, appropriate or excessive?

Although there are few Jewish legal objections to deriving the stem cells from adult or umbilical cord tissue, the problems arise with deriving stem cells from the embryonic tissue. Postimplantation embryonic tissue (an embryo already implanted into the uterine wall) is, after all, an early fetus; clearly, no sanction would be given to aborting a fetus in order to obtain stem cell tissue. Even were fetal tissue necessary to provide life-sustaining therapy for a patient, no sanction would be given to sacrifice an innocent fetus, even in the interest of saving another life. The only exception to this rule is the obligation to forfeit the life of the "non-innocent" fetus, when its continued existence constitutes a danger to its mother by virtue of the fetus's pursuer (*rodef*) status.

Even fetal life before the fortieth day of gestation, which is considered "mere water," could not be aborted in order to obtain stem cell tissue. Prior to forty days, a miscarried fetus does not trigger birth-related purity issues and therefore is of lesser status than a more mature fetus. (There is a large body of rabbinical writings regarding the forty-day status of a fetus.)

THE FUTURE

The prime source of embryonic stem cell tissue is embryos that have not been implanted into the uterine wall. As discussed earlier, they are usually the "by-products"—spare embryos left aside during in vitro fertilization in order not to dangerously overload the mother's uterus. The Jewish legal status of these nonimplanted embryos is somewhat unclear. Some rabbinical opinions suggest that in addition to the forty-day milestone, an embryo doesn't reach fetal status until it is implanted into the uterus. Prior to that, while still in a petri dish or other artificial medium, it cannot develop into a viable fetus. Therefore, such early embryos have no real-life potential at all, and they're not considered alive. Consequently, there would be no Jewish legal opposition to disposing of them, conducting research on them, or deriving stem cell tissue from them.

The status of preimplantation embryos has another potentially important Jewish legal consequence. Preimplantation genetic diagnosis (PGD) offers a promising approach to prevent the birth of genetically defective children. By studying embryos before implantation into the uterus, it is possible to identify those defective genes. By selecting only genetically intact embryos for implantation, the development of genetically defective fetuses would be avoided. Assuming the preimplanted embryo has not reached the level of a fetus, Jewish legal sanction may be possible.

The ethical issues raised by stem cell research and therapy are, of course, not only of interest to Jews. In an unprecedented national broadcast, President George W. Bush defined some fairly restrictive regulations. The administration also argued strongly in favor of banning all research into human cloning. Evidently, the crossroads of medical science and the generation of life itself raise fears and genuine concern in the minds of many thinking people.

It appears that Jewish legal concerns may be more permissive than is generally understood. Clearly, it behooves us, as Jews, to avail ourselves of whatever Torah and scientific knowledge we can, not only as we try to find the Jewish legal guidance for ourselves but perhaps, equally important, as we strive to fulfill our national mandate to be a Light Unto the Nations—to help shed light on these vexing issues for society at large.

Yoel Julian Jakobovits, M.D.

Chapter 65

Stem Cell Research in Jewish Law

Stem cell research is among the most promising and controversial technological breakthroughs of our time. Most cells in the human body are differentiated and, if they maintain the ability to divide at all, have the ability to form only cells similar to themselves. Stem cells have the unique property of being able to divide while maintaining their totipotent or pluripotent characteristics. Early in mammalian development, stem cells (under the proper conditions) have the ability to differentiate into every cell of the human body (totipotent), potentially forming an entire fetus. Stem cells derived from later stages of mammalian development have the ability to differentiate into multiple cell types but not into an entire organism. If we were able to manipulate the conditions controlling cellular differentiation, we might be able to create replacement cells and organs, potentially curing illnesses such as diabetes, Alzheimer's disease, and Parkinson's disease.

The ultimate promise of stem cell technology would be to combine it with cloning. Imagine a man dying of liver failure. If we could take a somatic cell from his skin and place the nuclear DNA into a denucleated egg cell, we would have created an almost exact copy[1] of that sick man's cell, capable of differentiating into his clone. Instead of allowing the cloned cell to develop into a fetus, we might place it (or its stem cells alone) into the appropriate environment that would cause it to differentiate into a liver that would be virtually genetically identical to the sick man's. If we could "grow" this liver to maturity, we could offer the sick man a liver transplant without the risk of rejection and without the need for antirejection drugs.

345

This sounds like a virtual panacea for many of man's ills. Yet we still do not know whether we are able to successfully clone a human; neither are we sure what practical value can be derived from stem cells. We are currently in the realm of fascinating speculation. It will require years of very expensive, labor-intensive research to determine the potential that stem cells hold for the treatment, palliation, and cure of human illness. Although stem cells have been isolated from adults and aborted fetuses, the best source is the "pre-embryo"—the small clump of cells that compose the early zygote only a few days following conception. Therefore, to best investigate the latent possibilities inherent in stem cells, scientists wish to use the approximately 100,000 "excess" frozen pre-embryos that are "left over" from earlier IVF attempts.

What is the halakhic perspective on such research, and what could the possible objections to such research be? There is little argument that the use of stem cells derived from adult somatic tissue pose few ethical problems. The issues raised by stem cell research involve the use of in vitro fertilized eggs that have not yet been implanted in a woman and the use of tissue from aborted fetuses.

 DID YOU KNOW?

The issues raised by stem cell research may be divided into several questions:

- Is in vitro fertilization permitted to begin with?
- What is the Jewish approach to abortion?
- Are pre-embryos included in the prohibition of abortion?
- May a very early embryo be sacrificed for stem cells that could save lives or at least cure disease?
- May we fertilize ova specifically to create an embryo to be sacrificed for stem cells?
- Need we make "fences" in the form of protective laws to protect fetuses from wanton destruction?
- May tissue from aborted fetuses be used for research or medical treatment?

IN VITRO FERTILIZATION

Artificial insemination has been dealt with at length by a spectrum of *poskim* (rabbis qualified to decide matters of Jewish law). Although artificial insemination by a donor is generally strongly condemned, the use of a husband's sperm for artificial insemination in cases of necessity was accepted by most rabbinical authorities.[2] The question of in vitro fertilization was dealt with later. A significant majority of authorities accepted in vitro fertilization under the same rubric and limitations as artificial insemination,[3] including the fulfillment of the *mitzvah* of procreation.[4] However, a fundamentally new question arose. What is the status of the "spare" embryos that are not implanted as part of the first cycle of IVF?[5] Must they be implanted in the mother as part of another attempt at pregnancy? May (or must) they be donated to another woman to allow the pre-embryo its chance at life? May they remain frozen indefinitely?[6] Most important to our topic, the question arose: May pre-embryos be destroyed? To answer this question, we must first generally examine the Jewish approach to abortion.

WHEN IS ABORTION ALLOWED IN JEWISH LAW?

To gain a clear understanding of when abortion is sanctioned, or even required, and when it is forbidden, requires an appreciation of certain nuances of halakhah (Jewish law) that govern the status of the fetus.

The easiest way to conceptualize a fetus in halakhah is to imagine it as a full-fledged human being—but not quite. In most circumstances, the fetus is treated like any other "person." Generally,

 DID YOU KNOW?

The traditional Jewish view of abortion does not fit conveniently into either of the major camps in the current American abortion debate. We neither ban abortion completely nor allow indiscriminate abortion on demand.

one may not deliberately harm a fetus, and sanctions are placed upon those who purposefully cause a woman to miscarry. However, when its life comes into direct conflict with an already-born person, the autonomous person's life takes precedence.

It follows from this simple approach that, as a general rule, abortion in Judaism is permitted only if there is a direct threat to the life of the mother by carrying the fetus to term or through the act of childbirth. In such a circumstance, the baby is considered tantamount to a *rodef*, a pursuer after the mother with the intent to kill her. Nevertheless, as explained in the Mishnah (*Oholos* 7:6), if it would be possible to save the mother by maiming the fetus, such as by amputating a limb, abortion would be forbidden. Despite the classification of the fetus as a pursuer, once the baby's head has been delivered, the baby's life is considered equal to the mother's, and we may not choose one life over another, because it is considered as though they are each pursuing the other.

Judaism recognizes psychiatric as well as physical factors in evaluating the potential threat that the fetus poses to the mother. However, the danger posed by the fetus (whether physical or emotional) must be both probable and substantial to justify abortion. The degree of mental illness that must be present to justify termination of a pregnancy is not well established, and therefore criteria for permitting abortion in such instances remain controversial.

Rabbi Moshe Feinstein, one of the greatest *poskim* in this century and the last, rules that even amniocentesis is forbidden if it is performed only to evaluate for birth defects for which the parents might request an abortion. Nevertheless, a test may be performed if a permitted action may result, such as performance of amniocentesis or drawing alpha-fetoprotein levels for improved peripartum or postpartum medical management. While most *poskim* forbid abortion for "defective" fetuses, Rabbi Eliezer Waldenberg (in his *Tzitz Eliezer*, vol. 9, chap. 51:3) is a notable exception. Rabbi Waldenberg allows first-trimester abortion of a fetus that would be born with a deformity that would cause it to suffer, as well as termination of a fetus with a lethal fetal defect such as Tay-Sachs up to the end of the second trimester of gestation.

The question of abortion in cases of rape, incest, and adultery is a complex one, with various legal justifications propounded on both sides. In cases of rape and incest, a key issue would be the emotional

> ### From the Sources
>
> As a rule, halakhah does not assign relative values to different lives. Therefore, almost all major rabbinic authorities forbid abortion in cases of abnormalities or deformities found in a fetus.

toll exacted from the mother in carrying the fetus to term. The same analysis used in other cases of emotional harm might be applied here. Cases of adultery interject additional considerations into the debate, which are beyond the scope of this short chapter.

In sum, the parameters determining the permissibility of abortion within halakhah are subtle and complex.

ARE PRE-EMBRYOS INCLUDED IN THE PROHIBITION OF ABORTION?

Although the practical aspects of the Jewish approach to abortion are relatively agreed upon, the exact source and nature of the prohibition is not. Depending on the origin of the prohibition, the application to the pre-embryo will differ. For instance, whereas most halakhic authorities consider the prohibition of abortion to be from the Torah, a few consider it to be rabbinic in nature. It is interesting to note that both the person who performs the abortion and the woman who voluntarily allows it to be done are culpable.[7]

The most obvious place to look for the biblical prohibition would be from the *aseret ha'dibrot* (Ten Commandments): "Thou shalt not murder."[8] This prohibition, called *retzicha*, usually carries a death penalty for transgression. Nevertheless, it appears the Torah itself teaches that killing a fetus is not equivalent to killing an adult. The Torah specifically states[9] that if, in the course of an altercation with a third party, a person causes a woman to miscarry, he pays only monetary damages, whereas if the woman herself were to die of her injuries, the aggressor would receive a death sentence. Rabbi Yehuda Ashkenazi, in his commentary on the Code of Jewish Law,[10] reasons from here that a fetus is not a full-fledged person, because, regarding the one who hits the woman, causing her to miscarry, "he pays the value of the child and we do not label him a murderer, nor do we execute him."

Notwithstanding the statement of Rabbi Ashkenazi, several *poskim* rule that abortion does represent murder, but without the punishment of death.[11] This law is similar to the law of one who kills a *treife*[12] (a specific type of terminally ill person), for whom there is a prohibition of murder but no death penalty.[13] If the pre-embryo is included in this prohibition, then very little short of the pre-embryo posing a threat to someone's life could justify its destruction. An independent threat to the life of a third party would not suffice to allow destroying the pre-embryo.

The argument regarding whether a fetus is included in the prohibition of murder is complicated and fascinating.[14] Both positions garner support from two sides of the same page of the Talmud. *Arachin* 7a states that the court should strike the abdomen of a pregnant woman to cause a miscarriage prior to her execution.[15] The life of the fetus seems inconsequential in that discussion. On the other hand, *Arachin* 7b states that the Sabbath may be desecrated for the life of a fetus—something that may only be done to save a life, or *pikuach nefesh*. This apparent contradiction is dealt with at length in the responsic literature.

But is the pre-embryo included in this prohibition? That question is best answered by evaluating the next possible biblical source for abortion. When Noah and his family exited the ark, God commanded them seven laws, which apply to all of humanity. The usual translation of one of these laws is: "Whoever sheds the blood of man, by man shall his blood be shed."[16] The Torah clearly demands capital punishment for murder. Although this prohibition appears straightforward, there is a fascinating twist.

The Talmud[17] attempts to prove that non-Jews, who are not obligated by most of the Torah's commandments given at Mount Sinai, are forbidden to perform abortions.[18] The Talmud brings the literal translation of the previously mentioned passage (with slightly altered punctuation), which is: "Whoever sheds the blood of man, within man, his blood shall be shed." It then asks: "What is the meaning of 'man within man'? This can be said to refer to a fetus in its mother's womb." This prohibition, as part of the Noachide laws, would apply to all people, Jew and non-Jew alike, although for technical reasons, the degree of severity would differ.[19]

Once the "standard" prohibition of *retzicha* (murder) is separated from that of killing a fetus, we may investigate how this difference might affect the status of the pre-embryo. From the Talmudic discussion of abortion, we might expect that pre-embryos are not covered by the prohibition of abortion, because they have never been implanted. The rationale for such a decision is based on the concept that a pre-embryo left in its petri dish will die. It is not even potential life until it is implanted in an environment in which it can mature.

Others derive the prohibition of abortion from the Torah's proscription of inflicting damage to one's self or others (*chavala*).[20] One may not wound one's self without a valid reason (such as a medical necessity as in surgery). Obviously, one may not damage someone else.[21] As a result, some claim that the prohibition of abortion arises from the prohibition of the woman wounding herself;[22] others feel that the derivation is from the prohibition against wounding the fetus.[23] Unlike murder, for which only a threat to the mother's life[24] could justify killing the fetus, the rationale of *chavala* allows greater leeway in allowing its abrogation. Particularly, if the wounding of the mother is the prohibition, her consent to being wounded might be considered a determining factor. Whether this prohibition applies to a pre-embryo is open to debate (albeit my personal opinion is that the prohibition of *chavala* does not apply at this level).

The last possible prohibition to consider is the Torah's forbidding of "wasting seed" (*hashchatat zera*).[25] This is the main prohibition involved in questions of male contraception (for example, using condoms), as well as the laws governing gathering of sperm for analysis, IVF, or artificial insemination. The prohibition forbids the "useless" emission or destruction of sperm that could create life. Some halakhic authorities have ruled that excess sperm from fertility treatments may be destroyed. Further, the emission of semen for analysis has been permitted as part of the process of procreation in those suffering from infertility.[26] (Nevertheless, according to most *poskim*, this prohibition does not apply once fertilization has occurred.) Because this ban may be waived for the sake of saving a life,[27] it is conceivable that destroying a pre-embryo to save someone's life (or potentially treat severe illness) would be permitted as part of the *mitzvah* of *pikuach nefesh*. (But on the question of treating severe illness, this would bring us into the complicated question of *v'chi omrim lo l'adam chatei bishvil sheyizke chaveirecha*—do we allow one to sin in order to save one's friend? This issue is beyond the scope of this chapter.)

Two positive biblical commandments bear on the obligation to save life (the obligation of *hatzala*). The Torah requires: "Do not stand idly by as your neighbor's blood is being shed."[28] This *mitzvah* is interpreted by the Talmud[29] to require one to expend positive effort and even money to protect an endangered person. Maimonides learns the whole commandment for a qualified individual to heal his neighbor from the obligation to return lost objects. Regarding a lost object, the Torah commands: "you should surely restore it to him."[30] From an extra letter in the sentence, Maimonides[31] derives that if one must return a lost object, he must certainly return someone's "lost" health.

Both of these positive commandments may apply, regardless of whether there may be any prohibition of abortion for a pre-embryo. But do these positive commandments apply to a pre-embryo? That is, do we have a positive obligation to protect the pre-embryo that is sitting in the freezer?

CAN WE BE MORE LENIENT EARLY IN GESTATION?

In our analysis, we must also evaluate whether we are more lenient with the destruction of an embryo prior to forty days' gestation. There is reason to argue that prior to forty days' gestation, the fetus lacks "humanity." The Mishnah[32] states that a miscarriage prior to forty days does not cause *tumat leida* (impurity due to childbirth).[33] The daughter of a *cohain* (priest) whose non-*cohain* husband has died may continue eating *trumah* (tithes) only if she has no children and is not pregnant. Rav Chisda[34] states that in a case where her non-*cohain* husband died soon after marriage, she may continue eating *trumah* for forty days. He reasons that if she is not pregnant, then there is no problem, and if she is pregnant, for up to forty days the fetus is *mayim b'alma* (mere water).

These sources suggest that a fetus prior to forty days' gestation is not considered to be an actual person, and we might extrapolate that destruction of such a fetus is not forbidden by Jewish law. If we now apply this reasoning to the possible sources for abortion discussed earlier, we note consistency on the part of the *poskim*.

Rabbi Unterman, former Ashkenazi chief rabbi of Israel, who ruled that a fetus is protected by the prohibition of murder (*retzicha*), rejects these sources as removing the early embryo from the prohibition of murder. He bolsters his opinion by quoting from *Toras Ha'Adam*,[35] a famous Jewish law book by Nachmanides (Rambam) that discusses medical issues. The Rambam quotes the Ba'al Halachot Gedolot, who asserts that one may desecrate the Sabbath for a fetus because, by desecrating one Sabbath, the fetus will be able to fulfill many Sabbaths in the future.[36] Thus the Ba'al Halachot Gedolot argues that saving the life of a fetus before forty days overrides the Sabbath; therefore, argues Rabbi Unterman, feticide is murder.

Rabbi Yair Bachrach, author of *Chavot Yair*, does not accept the "forty days" distinction because he derives the prohibition of feticide from wasting male seed, which is prohibited even before conception.[37]

Rabbi Yosef Trani (author of *Responsa Maharit*), who argues that abortion is forbidden as *chavala* (wounding) of the mother, does not specifically mention the forty-day cutoff. However, Rabbi Yechiel Weinberg (author of the *Responsa Seridei Aish*), clearly held that there is no prohibition of abortion before forty days, according to Rabbi Trani's opinion, as there is no "limb" to injure prior to formation of a recognizable fetus at forty days.[38] Rabbi Weinberg himself at first permitted abortion prior to forty days but later reconsidered his position.[39]

All of the approaches discussed so far apply only to Jews who are bound by Torah law. The prohibition of abortion for non-Jews devolves from the Noachide laws. Of course, non-Jews are forbidden to commit homicide. Yet according to many commentators, non-Jews are not bound by the commandment in Leviticus 19:16 to protect the lives of their comrades, since that was not commanded to Noah. The scope of their prohibition includes murder and "shedding blood of man within man." These obligations include only actual lives, not potential lives. Therefore, according to Rabbi Unterman,[40] there is no prohibition of abortion for a non-Jew, nor for a Jew to aid in such an abortion, before the fortieth day of gestation.[41]

MAY A VERY EARLY EMBRYO BE SACRIFICED FOR STEM CELLS?

Now that we have analyzed the possible ethical issues in destroying pre-embryos, what is the final outcome? For non-Jews, the issue appears most direct. The combination of the pre-embryo never having existed within a uterus and the generally accepted leniency toward abortion within the first forty days would strongly argue for a permissive ruling regarding the destruction of pre-embryos for stem cells.

Regarding Jews, the answer is more complicated. Because stem cell research is a new endeavor and cloning of humans has not yet occurred, there are no published responsa on the topic. We must, therefore, look to more practical cases that encompass our question to find an applicable ruling. We find such an issue with respect to the best course of action for couples who wish to avoid having children with Tay-Sachs disease when both partners are carriers of the Tay-Sachs gene. A similar problem arises in families where the wife carries a gene for a sex-linked disease, such as fragile-X.[42]

The most promising option for such couples is preimplantation diagnosis, in which a zygote conceived in vitro has a few cells removed to be tested for genetic defects before implantation. Only a zygote that is not homozygous for Tay-Sachs or not a male carrier of fragile-X would be implanted. Rabbi Yosef Shalom Eliyashuv, possibly the most influential *posek* in Israel today, has permitted preimplantation diagnosis and destruction of affected zygotes to prevent cases of fragile-X, even in a case of a woman with neurofibromatosis who only had skin lesions.[43] Rabbi Dovid Feinstein has taken a similar view as to the permissibility of discarding "extra" pre-embryos.[44] Preimplantation diagnosis, which is already accepted by some rabbinic authorities, is likely to be acceptable to most Jewish legal experts when used to prevent serious diseases in offspring.

Based on these rulings, it would seem that we now have a practical answer to our question of stem cell research. If the pre-embryo may be destroyed, it certainly may be used for research purpose and other life-saving work. In fact, Rabbi Moshe Dovid Tendler, in testimony for the National Bioethics Advisory Commission,[45] argued strongly in favor of the use of pre-embryos for stem cell research.[46] Nevertheless, it is important to realize that this conclusion is not unanimous[47] and that all these rulings are predicated on the understanding that the pre-embryo is not included in the prohibition of *retzicha*.

MAY WE FERTILIZE OVA SPECIFICALLY TO CREATE EMBRYOS TO BE SACRIFICED FOR STEM CELLS?

The creation of embryos for the purpose of taking their stem cells is a complex issue. Although no responsa yet exist specifically dealing with this question, it is likely that rabbinic authorities will not favor such a leniency. The mere existence of already-created pre-embryos creates a need to decide the halakhic ramifications of their destruction. We therefore may decide that such research is permitted *bedieved* (ex post facto), once the pre-embryos exist. However, since there are *poskim* who forbid abortion even within the first forty days,[48] it is much harder to argue *lichatchila* (a priori) that creation of pre-embryos with the intention of destroying them is permitted.

There are additional questions that we as a society must ponder. May we (or should we) deliberately create pre-embryos in order to destroy them?

DO WE PUT "FENCES" AROUND THE LAW AND THE USE OF STEM CELLS AND ABORTED FETAL TISSUE?

The rabbis often create protective edicts (*gezerot*) to prevent the desecration of Torah law. In addition, the rabbis may promulgate decrees intended to protect Torah values by preventing untoward behavior that is not already prohibited by the Torah itself. For example, more than a thousand years ago, Rabbenu Gershon enacted *gezerot* (rabbinic decrees) banning polygamy and opening the mail of others, despite the absence of actual Torah prohibitions for either of these two actions.

The protection of life is a strongly held Torah ideal. Although the destruction of pre-embryos in the course of fertility treatments or to prevent disease may be permitted, this does not mean that pre-embryos may be destroyed without compunction. To avoid the proverbial "slippery slope," should we ban stem cell research on embryonic stem cells as a dangerous encroachment on the sanctity of life? That is, even if pre-embryos may be destroyed, should we enact preventive laws barring stem cell research that requires the destruction of potential lives to avoid cheapening life by treating the process of creating humans as another scientific process, stripped of its miraculous underpinnings? In his testimony, Rabbi Tendler summed up the issue of protective enactments as follows:

> Jewish law consists of biblical and rabbinic legislation. A good
> deal of rabbinic law consists of erecting fences to protect biblical
> law. Surely our tradition respects the effort of the Vatican and

fundamentalist Christian faiths to erect fences that will protect the biblical prohibition against abortion. But a fence that prevents the cure of fatal diseases must not be erected, for then the loss is greater than the benefit. In the Judeo-biblical legislative tradition, a fence that causes pain and suffering is dismantled. Even biblical law is superseded by the duty to save lives, except for the three cardinal sins of adultery, idolatry, and murder. . . . Life-saving abortion is a categorical imperative in Jewish biblical law. Mastery of nature for the benefit of those suffering from vital organ failure is an obligation. Human embryonic stem cell research holds that promise.

Human embryonic germ cells may also be derived from gamete ridge tissue removed from first-trimester aborted fetuses (at approximately eight weeks of gestation). Although abortion of fetuses is a grave offense, it is difficult to justify prohibiting the use of life-saving tissue from these aborted fetuses for fear of encouraging or condoning abortion. This is another case where the cost of a preventive enactment might be the avoidable death of human beings.[49,50]

❧ *Daniel Eisenberg, M.D.*

Notes

1. Although the nuclear DNA would be identical to the donor skin cell, the mitochondrial DNA would be that of the donor egg.
2. See "Artificial Insemination in Jewish Law," *Maimonides*, 1999, 5(1).
3. Important exceptions are Rabbi Ovadia Yosef, who forbids it and rules that it does not fulfill the obligation of fathering children; *Tzitz Eliezer* XV, no. 45; and Rabbi Moshe Sternbach, who denies paternity to the sperm donor and forbids the procedure.
4. The use of sperm for IVF once the *mitzvah* of procreation has been fulfilled is more controversial.
5. See Rabbi Yitzchok Breitowitz, "The Preembryo in Halacha" (http://www.JLaw.com/Articles/preemb.html).
6. The development of cryogenic techniques to freeze pre-embryos only pushed off the crucial question of whether pre-embryos could be destroyed. Prior to cryogenic techniques, several rabbinic authorities

ruled that all fertilized embryos must be implanted. This severely limited the availability of IVF to Torah-observant Jews because of the great expense and low yields of each IVF attempt (necessitating fertilization of many ova), and the inherent risk of implanting many embryos. With the advent of cryogenic techniques, many ova could be fertilized, with only a few implanted. Nevertheless, the question remains of disposition of these "frozen" pre-embryos, which now number approximately 100,000.

7. *Nishmat Avraham, Orach Chaim* 656:1, p. 92.

8. Exodus 20:13.

9. Exodus 21:22–23.

10. *Be'er Hetiv, Choshen Mishpat* 425:2.

11. See Rabbi I. Y. Unterman, *Responsa Shevet M'Yehuda*, vol. 1, p. 29, and *Noam* 6 (1963): 1–11.

12. A *treife* is a person with an organic illness that is expected to be fatal within a year.

13. See *Igrot Moshe, Choshen Mishpat* II, 69B.

14. For more extensive treatment of this debate, see *Jewish Ethics and Halakhah for Our Time: Sources and Commentary*, vol. 1, by Rabbi Basil F. Herring.

15. To spare her the embarrassment of bleeding during her execution.

16. Genesis 9:6.

17. *Sanhedrin* 67b: "In the name of Rabbi Yishmael they said: A ben Noach [is liable] even for killing a fetus. What is the reasoning of Rabbi Yishmael? Because it is written [in Genesis 9:6]: 'Whoever sheds the blood of man by man [literally "in man"], his blood shall be shed.' What is the meaning of 'man in man'? This can be said to refer to a fetus in its mother's womb."

18. Because the Torah was given to the Jews at Mount Sinai, only they are bound by its commands. Nevertheless, all laws given to Noah, the father of all nations, are binding on non-Jews.

19. *Tosofot, Chullin* 33a, (d.h. *"Echad oveid kochavim"*), *Tosofot, Sanhedrin* 59a (d.h. *"Layka"*)

20. *Bava Kamma* 90b is based on Genesis 9:5 ("the blood of your lives I will surely require"). See *Responsa Maharit* 97 and 99. See also *Responsa Seridei Aish*, vol. 3, no. 127 (originally published in *Noam* 9:193–215).

21. The laws of damage in halakhah are extensively discussed in the Torah, Talmud, and codes of Jewish law.

22. See *Responsa Seridei Aish*, vol. 3, no. 127, p. 249.

23. Rabbi J. David Bleich, *Contemporary Halakhic Problems*, vol. 1, p. 341.

24. As noted, the fetus would be classified a *rodef*.

25. See *Nida* 13b and *Responsa Chavot Yair*, no. 31. *Responsa Sheilot Yaavetz*, no. 43, argues that once the sperm has been deposited in the woman, the primary prohibition of *hashchatas zera* no longer applies.

26. *Igrot Moshe, Even HaEzer* 1:70, 3:14.

27. Generally, all Torah prohibitions except for murder, idolatry, and forbidden sexual relationships are waived to save a human life.

28. Leviticus 19:16.

29. *Sanhedrin* 73a.

30. Deuteronomy 22:1–2.

31. Maimonides, *Commentary on the Mishnah, Nedarim* 4:4.

32. *Nidda* 30a.

33. *Tumat leida* is the impurity that is created by the birth process, whether live or by miscarriage.

34. *Yevamot* 69b.

35. Torat HaAdam (in *Mosad HaRav Kook Kitvei Haramban*, vol. 2, p. 29).

36. This line of reasoning is brought in Talmud *Yoma* 85b as one possible reason for why saving a life overrides the Sabbath.

37. See *Responsa Sheilot Yaavetz*, no. 43, where Rabbi Yaakov Emden argues that "wasting seed" only bars preventing the semen from reaching the woman's uterus. He nevertheless forbids abortion prior to forty days for other reasons.

38. *Seridei Aish*, vol. 3:350, no. 7.

39. *Seridei Aish*, vol. 3, no. 127, p. 249.

40. *Responsa Shevet M'Yehuda*, vol. 1, 9, and *Noam* 6:4.

41. Rabbi Chaim Ozer Grodzinski (*Responsa Achiezer*, 3, 65:14) even entertains the possibility that there may be no biblical prohibition of abortion before forty days. See also: *Tzofnat Paneach* 59; *Responsa Bet Shlomah, Choshen Mishpat* 162; *Torat Chesed, Even Ha'ezer*, 42:33— all of which discuss the decreased stringency of abortion within the first forty days.

42. Males with a single gene for a sex-linked disease will be affected by the disease.

43. Personal correspondence with Dr. Avraham Steinberg.

44. Personal correspondence with Rabbi Sholom Kamenetsky.

45. "Stem Cell Research and Therapy: A Judeo-Biblical Perspective," *Ethical Issues in Human Stem Cell Research*, vol. 3: *Religious Perspectives*,

1999, pp. H3–H5. The full text may be downloaded from the National Bioethics Advisory Commission Web site at http://bioethics.gov/pubs.html.

46. "The Judeo-biblical tradition does not grant moral status to an embryo before forty days of gestation. Such an embryo has the same moral status as male and female gametes, and its destruction prior to implantation is of the same moral import as the 'wasting of human seed.' After forty days—the time of 'quickening' recognized in common law—the implanted embryo is considered to have humanhood, and its destruction is considered an act of homicide. Thus, there are two prerequisites for the moral status of the embryo as a human being: implantation and forty days of gestational development. The proposition that humanhood begins at zygote formation, even in vitro, is without basis in biblical moral theology." Testimony of Rabbi Moshe Dovid Tendler, Ph.D., in ibid., p. H3.

47. For example, Rabbi J. David Bleich has voiced opposition to the destruction of pre-embryos and their use in stem cell research.

48. *Responsa Seridei Aish,* vol. 3:350, no. 7; *Responsa Shevet M'Yehuda,* 1:50; *Responsa Maharash Engel,* 7:85; and Rabbi Moshe Yonah Zweig, *Noam* 7:48.

49. "In stem cell research and therapy, the moral obligation to save human life, the paramount ethical principle in biblical law, supersedes any concern for lowering the barrier to abortion by making the sin less heinous. Likewise, the expressed concern that this research facilitates human cloning is without merit. First, no reputable research facility is interested in cloning a human, which is not even a distant goal, despite the pluripotency of stem cells. Second, those on the leading edge of stem cell research know that the greater contribution to human welfare will come from replacement of damaged cells and organs by fresh stem cell products, not from cloning. Financial reward and acclaim from the scientific community will come from such therapeutic successes, not from cloning." Testimony of Rabbi Moshe Dovid Tendler, op. cit., p. H4.

50. Other issues applicable to stem cell research are generic and apply equally to all research. Full informed consent, careful risk-benefit analysis, allocation of scarce resources, and the role of financial gain and remuneration in research have all been dealt with in Jewish law and are beyond the scope of this chapter.

Organ Donation

Chapter 66

Judaism and Organ Donation

All four branches of Judaism (Orthodox, Conservative, Reform, and Reconstructionist) support and encourage donation. According to Orthodox Rabbi Moses Tendler, chairman of the Biology Department at Yeshiva University in New York City and chairman of the Bioethics Commission of the Rabbinical Council of America, "If one is in the position to donate an organ and to save another's life, it's obligatory to do so, even if the donor never knows who the beneficiary will be. The basic principle of Jewish ethics—the infinite worth of the human being—also includes donation of corneas, since eyesight restoration is considered a life-saving operation." In 1991, the Rabbinical Council of America (Orthodox) approved organ donations as permissible, and even required, from brain-dead patients.

The Reform and Conservative movements strongly encourage organ and tissue donation. Rabbi Richard Address, director of the Union of American Hebrew Congregations Bio-Ethics Committee and Committee on Older Adults, states that Jewish traditions "provide a positive approach and by and large the North American Reform Jewish community approves of transplantation." According to Jewish tradition, the duty of saving an endangered life (*pikuach nefesh*) suspends the operation of all the commandments in the Torah, with the exception of three prohibitions: no one is to save one's own or another's life at the price of murder, incest, or idolatry. The sages of the Talmud interpret the words "he shall live by them," in Leviticus 18:5, to mean that the *mitzvot*—the divine commands— are to be a means of life and not of death. The sages specifically state that the duty of saving a life supersedes the Sabbath laws. From a Jewish point of view, it is sinful to observe laws that have been superseded because of a danger to life. One may do any work on Sabbath to save a life (Talmud, *Ketubot* 5a). "The Sabbath has been given to you, not you to the Sabbath" is a well-known statement from the Talmud (*Yoma* 85b). It has been noted that the German pessimistic philosopher Schopenhauer could not forgive Judaism for its affirmation of life.

In *Mishneh Torah*, Maimonides discusses the duty to profane the Sabbath when failure to do so is certain to endanger human life.

> The commandment of the Sabbath, like all other commandments, is set aside if human life is in danger. Accordingly, if a person is dangerously ill, whatever a skilled local physician considers necessary may be done for him on the Sabbath . . . when such things have to be done . . . they should rather be done by adult and scholarly Jews. . . . Similarly, if a ship is storm-tossed at seas, or if a city is surrounded by marauding troops or by a flooding river, it is a religious duty to go to the people's rescue on the Sabbath and to use every means to deliver them. (*Shabbat* 2:2–3)

℮ *UAHC Committee on Bio-Ethics*

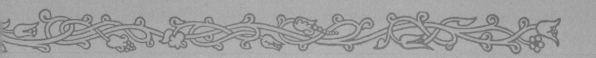

Chapter 67

The Gift of Life

In the space of one week I went from a perfectly healthy thirty-five-year-old woman to a liver transplant recipient. You think it can never happen to you, but your life can change in an instant.

Unlike many people who need a transplant, there was never any indication that anything was wrong with me until the night I got the flu. At least, I thought it was the flu. It was a Wednesday night when I went to bed with a fever and chills. The next day I awoke with the rest of the symptoms usually associated with a stomach flu—body aches, vomiting, and diarrhea.

By Friday I was growing steadily sicker. That evening, my husband and my mother-in-law, Miki Schulman, took me to the emergency room at our local hospital for what was supposed to be a quick visit for intravenous fluids. "It will probably make you feel better," my internist said.

Once there, my family received the startling news: I was suffering from complete liver and kidney failure. I was quickly moved to the intensive care unit as my condition rapidly deteriorated and my kidneys shut down. To this day, no one knows the reason for my illness.

At this point, my family received a crash course on what it would take for me to survive this ordeal. They were told that I had to have a liver and possibly a kidney transplant in the next forty-eight to seventy-two hours if I was going to live. Before Friday evening was over, I was transferred by ambulance to the organ transplantation center at New York University Hospital.

My sister-in-law, Kimi, all but moved in to care for my children, Joshua, who was then five, and my eight-month-old baby, Ashley

Rose. Josh seemed to grasp the severity of the situation. Told by his school's rabbi that he could ask for anything after saying his bedtime *Shema*, he began asking God to make "Mommy get better."

Perhaps someone was listening, because thankfully this story has a happy ending. By Monday evening we learned that donor organs, which turned out to be a perfect match, were available. Early Tuesday morning, October 26, the eleven-hour transplant procedure began. During the course of the operation, the surgical team concluded that my kidneys would probably start functioning once the new liver was in place, and the decision was made not to remove them. Fortunately, they were right, and within a few weeks my new liver and my old kidneys were working normally.

 Hadassah Policy Statement on Organ and Tissue Donation

Hadassah, the Women's Zionist Organization of America, is committed to the tenet that "he who saves a single life is as if he has saved an entire world." Organ and tissue donation is a direct extension of this message. In contrast to popular belief, all streams of Judaism hold that individuals may, and are encouraged to, donate potentially life-saving organs.

We are proud that the Hadassah Medical Organization is one of Israel's major organ transplantation centers, having been designated by the Israel Ministry of Health as a national center for bone marrow, heart, liver, kidney, and pancreas transplants.

In the United States, more than 60,000 people are on the national organ waiting list and on average thirteen people die each day while waiting for an organ. Thousands of missed opportunities for organ donation mean that not enough organs are available for those who need them.

Hadassah encourages all Americans to discuss with their families and medical professionals, in advance, organ donation and other end-of-life decisions so that more life-saving organs will be available to those in need. In this effort to save lives, Hadassah pledges to increase its efforts to raise awareness about the importance of donating organs and tissue.

A family I have never met but will be eternally grateful to made the difficult decision to have their loved one live twice. Her liver saved my life, and she lives within me. Because of this wonderful family in Buffalo, I was able to walk out of the hospital three weeks later with the expectation of living a long and healthy life.

For me, the last year has been spent recuperating. The year has been filled with emotional and physical pain; I still cannot believe what happened. But make no mistake. It is because of a family's foresight and generosity that I am here today to write my story. My greatest joy is the ability to raise my children and take care of my family. I have become a staunch advocate of organ donation awareness. I appreciate my second chance at life every single day. I am extremely fortunate and no longer take anything for granted.

Fifteen months ago I would have immediately dismissed the notion that I could ever need an organ transplant. I am sure you are thinking something like this could never happen to you or someone in your family. Let me assure you, you are wrong. I am living proof that it can happen. I implore you and your family to openly and seriously discuss becoming a potential organ donor. My donor and her family saved Joshua and Ashley's mommy. You never know whose life you may save.

Ellen Schulman

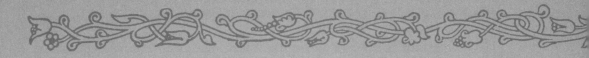

Chapter 68

The Myth of Organ Donation.

During her senior year of college, Hadassah member Karen Tishler found that she was increasingly out of breath. After being rushed to the hospital one night, tests revealed that she was in end-stage heart failure. Her only option was a heart transplant, if one became available in time. "You could live twenty years or you could die tonight," she was told. Fortunately for Karen, after just two days on the heart transplant waiting list, she received a donated heart from a seventeen-year-old male.

"One family's selflessness gave me back my life. Your agreement on your donor card or license and more importantly your discussion of organ donation with your family might mean just as much one day," recalls Karen, now a healthy, active high school history teacher in Birmingham, Alabama.

Unlike many people in need of an organ, Karen Tishler is one of the lucky ones. In the United States today, 61,000 people are on the waiting list for an organ transplant, sometimes for years, for only 20,000 transplants are conducted annually as demand far exceeds supply. As a result, 4,000 people die each year while waiting for an organ.

RELIGIOUS VIEWPOINTS

It is commonly assumed that Judaism does not permit organ donation. Contrary to this myth, every denomination—Orthodox, Conservative, Reform, and Reconstructionist—supports, if not encourages, organ donation.

According to Jewish law, using an organ to save a life is permissible and encouraged. "Whoever saves one soul, it is as if he saved an entire universe," says the Talmud (*Sanhedrin* 37a). Rabbi Moshe Tendler, a leading American Orthodox medical ethicist, frequently emphasizes, "If one is in the position to donate an organ to save another's life, it is obligatory to do so." In fact, the *mitzvah* (commandment) of saving a life outweighs any other Jewish concerns commonly believed to prohibit organ donation.

As part of our commitment to saving lives, Hadassah is now working to increase organ donation in the United States. By working to dispel the myth that Judaism prohibits organ donation and by increasing awareness about the importance of this *mitzvah*, we hope to encourage more Americans to take part in this vital effort.

BECOMING A DESIGNATED DONOR

Today, only 20 to 30 percent of *potential* donors actually make organs available. To help change this, hospitals, under a policy called "required request," must ask the next-of-kin if they are interested in donating their deceased relative's organs. This policy enables hospitals and health care professionals to play a key role in increasing donations, as families might not otherwise be aware of their right to donate.

Thus having a family discussion about organ donation well in advance of an emergency will make the decision easier should the time come. Otherwise, a decision may have to be made during an emotional time of crisis and without knowing each other's wishes.

LEGISLATIVE HISTORY

As the demand for organ transplants increased, the U.S. government recognized that guidelines were needed to ensure equity, safety, and access to organs. As a result, Congress passed the 1984 National Organ Transplant Act classifying human organs as a national resource not subject to compensation or sale.

The act also created a national organ allocation system. Through this system, when organs become available, they are distributed to those on waiting lists. The national system is broken down into eleven geographic regions, sixty-two local areas, and hundreds of Organ Procurement Organizations (OPOs). OPOs coordinate activities relating to organ procurement in a designated service area. They also evaluate potential donors, provide information about donation to family members, and arrange for the surgical removal of donated organs. OPOs are also responsible for preserving organs and making arrangements for distribution according to national organ sharing policies.

It is our hope that more life-saving organs will become available to those in need. To that end, Hadassah encourages all Americans to discuss, in advance, organ donation and other end-of-life decisions with their families and medical professionals.

A CALL TO ACTION

In addition to discussing organ donation with your family, there is another way to make a difference: through advocacy. Critical bipartisan legislation to eliminate the three-year time limitation on benefits for immunosuppressive drugs under the Medicare program is currently pending in Congress.

Organ transplant recipients must take immunosuppressive drugs daily, for the rest of their lives, to prevent their bodies from rejecting their new organs. A patient who is fortunate enough to receive a transplant is often faced with the dilemma of how to pay for the drugs necessary to keep his or her organ functioning properly. At a cost of more than $1,000 per month, these drugs are often only one portion of a patient's total medical costs. This strikes the poor and those on a fixed income the hardest.

The Immunosuppressive Drug Coverage Extension Act (H.R. 1115) is sponsored by Representatives Charles Canady (R-Fla.) and Karen Thurman (D-Fla.), and the Immunosuppressive Drugs Coverage Act (S. 631) is sponsored by Senator Mike DeWine (R-Ohio). In addition to the support of thousands of organ recipients and their loved ones, the legislation enjoys substantial cosponsorship in the House of Representatives and the Senate.

Check the Legislative Action Center by selecting "Make Your Voice Heard" on Hadassah's Web site (http://www.hadassah.org) to see whether your congressional representatives are cosponsors. Then be sure to take action—directly from our Web site—either to urge your members of Congress to cosponsor the bill or to thank them for their support.

For more information on Hadassah's organ and tissue donation program, contact the Department of Women's Health at (212) 303-8094 or womenshealth@hadassah.org.

✑ American Scene, *"It's in the Genes"*

Chapter 69

Tradition, Transcendence, and Transplantation

One of the great advances of modern medicine has been the successful development of organ transplantation surgery. People in previous generations either lost their lives or saw their lives severely impaired as a result of a faulty heart or diseased kidney. Now they can look forward to a normal and functioning lifespan, if surgery is successful.

But you can only transplant an organ if an organ is available. And the number of healthy hearts, for example, is tiny. You must harvest the heart from someone who is no longer using it (since she has died) but before deterioration of the heart after death. In addition, there is frequently a delay in obtaining permission from potential donors, which may adversely affect the organs' viability. Some patients, as a result, spend years on waiting lists before receiving a transplant. Sadly, some do not survive long enough to reach the top of the list.

Why does it take so long? That's because the patient's body tissue must be matched with the organ for biochemical compatibility. The more compatible, the more likely the transplant and the attendant medication will be able to overcome the body's natural tendency to reject the foreign invasion. Obviously, the more people willing to donate organs, the quicker and more successfully we can treat those people in need.

But many Jews object to organ transplants. Shockingly, while approximately 60 percent of the U.S. population agrees to be organ donors when asked, only about 5 percent of Orthodox Jews do so, and the record of Conservative and Reform Jews is not much better.[1] Over 40,000 people remain on waiting lists, desperate for organs.

Sometimes people are unwilling to donate because they are concerned about their own health, but very often their unwillingness stems from mistaken ideas about Jewish law or folklore. There is a commonly held presumption that Orthodox Judaism opposes all transplantation. Yet this is not the case. We must address all the myths surrounding organ donation to encourage more Jews to donate their organs.

If there are objections, they are raised at the time of donation—not when one is waiting to be a recipient. Though it sounds selfish, according to Jewish law one can always use a harvested organ to save a life, even if present medical practice were in complete violation of Jewish law. The imperative to save a life takes over at that point, whereas the moral violation is to be dealt with as soon as possible in the future.

Myth: I can't donate an organ because it violates Jewish law.

Reality: There is a mandate in Jewish law that prohibits desecration of the dead: *nivul hameit.* The body deserves respectful treatment; therefore, any mutilation of the body that may occur with the removal of organs or an autopsy is forbidden. However, a landmark rabbinic decision in the eighteenth century took into account the principle of *pikuach nefesh,* saving a life: Rabbi Ezekiel Landau declared that if there is a patient before us who is ill and could directly benefit from the autopsy of a deceased person who succumbed to the same illness, then the autopsy could take place to save the life. But if the purpose of the procedure is only to advance medical research to assist future patients and not to help a specific patient right now, then the autopsy is not justified. So too with organ donation: if the organ is given to a recipient in need, the prohibition of *nivul hameit* is lifted, and the act of organ donation becomes permitted—even meritorious.

This leniency does complicate current practice. Universal donor cards associated with driver's licenses do not restrict medical officials from using donated organs in any way they choose. This may include research, experimentation, or physician training. Such uses do not suspend the biblical prohibition against autopsy, delayed burial, and defiling the dead. One therefore must make arrangements to ensure that one's organs will be used only in direct transplantation and not for these other purposes. There are mechanisms, such as advance directives, available to accomplish this goal. Organizations such as Hadassah should help make these options available or, at least, guide people to them.

Myth: I can't donate an organ because I don't want to inhibit my bodily resurrection, which will occur in the messianic era.

Reality: This is a common concern with no basis in Jewish law, though it does exert a powerful pull on folk imagination. And even if this concern were legitimate, it would never stand before the possibility of saving a life or even of enhancing its quality significantly.

Some people insist that severed body parts (for example, from an amputation) be buried, preferably where the rest of the body is or will be buried, but one does not hear stories of great expenditures of time, effort, and resources to accomplish these ends. I know of no heroic story in our literature of someone conquering great obstacles to restore a limb to its body. It would seem that a God who can resurrect the dead can take care of the administrative details of ensuring that those who are resurrected come to life with the requisite parts of the body intact.

Myth: I can't donate an organ because then my death would be hastened.

Reality: This is a serious concern related specifically to heart transplants. Once the heart ceases functioning, it is useless for transplant. But in order for a heart donation to be possible, the donor must be considered deceased. How is this possible? When the patient's brain functions have ceased. This criterion for death, however, has been contentious.

Before the first heart transplant experiments in the 1960s, death was generally declared when the patient had stopped breathing. However, the cessation of respiration caused the cells of the heart to die, rendering it unusable for transplant. There was legitimate concern among rabbinical authorities about ethics violations—that hearts were being taken from patients who were merely "brain-dead" and who, therefore, may not have been finished using them. As a result, some Orthodox rabbinic leaders signed ads in the *New York Times* and other newspapers condemning the practice. Unfortunately, these ads reinforced the misunderstanding many Jews have that transplantation is always against Jewish law.

But ultimately, in 1988, the Chief Rabbinate of Israel approved heart transplantation, effectively agreeing that a patient who is brain-dead cannot independently breathe or produce a heartbeat. In these circumstances, a respirator can preserve the heart, while harvesting and transplantation may occur. Many Orthodox authorities interpret complete brain death as death, and transplantation is then permissible. Once the brain ceases functioning, the patient is no longer alive.

The early heart transplants were done before the discovery of antirejection drugs. As a result, recipients of these hearts were certain to die relatively quickly. It is not surprising, therefore, that the ads signed by the rabbis condemned the practice as the legal and medical murder of both the donor and the recipient.

Today, antirejection drugs have allowed the five-year success rate of heart transplants to surpass the 70 percent mark. Though still somewhat risky, the success rate is well within a range that would allow us to support such a procedure. If someone's health is seriously compromised, the dangers of surgery are acceptable, given the possible benefits that may well accrue.

Finally, we must point out the positive side of being a donor. Whether one accepts the "brain death" definition described here, which gives license to harvest a wider range of organs, or whether one rejects that definition and is therefore more restricted, there are many organs that one can donate. To do so is to fulfill one of the great *mitzvot* (positive acts). "Whoever saves one soul, it is as if he saved an entire universe," says the Talmud (*Sanhedrin* 37a). Each person is a unique, infinitely valuable, eternally irreplaceable entity; to restore life to such a being is among the greatest acts one can perform.

We are part of a global family. If we wish organs to be available to those we care about, we must help make them available to others. Although Jewish law cannot and should not mandate one's personal decision in such a sensitive and personal area, it can and does encourage us to do what we can to preserve and enhance people's existence. To do otherwise is to deny our commitment to the sanctity of life.

✍ *Rabbi Barry Freundel*

Note
1. E. N. Dorff, *Matters of Life and Death: A Jewish Approach to Modern Medical Ethics* (Philadelphia: Jewish Publication Society, 1998), p. 230.

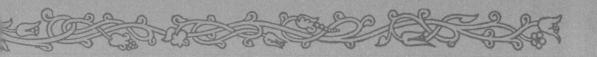

Chapter 70

Jews and Organ Donations

All Take and No Give?

Dr. Joel Rosh, a pediatric gastroenterologist and Orthodox Jew who for six years codirected the liver transplant program at New York's Mount Sinai Hospital, tells a story of an Israeli girl who flew with her family to the United States for a liver transplant.

On the plane, the young girl, while on life support, was declared brain-dead. The team that had been assembled to try to save her life now turned to her family and asked if they would donate her remaining healthy organs. They said no.

"The Israeli family explained, 'We feel for the other families and we want to help, but we have asked our rabbi and he has said that it is not permitted under Jewish Law.'"

That's one story about Jews and organ donations. Here's another:

Alisa Flatow, twenty, a Brandeis University junior, took the year off to study in a Jerusalem yeshiva, deciding before Passover to travel by bus with a few friends to a hotel at Gush Katif—a Jewish settlement in the Gaza Strip. She never made it. A Hamas suicide bomber drove his van into the bus, mortally wounding her and many Israeli soldiers, seven of whom were killed instantly.

Arriving from his home in West Orange, New Jersey, at Sorokin Hospital in Beersheva, Steven Flatow confirmed that the brain-dead young woman on life support was his daughter. The staff asked him a question: Would he be willing to donate his daughter's

This article was originally published in *Moment*, August 1995/Av 5755, pp. 32–35, 58–59. Reprinted by permission of Adena K. Berkowitz.

organs? After consulting with his wife and making a conference call with their rabbi, Alvin Marcus, and to Rabbi Moshe D. Tendler of Yeshiva University, an authority on Jewish medical ethics, Alisa's parents decided to donate her organs to six people on a waiting list who were clinging to life.[1]

"People have called it a brave decision, a righteous decision, a courageous decision. To us it was simply the right thing to do at the time," says Flatow. "I didn't know what all the media attention was about. As I was leaving Israel, at the airport, I mentioned this to a journalist who said to me, 'You really don't understand, do you?'"

What Flatow didn't understand was the emotional impact his family's gesture had on a grieving Israel—an impact captured by Prime Minister Yitzhak Rabin, when he told American Jews that "Alisa Flatow's heart beats in Jerusalem." But the Flatows' decision also drew attention to a painful issue—a perception that Jews—Israeli and American, religious and secular—are more reluctant than most to donate their organs after death. Citing "religious objections," some Jews have allowed organ donation to become an exception to their well-deserved reputation for generosity.

For close to thirty years, transplants have been performed in the United States and Europe with ever-increasing success for kidneys, livers, hearts, pancreases, and lungs, as well as bone marrow. But not enough people donate organs. To date, over 40,000 people remain on waiting lists in the United States, desperate for organs. According to the United Network for Organ Sharing (UNOS), 40,233 people were registered for organs in 1994, but only 18,251 transplants were performed; 3,098 people on the waiting list died. Every month, 2,000 people are added to the UNOS register.

With few exceptions, the only viable organ donations are from brain-dead donors whose breathing and circulation are being maintained artificially. Although polls show most Americans are willing to become donors, too few families actually give their consent when a tragedy occurs; only 5,000 donors are available each year, out of a potential pool of 10,000 to 15,000 donors. Such shortages fuel frustration and suspicion, as when doctors for the ailing Mickey Mantle were erroneously criticized for giving the former Yankee star special treatment in his successful search for a new liver.

In the general community, families voice a number of familiar objections to donation. According to Jeffrey Prottas of Brandeis

University, the former chairman of the Organ Donor and Procurement Committee of the National Task Force on Organ Transplantation, these include misconceptions that the donating process will mutilate a loved one's body and an erroneous but persistent belief that the donor's family will be charged for the procedure. Others simply are unaware of their loved one's desires to become a donor.

For many Jews, particularly the Orthodox, this reluctance is compounded by several factors: concern about violating halakhic, or Jewish legal, strictures against desecrating the dead or benefiting from a dead body (see Responsa, *Moment,* June 1995); the traditional view that the deceased be buried whole, and disagreement over whether to accept brain death as a halakhic definition of the end of life.

Organ banks do not keep track of donors based on religious identity, but my discussions with medical ethicists, experts, rabbis, and doctors across the country support the view that too many Jews are reluctant to become organ donors. Isaac Newman, an Orthodox Jew and coordinator of the New York metropolitan area's organ procurement program, says that only about 5 percent of Orthodox Jews asked to be donors consent; as a group, Jews are only slowly beginning to match the general population's 60 percent consent rate. Many non-Orthodox and nonobservant Jews, who often tend to demur to Jewish tradition on end-of-life issues, are also reluctant to give. At Conservative and Reform congregations where I have spoken, I have often been told by members of the audience that Jewish law absolutely forbids being an organ donor.

In 1987, Dr. Thomas Starzl, an American pioneer in transplant surgery, warned at a transplant conference in Israel that if Jews do not start giving, they will not get organs (of course any attempt to bar an ethnic group from receiving organs would be challenged legally). Sure enough, in 1992, French health authorities barred all their hospitals from performing organ transplants on Israelis, mostly because of Israel's "organ deficit" in Eurotransplant—the European transplant coordinating body. (Israel and members of the European Community previously had joint agreements on health care; most Israelis seeking liver transplants traveled to France.) And while France and Israel signed a two-year agreement to allow Israelis to receive liver transplants under certain conditions, most other European countries still do not accept Israelis for transplant.

In 1994, fifty Israeli patients needed heart transplants, and only twelve hearts became available; 700 people were on lists for kidneys, but only twelve received transplants from people who had died. While 700,000 Israelis have signed donor cards this seems to have little impact on their surviving relatives. "I can only remember one or two cases in which donors actually had signed a donor card," says Nurit Shimron, national coordinator of the Israel Transplant Association.

This reluctance comes, despite statements by rabbinic organizations representing the major denominations endorsing the concept of brain death and encouraging donations. In 1990, the Rabbinical Assembly passed a resolution urging all Conservative Jews to become donors. The Union of American Hebrew Congregation's 1991 health care proxy—a medical living will—likewise encourages Reform Jews to become organ donors.

The Orthodox Rabbinical Council of America's "Health Care Proxy" gives physicians permission to remove the signee's corneas, kidneys, lungs, heart, liver, and pancreas "for the sole purpose of transplantation." The directive also stipulates that physicians obtain the "concurrence" of an Orthodox rabbi or a member of the RCA's Bioethics Commission.

"People come up all the time and say, 'I thought Judaism opposed this because of resurrection of the dead and the need to be buried complete,'" says Judith Abrams, a Reform rabbi in Missouri, Texas, who has written widely on medical ethics (see Responsa, *Moment*, December 1994). "I reassure them that most Orthodox authorities permit organ donations if the [standard] brain-death criteria are met. What's more, if you do this incredible *mitzvah*, God will somehow make it up to you in the world to come."

Rabbinic authorities are not, however, unanimous on the "brain death" standard. Agudath Israel, the ultra-Orthodox organization, does not recognize brain death and does not endorse organ donations. In Israel, prior to the Flatow tragedy, the *haredi* (right-wing Orthodox rabbinate) opposed donations by Jews (a ruling by the late, revered Rabbi Shlomo Zalman Auerbach on brain death was considered ambiguous).

However, those who oppose donations do not prohibit Jews from *receiving* organs, a distinction that drives many ethicists and rabbis to distraction. "If a person is not dead by *our* halakhic definition when he is brain dead, then to go and take an organ from a non-Jew means you are killing a non-Jew to save a Jew!" fumes Tendler. "I cannot imagine a more horrendous ruling." In 1992, Rabbi Marc Angel, then president of the RCA, called the all-take no-give policy "morally repugnant."

Those who reject the "brain death" definition to permit donating but sanction receiving transplanted organs, including Rabbi Aaron Soloveitchik of Yeshiva University's Rabbi Isaac Elchanan Theological Seminary, see it differently. In their view the gentile donating the organ would do so anyway; the recipient is not responsible for this decision or the organ's removal and thus is in no way prohibited from benefiting from it.

The Alisa Flatow case may have broken the logjam on this issue. Within a few weeks of her death, a statement was issued by Rabbi Yehoshua Scheinberger, the "minister of health" for the Eidah Haharedit—an umbrella body for Israel's ultra-Orthodox. It allowed ultra-Orthodox Jews to accept the brain-death definition and donate organs, but with several conditions. It is forbidden, he declared, to transplant Jewish organs into the bodies of "non-believers"—gentiles or Arabs who hate Israel. (Most secular Israelis, he said, would not fall under the category of nonbelievers.) In addition, he insisted that an Orthodox rabbi sit on the committee that approves the transplants. Both conditions were rejected by the Israel Transplant Association, but negotiations are under way.

Scheinberger's conditions were widely criticized. Rabbi David Feldman of the (Conservative) Jewish Center of Teaneck, New Jersey, and an expert on Jewish medical ethics, said Scheinberger was not speaking as an authority, and even if he was, "he was wrong. There is no basis in halakha or in Jewish morality to support limiting a donation to a Jewish or an observant Jewish recipient, and it is important that people be disabused of the idea." Tendler regards Scheinberger's statement as an error "halakhically, emotionally and sociologically" and a *"hillul ha'Shem"*—a desecration of God's name. Nevertheless, he calls Scheinberger's positive ruling on brain death "a great thing."

Israeli transplant experts like Nurit Shimron, however, say it is too early to tell what practical impact Scheinberger's views will have on donations. Dr. Mordechai Kramer, an Orthodox Jew and coordinator of the lung transplant program at Hadassah Hospital, believes that donations continue to lag because of misconceptions about brain death. "If you ask people on the street, will they give, the majority say yes. But when it comes to their family members, most are not ready to do it. With a brain-dead patient, people think he will get better. And that isn't only the *haredim* but non-Orthodox as well."

In the United States, a number of rabbis report an increased awareness of donations since Alisa Flatow's death. "People have been talking about it a lot and it has brought another level of consciousness to the debate," says Rabbi Zahara Davidowitz-Farkas, coordinator of Jewish chaplaincy at New York-Cornell Medical Center.

"I was able to convince people who previously had said 'Isn't this forbidden?' to realize what Jewish tradition says about donating organs," says Rabbi Brian Zimmerman of Temple Beth Ami in Rockville, Maryland.

Those who continue to reject brain death are also being urged to remember another halakhic concept, *mishum aivah*, "because of enmity," which holds that certain Torah laws can be suspended to prevent hatred between Jews and non-Jews. I don't believe that in our own age we have to worry about anti-Semitic outbreaks because of low organ donations from Jews. But we do have to reexamine our commitment to the larger community.

Jewish organizations should seize the momentum of the Flatow example and redouble their efforts to encourage donation. At the same time, they should help transplant teams make sure that Jewish law is followed, that *kevod ha'met* (respect for the deceased) is upheld, that the body of the donor is draped properly, and that all blood and tissue is buried with the body in accordance with Jewish law.

The public has to be reassured that donating an organ doesn't mean death will be hastened in any way (for example, doctors involved in removing a patient's organs for transplantation are prohibited by law from certifying the patient's death).

Most of all, families need to talk to one another. For even if an individual signs a donor card, it is the family that makes the ultimate decision to participate in a lifesaving venture.

Says Rabbi Tendler, "Alisa Flatow will not only get credit in heaven above for the four people alive, walking around with her organs, but the many hundreds who will be saved because other people will be inspired to follow her example."

&℘ *Adena K. Berkowitz*

Note

1. Of the six, two are known to have died following the operation: Serena Shmuelevitz, forty (kidney and pancreas), and Shabtai Rehamim, twenty-three (liver). The known survivors include Malka Nir, forty-eight (lung), and Jacob Salinas, fifty-six (heart). Alisa's corneas were saved for later transplantation.

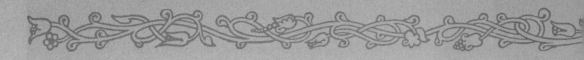

Chapter 71

When Is Death?

The trend in Jewish legal tradition favors actions that lead to *pikuach nefesh* (saving a life) over prohibitions protecting the sanctity of the body. Nevertheless, the rabbinic acceptance of organ donation was slowed by disagreements over whether to accept "brain death," a concept that emerged only in the late 1960s.

In all but brain death, earlier rabbinic authorities had paved the way for organ donation. Rabbi Ezekiel Landau, the famed eighteenth-century halakhic authority known as the Node B'Yehudah, was asked whether an autopsy could be performed on a patient who had died of a kidney stone, in hope of finding a way to prevent such cases in the future. Landau weighed the Talmud's prohibitions against mutilating the dead (*Hullin* 11b; *Bava Batra* 154a) against the possibility that information gleaned from an autopsy could save another's life. Landau held that if there is a *choleh lefaneinu*, an ill patient before us, then the usual ban on autopsies could be overridden for the sake of *pikuach nefesh*.

The "patient before us" principle could be interpreted narrowly, but countless rabbis have since cited this requirement as justification for a more universal perspective on human suffering. In 1965, for example, the Israeli rabbinate and Hadassah Hospital entered into an agreement that allowed autopsies not only for immediate lifesaving but also to aid in detecting hereditary illnesses and gathering criminal evidence. Similarly, potential organ donors are assured that their organs will be used immediately and not stored in a "bank."

In the late 1960s, *pikuach nefesh* was applied to allow transplants of the cornea. Then-Ashkenazi Chief Rabbi I. Y. Unterman held that, given all the dangers that blind people might face, such an operation could literally save their lives. But would the ruling apply if the transplant recipient was blind in only one eye? Would this then violate the prohibition of "benefiting" from the dead or allowing the deceased donor to be buried without all body parts? Unterman responded that a cornea ceases to be "dead" once it is transplanted and revived. Desecration, meanwhile, applies only to a visible incision or removal of a visible, external organ: The eye can be removed and the eyelids of the deceased closed.

Transplant technology requires that organs be "harvested" from bodies whose cardiac and respiratory functions may be maintained only by mechanical means. Traditionally, death was defined as the cessation of the heartbeat. In 1968, an ad hoc committee at Harvard Medical School urged that death be defined as the irreversible cessation of all functions of the brain, including the brain stem. The Harvard criteria have been adopted by the medical establishment (a President's Commission on medical ethics endorsed the criteria in 1981).

The cessation of breathing was considered absolute evidence of death in the Talmud (*Yoma* 85a)—a view later adopted by the twelfth-century sage and physician Maimonides and in *Shulchan Aruch*, the Code of Jewish Law. Later rabbinic authorities, such as the Hatam Sofer (1762–1839), added cessation of cardiac activity to cessation of respiration as conclusive evidence of death.

Brain death defied both of these criteria. Initially, the late Rabbi Moshe Feinstein (1895–1986), the preeminent American Orthodox rabbinic authority of his time, resisted the concept of brain death.[1] In a responsum written in 1968, he called the person who removed the heart of a brain-dead patient a murderer. But in a later responsum, written in 1976, he appeared to accept the "brain death" definition (*Ig'grot Moshe, Yoreh De'ah,* vol. 3, no. 132). As Feinstein wrote that year to the chairman of the New York State Assembly's Committee on Health, "The sole criterion of death is total cessation of *spontaneous* respiration. In a patient representing the clinical picture of death, i.e. no signs of life such as movement or response to stimuli, the total cessation of independent respiration is an absolute proof that death has occurred" (emphasis added).

Rabbi Tendler of Yeshiva University, Feinstein's son-in-law and a professor of Talmud and biology, expanded on Feinstein's thinking to

Resources for Organ Donors

To receive an advance directive (living will) and other information on organ donations, contact the following:

Rabbinical Council of America (Orthodox)
Commission on Medical Ethics
278 Seventh Avenue
New York, NY 10001
(212) 807-7888

Rabbinical Assembly (Conservative)
Contact your local rabbi.

Union of American Hebrew Congregations (Reform)
Committee on Bio-Ethics
117 South 17th Street, Suite 2111
Philadelphia, PA 19103
Contact: Rabbi Richard Address
(212) 563-8183

Reconstructionist Rabbinical Association
Bio-Ethics Committee
Church Road and Greenwood Avenue
Wyncote, PA 19095
Contact: Yael Shuman
(215) 576-5210

National Institute for Jewish Hospice
8723 Alden Drive
Los Angeles, CA 90048
(800) 446-4448

become the chief proponent of the halakhic acceptability of brain death. He invokes Rabbi Feinstein's later responsum on heart transplantation, which begins with a discussion of decapitation. Feinstein, quoting Maimonides, argues that an animal is to be considered dead, even if its limbs continue to move after it is decapitated. Tendler compares brain-stem death, or what he calls physiological decapitation, to this physical decapitation and regards it as a halakhically acceptable definition of death. In 1986, the Israeli Chief Rabbinate accepted the halakhic validity of brain death to permit heart transplants in Israel, but the rabbis required certain tests to determine whether there is brain activity.

A leading critic of the acceptance of brain death in Jewish law has been Rabbi J. David Bleich, professor of Talmud and Jewish Law at Yeshiva University and Cardozo Law School. Bleich also sites Feinstein in his response, and questions the validity of tests performed to determine total cessation of brain stem activity and sticks to the traditional definition of death: cessation of all respiratory and cardiac activity.

    Adena K. Berkowitz

Note

1. At one point Rabbi Feinstein reasoned that a heart transplant was a "double murder"—its victims the "patient" whose organs were removed, and, because early success rates were low, the recipient.

Chapter 72

Coordinating *Mitzvah* and Miracle

It usually begins with a phone call. "Hello. This is the national transplant center. We have a potential liver donor. He's sixty-nine years old and has some underlying disease. His blood group is AB, and I know you have two ABs on your waiting list. Is this any good for you?"

Yehudit Vaknin, R.N., holds the phone in one hand and rapidly notes the details with the other. "Let me check with the doctors," she says. "I'll get back to you."

This time it doesn't work. Dr. Yaron Ilan of Hadassah's Liver Institute turns down the organ on grounds of the donor's age.

"I get very hopeful every time," says Jerusalem-born Vaknin, forty-one, who became transplant coordinator at the Hadassah-Hebrew University Medical Center at Ein Karem after thirteen years as an emergency-room nurse.

Sometimes, however, the excitement is justified, and Vaknin began her job as coordinator with just such an early success. As usual, it started with a phone call, this time as she sat down to Friday night dinner in her Kiryat Yovel apartment with her husband, their two teenage daughters, and their six-year-old son.

"The call was from the head of Hadassah's trauma unit, Dr. Avi Rivkind," she says. "He told me 'We have a road accident victim here, a young Arab woman I have no doubt will be declared brain dead. I think you should come.' I went at once, of course."

Together with the trauma unit's duty physician, Vaknin went to the stricken family. As gently as he could, the doctor told the young woman's waiting father, brothers, and uncles that she would not recover.

Meanwhile, Vaknin informed Dr. Avi Israeli, HMO director general, that there was a potential donor in the hospital, submitting to him the formal request to summon an official medical committee to establish brain death.

"There are very specific tests the committee must perform to satisfy themselves that the patient is brain dead," Vaknin notes. "Once the committee was convinced, they signed the formal declaration and I went back to the grieving family."

"'You've lost your daughter, your sister, your niece,' I told them. 'Your grief must be boundless. But you've told me what a wonderful young woman she was, how all she ever wanted to do was help others. If you could ask her now, don't you think she'd take this chance to help?'"

They were an educated Muslim family, and they asked for time to think. Within hours, they consented to give their daughter's heart, lungs, kidneys, liver, pancreas, and corneas for transplant—organs that went to nine different patients. Her bones and skin went to Israel's Bone and Skin Banks at Hadassah.

"One thing we can assure the families of potential organ donors is that we've acquired expertise in the complex surgery and aftercare, and our record easily matches those of all good transplantation centers," says Dr. Ahmed Eid, Hadassah's senior surgeon in charge of organ transplantation.

Entering the field when it was relatively young and before it was transformed by the antirejection drug cyclosporine, Dr. Eid specialized in transplantation surgery at the Mayo Clinic on a Hadassah fellowship. "It's a very exciting field," he says. "It enables us to give life to patients with a hopeless disease. The bottleneck in Israel, as elsewhere, remains the availability of donated organs."

Organ donation has been slow to catch on among Israel's observant Jews and traditional Muslims, but the country's sluggish record is improving. At Hadassah, where no organs at all were donated through 1996 and most of 1997, there are now several donors each year, a slow but promising start.

One reason for the increase is the ongoing education-information efforts by individuals, groups, and hospitals. Another is the health ministry's centralization and coordination of this effort; since 1997 it has provided for the appointment of transplant coordinators in every hospital in the country, and they run ongoing seminars to help these coordinators function effectively.

"I go to transplant center workshops once a month, and I find them very helpful," says Vaknin. "The computerization of patients waiting for organs also makes an important difference. In August, for example, a kidney, a liver, and a heart were transplanted into three Hadassah patients, all coming through the center."

Hadassah has made its own contribution to increasing the number of donors by selecting an experienced nurse as its transplant coordinator.

"At first the thinking was that persuading a family to donate the organs of a loved one is a job for social workers," says Sari Gotthold, who preceded Vaknin and was the first registered nurse to hold the job at Hadassah. "But we've seen that the work is essentially that of a nurse, supporting families through their ordeal. In my second month on the job, nine potential donors were admitted. One fortunately recovered; one went into a vegetative state; in another, brain death was never established.

"I spent days with the relatives, introducing myself as a nurse who works with families of the severely ill. I went with them into the intensive care unit, stayed with them while they spoke to the doctors. I brought them coffee, showed the observant where to go for a minyan. What I did was build a human connection. Yes, I had an ulterior motive, but I also did it for its own sake. That's part of what my job is."

Vaknin concurs. "You are there to help people in extreme circumstances. It's a job with a high burnout rate. You're constantly on call and constantly working with people living through some of life's hardest moments. But then there are the successes."

One of these was fifty-one-year-old Yaakov Yarden, a teacher from Shilo. For him, his renewed life began the usual way. "It was three in the morning on Friday, July 2," he recalls. "The phone rang. It was Hadassah. 'We have a donor; be here in three hours.'"

For this father of seven, this was the first link in what he now calls his chain of miracles. "I'd been ill for thirteen years," he says, "and my illness had damaged my liver. I managed pretty well through much of that time, but earlier this year I began to deteriorate badly. On July 1, the doctor at Hadassah told me that if no donor came through in the next two or three months, I should go abroad with a lot of money in my pocket. I nodded, but I'd already decided I'd stay in Israel with my family, no matter what. Hours later, the phone rang."

Another link in Yarden's chain was that he was assigned this particular liver because, despite the urgency of his case, he did not top the recipient list. "There was another patient ahead of me, but he was running a fever that night," Yarden says. "Luckily, he got a donor shortly afterward and is doing well. My good fortune was that I got the liver of someone who had been young and healthy. I didn't come around from surgery for three and a half days, and it was only because the donor liver was so strong that I survived."

It is the successes that energize Vaknin. "I approach the family of every candidate, including those least likely to donate, such as ultra-Orthodox Jews and Muslims," she says. "I talk to them about the *mitzvah* of giving life and ask them what they suppose the potential donor would feel about giving his organs."

Desperate though the need for organs is, Vaknin, like her predecessor, tries to secure agreement from the widest swath of family possible to prevent destructive recriminations later. "Even if the brain-dead patient has a signed organ-donor card, I still seek the family's consent. I say, 'Look, he wanted to give.' But if they refuse, we don't take the organs."

Vaknin herself is among the 130,000 Israelis with signed donor cards. "It's something I believe in passionately," she says. "I have seen how sudden tragedy can give life to others. I think my total conviction helps me persuade others."

ೋ *Wendy Elliman*

PART ELEVEN

Jewish Views on AIDS, Smoking, Abortion, and Eating Disorders

Chapter 73

AIDS

✑ *The Basics from the Jewish AIDS Trust*

Established in England as a charity in 1988 to provide the Jewish community with HIV education, counseling, and support, the Jewish AIDS Trust (JAT) extended its work to include education and awareness-raising of all sexual health matters, including HIV.

 DID YOU KNOW?

What is the difference between HIV and AIDS?

HIV stands for *human immunodeficiency virus*. It can be transmitted from one person to another. A person who is infected is said to be "HIV-positive."

AIDS stands for *acquired immune deficiency syndrome*. It is not something we catch. AIDS is caused by HIV and is a description that is given when certain diseases or symptoms are seen, not an illness in itself. Because AIDS occurs when a collection of symptoms appears in the patient, it is common practice for people working in the sexual health field to refer to it as "symptomatic HIV."

Generally, a doctor makes the decision about when HIV has become symptomatic HIV. A person can be HIV-positive for many years without having symptoms that are considered to be HIV-defining illnesses.

HOW HIV IS TRANSMITTED

There are three distinct ways to transmit HIV:

1. Having penetrative sexual intercourse without using protection (a condom)
2. Sharing needles and syringes when injecting drugs
3. Passing the virus from mother to baby during pregnancy or childbirth or through breast-feeding

Pregnant mothers in Britain today are encouraged to have an HIV test. Knowledge of HIV status can reduce the risk of transmission from mother to baby to just 1 percent—as long as the mother takes special medication, the baby is born by caesarean section, and the mother does not breast-feed. Knowledge of HIV status will also prolong the mother's life by giving her access to full medical services and medications as it becomes necessary to do so.

Is there an easy way to remember all this? Yes. Remember the QQR model: *quality, quantity, route:*

Quality: The HIV virus must be of good quality in order to infect someone. Outside the body it deteriorates quickly and is easily destroyed by heat, water, detergent, and so on.
Quantity: You need a certain amount of the virus to be at risk. Visible amounts of fresh blood, semen, vaginal fluid, and breast milk all contain sufficient levels of the virus. Sweat, saliva, urine, and all other body fluids do not.

 DID YOU KNOW?

When is HIV *not* transmitted? It's *not* transmitted by kissing, touching, hugging, or sharing the same cutlery or Kiddush cup. It's *not* transmitted from a toilet seat or by mosquitoes. All normal day-to-day activities are perfectly safe. It is also *not* transmitted via saliva, vomit, tears, urine, feces, or sweat.

Route: To become infected, good-quality virus in sufficient quantity has to enter your bloodstream. Having unprotected sex and sharing needles are two ways entry is provided; cuts and cold sores do not because they are either bleeding outward or they have scabbed over.

Without these three links, the chain of infections is broken, and HIV cannot be transmitted.

TESTING FOR HIV

The HIV test is a blood test that looks for the presence of HIV antibodies. These are produced by the immune system in response to HIV and are used as markers to show that HIV is in the blood.

You can get a test at any genitourinary medicine (GUM) clinic or at an HIV clinic. These are listed in the phone book (GUM clinics may also be called STD clinics; STD stands for *sexually transmitted diseases*). These clinics offer a confidential service and will also usually offer pretest and posttest counseling. You need not tell the clinic who your general practitioner is. Indeed, you need not give your real name. Some clinics test and give the results the same day; others might take one or two days, or up to a week, to get the results.

You can also ask your doctor about a test, but this is not always the best option. Some general practitioners do not know all the facts around HIV, and the result of the test will go on your medical record, which might form part of a report your doctor writes about you.

A word of caution: It can take up to three months after HIV infection for the antibodies to show up in the blood. During this period, it is possible for the person who is infected to pass the virus on, even though a test might wrongly suggest that the virus is not present. Therefore, it is important to wait for three months before having a test if you think you might have been infected.

SOURCES OF INFORMATION

Some of the information in this chapter was taken from the Terrence Higgins Trust's booklet *Testing Issues.* You can get a copy from the trust or have a look at its Web site (http://www.tht.org.uk).

DID YOU KNOW?

Treatments are divided into two categories: treatments for illnesses that arise because of HIV and AIDS, such as pneumonia and diarrhea (for more information about these, go to one of the HIV sites listed on our links page at http://www.tht.org.uk); and treatments that are designed to fight the HIV itself.

TREATMENT AND PROGNOSIS

Since 1996, treatments to fight HIV have come on in leaps and bounds, and the development of new drugs continues. You may have heard the phrase "combination therapy." All this means is that people are given three or four different drugs together, as this is much more effective against HIV than using one drug by itself. Work here is ongoing, and new discoveries are being made all the time.

Although many people have benefited from combination therapy, others have not. Even for those who have found them helpful, the drugs are very difficult to take. They have to be taken at all hours of the day and night; some cannot be taken with certain foods. Resistance to the drugs (when the drugs are no longer effective against HIV) often occurs. It is not known how long any beneficial effects might last, and, most important, the drugs are not a cure. Even people who are feeling better still have HIV and are still infectious.

JEWISH VALUES

Pikuach Nefesh

Pikuach nefesh (the saving of a life) is probably the highest value in Judaism. Lifesaving is, indeed, a *mitzvah* so important that it must be pursued relentlessly, even if other religious mandates have to be set aside. Thus in order to save life we are not merely permitted, we are even obliged to break the Shabbat; our rabbis assert that any act devoted to saving a life is to be prized above all.

The HIV and STD epidemic represents an unparalleled challenge to the Jewish commitment to *pikuach nefesh*. HIV infection and AIDS have made death and dying a reality in the lives of individuals, families, and communities. STDs can cause irreparable damage such as miscarriage, infertility, and ectopic pregnancy. We may feel overwhelmed by the enormity of this epidemic. We feel powerless. What can we do?

We remember the saying, "Prevention is better than cure." *Pikuach nefesh* can be deemed to start from this point. We remember that by preventing the transmission of syphilis we prevent the risk of stillbirth. By preventing the transmission of chlamydia we reduce the risk of ectopic pregnancy, which is life-threatening to both mother and child. And by preventing HIV transmission we reduce the number of those living with an incurable illness.

Educational campaigns are a vital way of informing people about HIV/AIDS and general sexual health. Make this your personal contribution to *pikuach nefesh* by encouraging your friends, relatives, acquaintances, and children to think about safe-sex practices. Truly safe sex means no sexual activity at all, which relates to the Jewish value of *shomer negiah* (no touching) before marriage.

In all sexual relationships outside marriage, "safer sex" must be practiced. Safer sex entails using condoms correctly and ensuring that both you and your partner are tested at a National Health Service Sexual Health (GUM) clinic before engaging in any sexual activity.

If you feel that you are unable or unwilling to become personally involved in such a way, your support for those who are involved is vital. Government provision for sexual health and HIV is inadequate, and voluntary organizations are always hungry for money. A donation to JAT could be your contribution to *pikuach nefesh*.

Shituf Betsa'ar

Jews, in response to the requirement of *shituf betsa'ar* (empathy) are encouraged to make a leap of the imagination so as to place themselves temporarily in the interior world of another person. This is what is meant by the act of empathy.

It is usually easy enough to be aware of and responsive to the feelings of people who resemble ourselves very closely—those with whom we share, for example, characteristics such as age, gender, social class, and so on. When it comes to people who are different from our-selves, empathy becomes much harder. How difficult it can be, for example, simply to enter and respect the interior world of our own child! And the further we move away from people who reflect our-selves and encounter people from alien backgrounds and ways of life, the more we may be tempted to respond to them, not as individuals but as a "type." *Shituf betsa'ar* obliges us to remember always that other person—that sometimes strange and threatening person—is, above all, a person whose individuality is to be prized as much as we would wish him or her to prize our own individuality.

Sometimes, a person living with HIV infection or AIDS can seem very different indeed from ourselves. We wonder if this person may have been unfaithful or may be supporting a drug habit or prosti-tuting themselves. But in the end, he or she is still as much a human being as we are.

Shituf betsa'ar requires us to remember this and to be aware of the additional suffering we may cause by our carelessness, our dis-missive attitudes, and our fear and hatred. It requires us to be sensi-tive to these dynamics and to treat people with HIV/AIDS as we ourselves would wish to be treated if we were in their position.

Chesed Ve'emet

The biblical concept of *chesed ve'emet* (responding with loving-kindness) requires us, as Jews, to respond to our fellow human beings with loving-kindness and truthfulness, or integrity. This obligation has special significance in the worldwide HIV and STD epidemic.

Emet (the principle of truthfulness and integrity) requires us to confront the facts of life, however difficult or painful these may be. And first of all, we must be honest with ourselves. It is dishonest to assert that STDs and HIV are not issues for the Jewish commu-nity. This is to indulge in wishful thinking to the effect that there are no Jewish gays or drug-takers, that heterosexual Jews never have "illegitimate" sexual relationships, or that we are somehow pro-tected from STDs and HIV by our status as God's chosen people. *Emet*—honesty—not only forces us to acknowledge that the real lives of Jewish people can often fall short of Jewish ideals but that "holier than thou" does not mean "healthier than thou." The righteous also suffer, as the Book of Job attests. STDs and HIV are no respecters of religion, or "religiosity," let alone age, sex, race, nationality, or sexual orientation. It is not who you are that puts you at risk from infection. It is what you do.

The principle of *chesed ve'emet* indicates the attitude toward people with STDs and HIV that we, as Jews, ought to adopt. We are required to be humane, compassionate, and caring and to eschew expressions of fear, hatred, condemnation, and disgust. It helps if we can resolve to regard STDs and HIV as illnesses rather than as a disgrace. *Chesed* imposes on us the obligation to treat people with STDs and HIV in precisely the same manner as we would treat people with other illnesses—to ameliorate their suffering, to provide consistent and loving support, and to do all we can to ensure that they are not additionally burdened by individual or social prejudice and discrimination, including our own.

Chesed ve'emet requires us to inspire our society with a perspective on STDs and HIV that reflects the eternal Jewish principles of compassion and truth.

Kol Yisrael Arevim Zeh Bazeh

Kol Yisrael arevim zeh bazeh (each Jew is responsible for every Jew) is a value that Jewish people are taught, and the rabbis also remind us that this *mitzvah* should shape our relations, not only with our fellow Jews but with humanity in general.

In the sexual health context, the principle of mutual responsibility requires two things: (1) an informed awareness about STDs and HIV and (2) informed behavior in the face of the STD and HIV epidemic. Each adult is responsible for making him- or herself aware of up-to-date facts about STD and HIV transmission and treatments. Such information is vital in terms of health education, and it can also be the basis for constructive and meaningful relationships with others.

We are all responsible for our own behavior. The message of "safer sex" stresses the importance of taking responsibility, not only for our own health but also for our partner's. This means that we may have to grapple with our traditional aversion to the use of condoms and ask ourselves whether, in the light of the *mitzvah* of *pikuach nefesh*, their use for the prevention of infection in sexual intercourse can represent responsible behavior in the STD and HIV epidemic.

As adults, we also face a responsibility to our children. As Jews we pride ourselves on the strength of our family lives, and we endeavor to instruct our children in the responsibility of loving relationships.

Now we must also teach them about STDs and HIV, both to protect them and as part of their education as responsible people. Our instruction in this area needs to be calm, dispassionate, and objective, for in this way we convey our regard for our children as responsible young people. If we make it mysterious, anxious, angry, threatening, or guilt-provoking, we run the risk of encouraging disobedience and irresponsibility; too firm a "Thou shalt absolutely not!" often invites the response of "I jolly well shall!"—the last thing we want!

Bikkur Cholim

Bikkur cholim (caring for the sick) is one of the most important obligations in Judaism; indeed, our daily liturgy includes this *mitzvah* on its list of commandments that promise continued reward. It implies, above all, the value of active caring for another person, as opposed merely to the intention to care.

HIV/AIDS can be a particularly isolating condition. Too often, it is accompanied by rejection—by families, friends, and colleagues. But people can be rejected indirectly as well by a family's denial that a person has HIV or AIDS or by the difficulty they experience in speaking about it. Sometimes, feeling scared or ashamed to speak about their condition, people with AIDS isolate themselves. Isolation is further increased by physical helplessness, reduced control over one's own body, and a loss of hope. All these can combine to create a physical and emotional environment in which *bikkur cholim* may be the most significant act of intervention from which a person with AIDS can benefit.

Bikkur cholim demonstrates unmistakably that AIDS has not isolated a person from the circle of his or her own community. Indeed, *bikkur cholim* is an extension of Judaism, for at an important level it represents a declaration of a Jew's obligation to imitate God's caring and compassionate nature.

The *mitzvah* of caring for a person with AIDS can generate feelings of stability and safety. For such a person, as well as for family members, friends, and caring visitors, the dependability of others can often be of vital importance.

As with all *mitzvot*, visiting the sick is not a one-time "good deed." The true reward for performing any *mitzvah* is the opportunity to do another. For the person with AIDS, the ability to rely on *bikkur cholim* as a continuing example of Jewish activism can result in a healing sense of belonging to a unique family: *Am Kedushah*, the Jewish people.

Tikkun Olam

Tikkun olam (repairing the damaged world) is required of Jews. Our Kabbalistic scholars tell us that at the beginning of time, God's presence filled all space with Divine Light. God was everywhere—the sum total of all that existed. But in order for there to be a space in which the creation of the physical universe would occur, it was necessary for God to limit himself. Consequently, he imposed upon himself a contraction or withdrawal in order to leave room for the universe. This process, bathed in Divine Light, resulted in the creation of our world.

But there was a price to be paid for God's beneficence. His Divine Light became fragmented, and its sparks are now scattered throughout the entire universe. The lifelong challenge to each and every individual is to gather these sparks together once again (*tikkum olam*) so that the Divine Light can be reunited.

Tikkun olam thus obliges Jews to repair our evidently imperfect world. But what does this mean in the context of HIV infection and AIDS? In fact, the AIDS epidemic presents us with a particularly demanding agenda. Perfection of the world must certainly include both the endeavor to make ourselves and our institutions as perfect, which means as compassionate and humane, as possible. Where there is ignorance, we are required to bring enlightenment. Where there is hatred or fear, we are obliged to bring love and courage. Where there is suffering and pain, we are required to bring relief.

HIV/AIDS is a stigmatized condition and, in many parts of the world, a death sentence. It becomes essential for Jews, in accordance with the obligation of *tikkun olam*, to take a leading role in advocating the legal, economic, occupational, and social rights of people with AIDS and those diagnosed with HIV infection, and to combat efforts to remove these rights.

The Jewish AIDS Trust

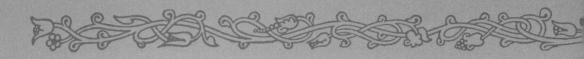

Chapter 74

AIDS: A Jewish Perspective

The spread of the virus, responsible for the dreaded and invariably fatal illness of AIDS, is one of the most serious public health crises of the century. Originally limited in the West to homosexuals and intravenous drug users, HIV has now spread to the heterosexual population as well. The proliferation of AIDS raises a host of legal and ethical questions and, as is true for all the pressing issues of the day, Judaism offers valuable insights and perspectives.

At the outset, one possible misconception must be dispelled. The argument is sometimes made that because AIDS is spread by conduct that both Judaism and Christianity regard as immoral, society should not be overly concerned. Let the sinners suffer the consequences of their sin.

This is an utterly fallacious argument for two reasons.

First, as noted, increasing numbers of people contract AIDS without engaging in homosexual activity or drug use. Many have contracted the disease from blood transfusions (particularly in the early 1980s, when blood screening was less developed); babies have contracted the virus in utero from their mother's placenta; at least some health care professionals have been infected from AIDS-carrying patients, and even some patients from health care workers (Kimberly Bergalis died of AIDS in 1989 after allegedly being infected with HIV by her dentist). Needless to say, the innocent, unknowing sexual partners of persons who contracted AIDS are at risk as well. The belief that AIDS only strikes "sinners" is simply false.

Second, the "sinner" argument is premised on a fundamental misconception. Even if every single case of AIDS were the product of sinful misconduct (which is decidedly not the case), this would in no way minimize our duty to alleviate illness, pain, and suffering. Any case of sickness, whether AIDS, cancer, or heart disease, may or may not be a divine punishment, but that is God's business, not ours. The Torah requires that we not stand by idly while others suffer, and this obligation extends to those who follow the Torah as well as those who do not. The Talmud in Tractate *Brachos* recounts that Rabbi Meir was once being persecuted by evil men and as a result prayed for their demise. His learned wife, Bruriah, rebuked him, citing the verse in Psalms where King David declares, "Let *sin* perish from the earth"—*sin*, not *sinners*. Rather than hope that sinners will die, one should pray that they will repent and see the light. This is exactly the attitude we must take in aggressively combating this fatal disease.

With regard to specific issues, one of the most controversial aspects in this area concerns proposals for mandatory AIDS testing for high-risk groups and disclosure of the results of that testing to past and present sexual partners. On one level, AIDS patients have an understandable desire to keep their status confidential. Disclosure could result in serious discrimination, loss of employment, termination of insurance (although illegal), eviction from housing, and severe social ostracism. At the same time, however, if the HIV-positive patient refuses to make disclosure on his or her own, innocent persons are put at great risk. Consider the HIV-positive patient who informs his physician, "I'm going to die anyway so I want to have a good time as long as I can. I refuse to abstain from sex, and I prohibit your disclosing my status to anyone." Or what if the patient is more subtle and doesn't openly declare that he will attempt to keep his status secret but the physician suspects that this is the case?

Halakhah normally accords great respect to confidentiality, even outside of the particular context of the doctor-patient relationship.

This is called *loshon hora* (evil speech) and puts severe constraints on even "harmless" social gossip. Nevertheless, the prohibitions of *loshon hora* are not absolute. Disclosure of negative information is permitted, and even halakhically required, if necessary to prevent physical, financial, or emotional harm to a third person. For example, if you plan to enter a business partnership with someone who I know is a convicted embezzler, I may (and must) inform you of that fact, notwithstanding the law of *loshon hora*. If a woman is about

DID YOU KNOW?

It is prohibited under Torah law to ever disclose derogatory or embarrassing information about one person to another, even if that information is true, unless very specific conditions are met.

to marry a man who has a history of psychiatric problems and abuse, disclosure is mandatory. Halakhah says I may not exaggerate. I may not state as fact that which I have heard only as rumor. I may not disclose the information to those who have no pressing need to know it. But confidentiality must yield when innocent third parties are put at serious risk. *A fortiori*, this consideration would apply to AIDS cases when nondisclosure may result in death, not merely financial loss. Halakhah would thus appear to support both compulsory testing and mandatory disclosure, at least on a need-to-know basis.

The matter becomes more complicated, however, when we consider long-range effects, as opposed to immediate short-term benefits. Many public health experts have argued that any policy that undermines confidentiality will result in fewer people being tested. (Even mandatory testing can be skirted. After all, how would the government be able to identify all homosexuals?) Consider a person who would be willing to submit to AIDS testing if the results of the testing were to be kept absolutely confidential. If such guarantees were forthcoming, such a person would come forward and be tested. If the results were positive, he could receive AZT treatments and may very well decide, on a voluntary basis, to disclose his status to past or present sexual partners or, at the very least, practice safe sex with a condom. If, on the other hand, confidentiality is not absolute, some persons would simply refuse to be tested at all. As a result, they would be deprived of early treatment opportunities and would continue to spread the virus unknowingly until such time as the AIDS symptoms become apparent. Thus some medical ethicists argue that confidentiality must be respected, *even at the expense of a particular person's life* because, in the long run, such a stance will save many more lives in the future.

The dilemma this issue poses is similar to one that reputedly confronted Winston Churchill during World War II. British intelligence had broken some German codes that indicated that the Nazis were going to firebomb the town of Coventry. Were Coventry to be evacuated, however, the Germans would realize that the codes were cracked and would have them changed. As a result, allied forces would have lost an invaluable source of information, possibly endangering the entire war effort and placing countless future lives in jeopardy. Should ten thousand specific and identifiable people be allowed to die in order to prevent the *possible* loss of thousands of unidentified future victims? Churchill answered in the affirmative.

This heart-wrenching dilemma is at the heart of the confidentiality debate. Space precludes a full consideration of this problem, but Rabbi J. David Bleich, a leading scholar, concludes that if it, indeed, can be established that greater confidentiality will, in the long run, promote the saving of lives (and he emphasizes that this has not been empirically established), halakhah would permit the consideration of the long term, even at the expense of the immediate victim.

Here are some other halakhic issues:

Use of condoms. Although Jewish law generally frowns on the use of condoms as a contraceptive, it would permit their use as a means to prevent the spread of a life-threatening illness. The Torah would not require an AIDS patient to practice lifetime abstinence. Whether condoms should be openly distributed to students in schools is a more difficult issue. Obviously, Judaism believes that sex should take place within the framework of a loving and committed marriage and frowns on any efforts that would openly legitimize alternative lifestyles and premarital affairs. At the same time, if adolescents are going to be sexually active, they should be aware of precautionary steps. The school must walk the tightrope of affirming abstinence and responsibility as the desired norms but making condoms available as a far distant second-best—an evil that is the lesser of two evils.

Physician endangerment. Under Jewish law, even a physician is not obligated to put his life in danger in treating patients with an infectious disease, though it is an act of piety to do so. Nevertheless, where the risks are relatively minimal or are no greater than those the physician customarily incurs for his own benefit (driving on the highway, piloting a plane), the physician may not shirk his duty by invoking the specter of an illusory danger. This is especially so when reasonable precautions can virtually eliminate the danger. In any event, even where a physician may morally refuse to treat high-risk patients, a hospital, as a legitimate incentive to encourage treatment, may deny staff privileges to any health care provider who refuses to treat admitted patients. (Whether this would be true for a physician who refused to perform abortions is another matter.)

Mikveh, tahara, milah. The AIDS virus does not survive in water, so there would be no reason to deny AIDS patients the use of the ritual bath (*mikveh*). Similarly, while members of the *Chevra Kadisha* (Burial Society) could conceivably contract HIV from the body fluids of the corpse that they are washing, if they are wearing gloves the risks are virtually nil. Unlike the case in surgery, there are no needles or sharp objects that can puncture the gloves. The consensus of most authorities is, therefore, that a *tahara* (ritual cleansing) should be performed. A final concern involves circumcision (*brit milah*). In the Orthodox rite, after making the incision, the *mohel* actually sucks the wound to draw out blood and promote clotting. Because babies can acquire the virus through their mothers, this creates a risk for the *mohel*. The AIDS virus, however, cannot survive a solution of 75 percent alcohol, so a quick swishing of 150-proof rum prior to the sucking will avoid all problems.

A final point: although we must relate to all victims of illness with concern and compassion and have no right to reject persons who need our assistance, it cannot be denied that God is trying to give us a message—a message that society refuses to learn. An illness that became virulent and rampant because of homosexuality and drug use (although presently not limited to those categories) is a vivid reminder that society cannot indefinitely engage in immorality with impunity. The breakdown of values carries serious costs, including the deaths of innocent victims. Our culture of moral relativism, situational ethics, sexual freedom, hedonistic materialism, and family breakdown brings in its wake tragic dimensions of crime, misery, and suffering. If we address AIDS exclusively as a medical problem, we are missing the boat. God has given us an early warning detection system to put our spiritual house in order. Let us be responsive to his call.

GAYS IN THE MILITARY

Judaism does not support discrimination against persons merely because they are homosexual or engage in homosexual activity. After all, the Torah requires that Jews observe the Shabbat and eat kosher, yet no one suggests that, even in a halakhic society, non–Shomer Shabbat persons should be denied employment. Essentially, in the absence of a temple or a Sanhedrin (high court of seventy-one rabbis), the level of a person's religious commitment is a matter between that person and God; it is not the business of the state. Even religious teachers are supposed to instruct, enlighten, and encourage but not coerce or persecute.

A similar approach should be taken with gays in the military. Sexual orientation or preference should simply be nobody's business. The question of sexual orientation should be dropped. Obviously, heterosexuals should not be forced to witness homosexual activity nor should the government make any statement putting its imprimatur on such activity. Provided, however, that such activity is private and nonintrusive, it is nobody's concern but God's and is essentially as irrelevant (for military duty) as one's level of kashrut observance.

Rabbi Yitzchok Breitowitz

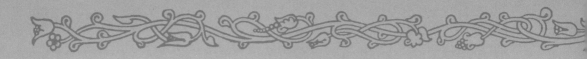

Chapter 75

Smoking: Is It Kosher?

Studies have linked smoking to a variety of illnesses, including heart disease, lung cancer, emphysema, and bronchial disorders. The health risks that smoking presents pose a halakhic question: Does halakhah permit smoking?

In Judaism, health is a religious concern. Maimonides notes that a sound mind requires a sound body, and for this reason it is a religious obligation to take care of one's health (Deuteronomy 4:1). There are many halakhic regulations enacted for health purposes (see *Shulchan Aruch* YD 116). In general, health regulations are treated with greater stringency than any other section of halakhah (*Hullin* 9b).

Although health and safety are halakhic obligations, it does not mean that every health and safety risk are prohibited. It is normal for people to accept certain safety risks in the course of their regular activities. Regular activities such as driving, flying in a plane, or giving birth to a child entail some risk. What needs to be determined is which risks are considered to be halakhically acceptable and which are not.

The crucial text for determining the criterion of acceptable risk is found in *Yebamot* 72a. The Talmud states, in the name of Rav Papa, that even though there is an obligation to avoid danger, when many people ignore a specific type of health hazard, it is halakhically permitted to ignore it because "the Lord watches the simple" (Psalms 116:6). There are several interpretations of Rav Papa's statement. To some, this means that even a demonstrated health hazard may be ignored if most people ignore it as well (*Ritva*, s.v. "*Shomer*"). This interpretation sees acceptable risk as subjective and socially determined: I cannot be more reckless than most other people in my society. One can conclude that, according to this view, if large groups of people ignore the health risks of smoking, it is not halakhically prohibited.

A different interpretation is offered by Rabbi Yaakov Etlinger (*Binyan Zion* 137). He explains that there is a difference between behavior that presents an immediate danger and behavior that may present a future danger. An action that presents immediate danger, such as entering a burning building, is prohibited. Something that may turn dangerous in the future, such as a long boat trip, is allowed because "the Lord watches the simple." Some argue that, according to Ettlinger's opinion, smoking, which does not present immediate danger to the smoker, would be permitted.

Others take a different view of the text. They say the dispensation of "the Lord watches the simple" only refers to cases where the danger is extremely small (*Achiezer* 1:23:2) or cases where the danger is "well known," but there is no empirical, scientific evidence to substantiate it (*Tzitz Eliezer* 15:39; cf. *Beit Yoseph* YD 262). According to this interpretation, any scientifically demonstrated health hazard is absolutely prohibited. Because of this, Rabbi Eliezer Waldenberg prohibited smoking, saying that there is unambiguous scientific evidence that cigarette smoking is dangerous. Rabbi Waldenberg says those who do smoke must make every effort to quit smoking.

More controversial is the view of Rabbi Moshe Feinstein (*Iggrot* CM II:76; dated June 10, 1981). While Rabbi Feinstein strongly discourages smoking, he writes that since many people who smoke do not suffer any health problems, and most who smoke are not endangered by it, one may say that smoking is permitted because "the Lord watches the simple." Due to Rabbi Feinstein's authority, many rabbis are loath to prohibit smoking. However, a ruling by the Rabbinical Council of America (available at http://www.rabbis.org/publications/smoking.pdf), which Rabbi Feinstein's son-in-law, Rabbi Moshe Tendler, coauthored, argues that in light of recent studies demonstrating the widespread danger cigarette smoking presents and the fact that there are considerably fewer smokers today, Rabbi Feinstein would today reverse his position and prohibit smoking.[1]

Like many questions in halakhah, there is more than one opinion as to whether smoking is permitted or prohibited. However, all authorities agree that taking good care of one's health is an important religious value and may not be overlooked.

✑ *Rabbi Chaim Steinmetz*

Note

1. Although, based on the published opinion just cited, Rabbi Moshe Feinstein did not prohibit individuals from smoking, it should be noted that in a letter to Rabbi Reuven Sofer dated *Tishrei* 5741, Rabbi Moshe specifically prohibited smoking in a *bet midrash* (study hall) and other public places where objections to smoking are raised. See generally *Smoking and Damage to Health in the Halachah*, by Rabbi Menachem Slae (Acharai Publications, 1990), pp. 53–56, which reprints the letter in its entirety. In a relevant part, Rabbi Moshe writes: "It is prohibited for smokers to smoke in the study hall if even one person is present who is discomforted from it, even if he is not injured and made ill, certainly if the possibility of illness and injury exists, even if the time lost from Torah study would be greater if the smokers would be prohibited from smoking, as the smokers are forbidden to smoke in the study hall and in any place (in general) where non-smokers are found who protest that the [smoke] injures them, or even if the smoke discomforts them."

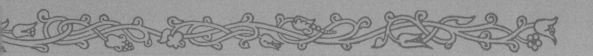

Chapter 76

Smoking: The Rabbinical Council of America Roundtable's Proposal

The Rabbinical Council of America's proposal can be summarized as follows:

1. Since it is an established fact that all tobacco smoke constitutes a definite and immediate danger to one's health, such activity is in violation of the Torah's injunction against harming oneself.
2. Since scientific research has shown passive smoking by those in the presence of nonsmokers to be equally dangerous, it constitutes a public danger and assault (*habalah*). Therefore, smoking must be banned in all public arenas such as synagogues, schools, *mikva'ot*, and all public functions.
3. Those who choose to continue smoking rely on *shomer peta'im hashem*. In light of contemporary medical knowledge, this idea no longer obtains.

Over the course of the past twenty-five years, it has become increasingly clear that the smoking (or ingesting) of tobacco constitutes a serious, inevitable danger to the user. The ingesting of tobacco smoke has been intrinsically linked to heart disease, stroke, lung cancer, pancreatic cancer, and dozens of other fatal and potentially fatal illnesses.[1]

Indeed, at present, it is the overwhelming opinion of the medical research community that tobacco smoke in any amount will render immediate damage to the human physiology.[2] Over the course of the past sixteen years, it has also been conclusively demonstrated that nonsmokers who inhale the smoke of other people's cigarettes are at real and significant risk of contracting the very same illnesses as the smokers themselves.[3] In recognition of this fact, an increasingly large number of governments and government agencies have banned smoking in the presence of or in proximity to nonsmokers, out of concern for the health rights of the latter. In light of this situation, it is both relevant and urgent that the halakhic dimensions of this question be reexamined.

PASSIVE SMOKE

It is axiomatic, according to Torah law, that one individual is not allowed to harm another. This point is discussed extensively in the Gemara[4] and summed up in the *Shulchan Aruch* as follows:[5] "It is forbidden for one man to strike his fellow, and if he does so, he violates a negative commandment" (Deuteronomy 25:3).[6]

And if the Torah was strict with regard to the striking of the wicked, *a fortiori* regarding the striking of the righteous, and he who raises his hand to strike his fellow, even though he does not do so, he is deemed to be a wicked person. In light of the already-cited scientific evidence, it is clear that the infliction of injury on another party by means of tobacco smoke constitutes assault. Indeed, even prior to the publication of the lion's share of the scientific evidence concerning "passive smoke," the great Rabbi Moshe Feinstein asserted that people harmed by the smoke of others were empowered by halakhah to sue for damages. As he himself wrote:[7]

> But the matter (i.e. the legal implications of "passive smoke") are far worse, since smokers actually commit assault. . . .And it is obvious that were the courts competent to adjudicate torts,[8] they would be empowered to enforce collection of their estimate of the suffering caused [by the smoke], and if [the complainant] had become ill therefrom, he would be entitled to compensation of medical expenses, even if he had not incurred direct damages due to absence from his employment.[9]

It might be objected, though, that such a conclusion is only germane when the damage done by environmental tobacco smoke (ETS) is substantial enough to warrant suit for damages. This, however, can hardly be the case in a short period of exposure to someone's smoke on an ad hoc basis.

Such a conclusion, however, cannot be maintained. For independent of the possibility of incurring financial damages, assault constitutes a forbidden action, according to the Torah, irrespective of whether there is significant damage inflicted or not.[10] The point is summed up in the *Shulchan Aruch*:[11] "If he struck his fellow with a blow which inflicted damage less than the value of a penny, receives stripes (*malkot*) [as punishment], since no monetary obligation is incurred thereby."

Because, as already noted, temporary exposure to ETS has immediate, deleterious effects on one's health, it is clear that it is forbidden to allow smoking in the presence of nonsmokers, even on a short-term basis. What is more, in light of the immediate effects of ETS on the physiology of the nonsmoker, it seems clear that even if he or she is not immediately irritated thereby, that he may not forgo his prerogative and allow another person to smoke (*mehilah*).[12] This is due to the well-known fact that an individual is not allowed to harm himself.[13]

Finally, the upshot of several key rulings in halakhic literature makes it clear that preventing the generation of ETS and its attendant damage to the health of those who inhale it is not simply the responsibility of the smoker and the nonsmoker but rather that of the community generally, and especially that of the court (*Bet Din*). For example, Rambam writes[14] that over and beyond the obligation to erect a fence around one's roof (*ma'akeh*),[15] the sages forbade many things that are injurious to one's health, "and anyone who violates them and says, 'I will place myself in danger and what business is it of other people [should I do so],' one inflicts him with 'Stripes of Rebelliousness' (*Makkot Mardut*)."

Upon this passage the *Aruch HaShulchan* comments that the Rambam does not intend to imply that since the punishment is rabbinic in nature, so is the crime. "For certainly this involves the violation of a Torah prohibition, it is only that one cannot receive normal stripes (*malkot*) for it, just as there are many Torah prohibitions for the violation of which no *malkot* are administered."[16]

And the Yaffe LaLev[17] adds that not only is the crime of injuring oneself punishable, this fact plainly establishes that it is the obligation of the court to ensure that such behavior is not pursued.[18] In light of all that's been said, it is clear that rabbis and communities are obliged by halakhah to ban smoking at all functions and meetings, buildings and facilities under their jurisdiction, pursuant to the sacred trust to secure the observance of Torah law and to protect the physical and spiritual welfare of their members.[19]

ACTIVE SMOKING

Based on the presentation here, it ought to be equally apparent that if ETS is forbidden according to halakhah, owing to its not only being a nuisance but actually constituting an immediate danger, the same must be said *a fortiori* of active smoking.[20] And indeed, this is the published opinion of both Rabbi Hayyim David HaLevi, the Sephardic Chief Rabbi of Tel Aviv,[21] and of Rabbi Eliezer Waldenberg,[22] both of whom are outstanding contemporary halakhic authorities. They both base themselves on the prohibition against harming oneself and on the explicit statement of the Rambam that the rabbis have the authority to ban any action that harms one's health.[23]

The one authority who consistently refused to prohibit "active smoking" per se, was the late Posek HaDor, Rabbi Moshe Feinstein. Although he strongly urged people to stop smoking and discouraged others from developing the habit,[24] he held tenaciously to the position that smoking could not be banned on purely halakhic grounds. In light of the preeminent position occupied by Rabbi Feinstein, any proposal to ban smoking on purely halakhic grounds must perforce address his objections thereto.

Rabbi Feinstein heavily based his inability to forbid smoking on the argument that when a specific action possibly entails an element of danger, and people are willing to take that risk (which albeit is only a risk), one cannot forbid people from that action for "the Lord protects the Simple" (*Makom SheDashu Bo Rabim, Shomer Peta'im HaShem*).[25] As he wrote in his last responsum on the subject:[26]

> To generalize the principle of "the Lord protects the Simple" which appears in Shabbat (129b) and in Niddah (45a) relates to two cases

where there is some risk of danger and [nevertheless] people are not careful [avoid them], though it certainly is true that in an average case of possible danger it is forbidden to rely on this principle . . . [nevertheless] it appears obvious that as regards something which does not entail any negative effects upon the health of a large number of people . . . even though it does exert harm upon a distinct minority, there is still no prohibition to eat them[27] as per the possible danger involved, since the majority are not harmed therefrom. . . . And cigarette smoking is akin to such things, since those who are accustomed to smoke enjoy it very much, and suffer from the lack of cigarettes more than the lack of certain types of good food, and even more than total food deprivation for an abbreviated amount of time. [What is more] the danger (*kilkul*) of becoming ill from this is in any case very small, *a fortiori* is the possibility of developing cancer and other life threatening illnesses exceedingly small . . . and in a risk like this one applies the rule, "the Lord protects the Simple."

The upshot of Rabbi Feinstein's presentation is that the rule of *shomer peta'im hashem* (the Lord protects the simple) applies when two conditions are present: (1) the activity in question only presents a possible danger to the individual, and (2) most people are willing to take the risk involved in pursuing that activity. At the time that Rabbi Feinstein wrote this responsum, both of these factors seemed to indicate halakhic license to smoke. Today, however, in light of the scientific evidence published in the decade since this responsum was written and based on Rabbi Feinstein's explicit definition, it is clear that neither of these considerations obtains any longer. First, the danger involved in smoking is not merely possible; it is inevitable. And although death from lung cancer may well only affect a minority of smokers, damage to the cardiovascular and pulmonary systems is immediate and inevitable. Thus we have entered into a situation in which smoking is a definite danger (*bari hezeka*).[28]

Similar conclusions may be reached regarding the second element in Rabbi Feinstein's equation, that is, the willingness of people to take the risk involved in smoking. Here there seems to have occurred a substantive change. Over the past ten years a large antismoking educational effort has been undertaken by the American Cancer Society and the Office of the Surgeon General of the United

States. The results of this campaign have been that large numbers of people have stopped smoking, while others have not cultivated the habit because of the risks involved. Clearly, then, smoking is no longer a *Davar SheDashu Bo Rabim*.[29] Each of these considerations, taken both separately and together, leads us to one ineluctable conclusion, namely, that based on present research and the stated argument of Rabbi Moshe Feinstein, the smoking of cigarettes constitutes a blatant violation of the Torah's commandment against inflicting harm on oneself and hence is absolutely prohibited according to Jewish law.[30]

CONCLUSIONS

As a result of our discussion here it is apparent that definite action must be taken in order to eradicate smoking from the Orthodox community. This is called for both out of consideration for the health of the smoker, as well as that of the innocent bystander assaulted and harmed by the smoke he generates. In both instances, the community (as represented by the Rabbinate and Batei Din) are responsible for the enforcement of halakhic norms regulating the general welfare. As practical steps toward the realization of a smoke-free community, we recommend that our colleagues take the following steps:

1. Smoking should be banned from all synagogues, synagogue functions, day schools, *mikva'ot,* and all other institutions and events under the supervision of the rabbi.
2. Rabbis should themselves cease to smoke and should publicly educate their congregations as to the medical and halakhic severity of smoking. This should include not tolerating smoking in their own homes and businesses, as this either facilitates or causes assault on others.
3. It must be pointed out that had the present-day research been available, scholars of previous generations who themselves smoked would not have sanctioned this conduct.

Rabbi Jeffrey R. Woolf, Rabbi Reuven Bulka, Rabbi Saul J. Berman, and Rabbi Daniel Landes, for the Rabbinical Council of America

Notes

1. S. A. Glantz and W. W. Parmley, "Passive Smoking and Heart Disease: Epidemiology, Physiology, and Biochemistry," *Circulation*, 1991, *83*, 1. (Thanks to Dr. Fred Rosner for providing us with the periodical literature behind this topic.)

2. Ibid., pp. 1, 4–5.

3. Ibid., pp. 1–12. See also J. Fielding, and K. J. Phenow, "Health Effects of Involuntary Smoking," *New England Journal of Medicine*, 1988, *319*, 1452–1460; M. R. Masjedi, H. Kazemi, and D. C. Johnson, "Effects of Passive Smoking on the Pulmonary Function of Adults," *Thorax*, 1990, *45*, 27–31; G. H. Miller, "The Impact of Passive Smoking: Cancer Deaths Among Non-Smoking Women," *Cancer*, 1990, *14*, 497–503; C. Humble and others, "Passive Smoking and Twenty-Year Cardiovascular Disease Mortality Among Non-Smoking Wives in Evans County, Georgia," *American Journal of Public Health*, 1990, *80*, 599–601; D. Janerich and others, "Lung Cancer and Exposure to Tobacco Smoke in the Household," *New England Journal of Medicine*, 1990, *323*, 632–636; S. D. Woodward and M. H. Winstanley, "Lung Cancer and Passive Smoking at Work: The Carroll Case," *Medical Journal of Australia*, 1990, *153*, 682–684.

4. *Baba Kamma* 91a–91b.

5. *Shulchan Aruch, Hoshen Mishpat* 420: 1. In an edifying pamphlet on the subject of smoking, Rabbi Menachem Slae enumerates no less than thirty-six commandments (both positive and negative) that are violated by smoking. Among these are the commandments: (1) not to murder, (2) causing injury to a fellow Jew, (3) not to curse one's fellow Jew, (4) not to lead one's fellow astray (*lifnei iver*), (5) desecration of God's name, (6) wanton destruction (*Bal Tashchit*), and (7) not to eat nonkosher food. See M. Slae, *Smoking and Damage to Health in the Halachah* (Jerusalem: Acharai Publications, 1990), pp. 26–33.

6. The Torah (Deuteronomy 25:3) sets a limit to the number of stripes a convicted criminal may receive. If the person administering them exceeds this number, he is himself liable for assault and the damages incurred thereby. See *Sanhedrin* 85a and *Ketubot* 36a.

7. Resp. *Iggerot Moshe, Hoshen Mishpat*, II, no. 76.

8. Contemporary rabbinical courts cannot address questions of criminal tort, as they lack the required level of rabbinic ordination (*semicha*). See *Shulchan Aruch, Hoshen Mishpat*, I:I and commentaries, ad loc.

9. Rabbi Feinstein underscores the immanency of the legal obligation engendered by damage due to ETS by noting a fundamental distinction

between torts (*habalot*) and fines (*kenasot*), even though adjudication of both requires a court possessed of full rabbinic ordination (*mumhim semuchim*). In the latter case, says Rabbi Feinstein, no liability exists for the accused, even where it is patently clear that were a competent court extant, he would be adjudged responsible for the fines in question. This is because in the case of *kenasot*, it is the court that not only collects the fine but also creates the obligation to pay via its rendering of judgment.

The instance of torts, however, is different. Here, it is the action of the defendant that generates the obligation to pay. The court merely clarifies the obligation and enforces it. In other words, the role of a court of *semuchim* is essential in the case of fines and a technicality in the case of torts. The difference, Rabbi Feinstein concludes, is in the instance of whether the defendant might be morally obliged to pay (*LaTzeit Yedei Shamayim*). In the case of torts, where a mere technicality prevents the collection of damages by the plaintiff, there is an obligation to pay. In the case of fines, however, since no competent court ever created the obligation to pay, no supererogatory requirement exists either. (Cf. *Baba Metzia* 91a; *Rashi*, ad loc, s.v.; *Rava; Tos.*, ad loc, s.v. *B'va*, and the important discussion in *Ketzot HaHoshen* 28:1.)

10. See the discussion in *Encyclopedia Tamudit*, XII, Jerusalem, 1978, pp. 679–746, s.v. *Hovel*.

11. *Hoshen Mishpat*, Sec. 420: 2. See also *Aruch HaShulchan*, op. cit., par. 3.

12. Earlier discussions of the question whether the nonsmoker had the right to waive his prerogatives were based on the assumption that smoking was merely an irritant, or only harmful in the long run. See *Tzitz Eliezer*, op. cit., and the discussion by Rabbi Y. Grubner, *Kunteres B'Issur Ishun, HaDarom* , 1984, 53, 71–83.

13. *Hoshen Mishpat*, op. cit., par. 21 and *Aruch HaShulchan*, op. cit., par. 43. Both are based on the discussion in *Baba Kamma* 90b. In his formulation, the Rambam makes it clear that the prohibition against injuring oneself is of equal force as that against hurting one's fellow (*Hil. Hovel u'Mazik* v:1). A similar position is adopted by the Rashba (*Responsa* I:616) and the *Rosh on Baba Kamma* (VIII:13). Others, however, assume that the prohibition is rabbinic in origin (for example, *Bet HaBehirah L'Baba Kamma*, ad loc). See Slae, p. 14 no. 24. This is a decidedly minority opinion, both in terms of the number and stature of those who espouse it.

14. *Hil. Rotze'ah U'Shmirat Nefesh*, XI: 4–5.

15. See *Sefer HaHinnukh*, nos. 538 and 567.

16. *Aruch HaShulchan, Hoshen Mishpat*, sec. 427 par. 8. Rabbi Moshe Feinstein, however, takes pointed exception to this interpretation of the Rambam and argues that the Rambam simply means to exhort people to abandon potentially deleterious habits and not to prohibit them outright. He does not, however, explain why the Rambam allows stripes to be administered.

17. Cited by Slae, p. 16, no. 42.

18. Of course this is besides the general obligation of the community to secure the general welfare and to rebuke those who violate the norms of the Torah.

19. Confirmation of the propriety of such action is found in the fact that such action was specifically and emphatically advocated by Rabbi Eliezer Waldenberg (see note 20). Similar actions have been undertaken by the Lubavitcher Rebbe, Rabbi M. M. Schneerson, the Gerer Rebbe, and the Rosh Yeshivah of the Ponevez Yeshivah, Rabbi Eliezer Menahem Shach. The positions of the former two authorities were published in Rabbi Y. Grubner (see note 11), pp. 80–83. Rav Shach's order that banned smoking, which appeared in the *Bet Midrash of Ponevez*, was published with an explanatory cover letter in Slae, op. cit., pp. 58–61.

20. Another issue related to the impact of smoking is its effect on the fetus during pregnancy. See the discussion in Slae, chap. 3.

21. *JTA Daily News Bulletin*, Nov. 28, 1976.

22. Resp. *Tzitz Eliezer*, XV, no. 39.

23. *Hil. Rotze'ah U'Shmirat Nefesh*, XI: 5.

24. At the conclusion of one responsum (*Iggerot Moshe, Hoshen Mishpat*, II, no. 76), Rabbi Feinstein writes that "it is nevertheless appropriate for every person, especially Bnai Torah, not to smoke, since it presents a potential danger to life (*Hashash Sakkanah*) and has no redeeming value." (See the remarks of Dr. Fred Rosner in the *Journal of Halachah and Contemporary Society*, 1990, *20*, 61–63.) A similar position was advocated quite strongly by Rabbi J. David Bleich in his "Survey of Recent Halakhic Periodical Literature," *Tradition*, 1976–1977, *16*, 121–123.

25. The concept is discussed in *Shabbat* 129b, *Yevamot* 72a, and *Niddah* 31a. See the extensive discussion by Rabbi Grubner (op. cit., pp. 73–77). Rabbi Moshe David Tendler is listed in the exact formulation of this phrase.

26. *Iggerot Moshe* (ibid.). The responsum is dated 8 *Sivan* 5741 (June 10, 1981).

27. Rabbi Feinstein is referring specifically to certain types of food that can harm the health of some people.

28. Similar conclusions were offered earlier by Rabbi Waldenberg (ibid.); Rabbi M. Halperin (in *Assia*, 1986, *5*, pp. 244ff.), and Rabbi Reuven Bulka (in *Proceedings of the World Conference on Smoking and Health*, Winnipeg, Canada, 1983).

29. This observation was originally made to us by Rabbi Moshe Tendler. This conclusion does not seek to ignore the large number of people who continue to smoke. At the same time, it appears to us that this population is no longer determinative. First, the issue of *Dashu Bo Rabim* is a question of societal sensitivity and not absolute numbers. Second, it is difficult to assess the element of free will involved in "taking the risk" in light of all that we know concerning the nature of nicotine addiction and the addictive personality. As a side issue, which transcends our discussion here, one might be moved to wonder whether, at present, offering a match to a smoker might not be a violation of *Lifn Iver Lo Toiten Mikhshol* or at least of being *Mesaye'a Yedei Ovrei Averah*. Also it would seem reasonable that synagogues ought no longer leave candles burning in their kitchens on Yom Tov, since in light of contemporary social realities, smoking is no longer a *Davar HaShaveh L'Chol Nefesh* and hence constitutes a prohibited activity (*melacha*) on Yom Tov.

30. This line of argument effectively removes Rabbi Bleich's objections to a purely halakhic ban on smoking as well (see note 23).

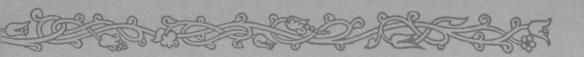

Chapter 77

Smoking: A Jewish Perspective

May an observant Conservative Jew continue to smoke cigarettes, in view of the fact that cigarette smoking is dangerous to one's health?

"The Surgeon General Has Determined that Cigarette Smoking is Dangerous to Your Health" is a notice that confronts us wherever we go. It is prominently displayed on all cigarette advertisements. It is printed on every package of cigarettes. It is repeated on radio and television. Nevertheless, the smoking of cigarettes continues here and abroad. Judaism expresses attitudes and values that are relevant to the question of cigarette smoking. There are definite directives about substances that are "dangerous to your health."

THE PRESERVATION OF HEALTH IS A *MITZVAH*

It is important, first of all, to explain the biblical attitude toward the maintenance of our own health. The basic attitude is expressed in Deuteronomy 4:15: "Take good care of your lives." This reflects the understanding basic to all biblical faiths—that life is a gift, a privilege

This chapter was written by the late Rabbi Seymour Siegel, who was the Ralph Simon Professor of Ethics and Theology at the Jewish Theological Seminary of America and for many years chaired the Committee on Jewish Law and Standards (CJLS). It is reprinted here with the permission of the Rabbinical Assembly. The CJLS is composed of members of the Rabbinical Assembly and the United Synagogue of Conservative Judaism and is responsible for the halakhic policies and decision making of the Conservative movement.

given to us by the Creator. This means that we are bidden to guard, preserve, and enhance our lives and the lives of others. To neglect our health—to willfully do something that can harm us—is not only to court disaster for ourselves but is also an affront to the One who gave us life. Therefore, the preservation of health is a *mitzvah*.

This idea is expressed most concisely by Moses Maimonides (1135–1204), who is considered one of history's greatest physicians. Maimonides is accepted as one of Judaism's greatest scholars. Maimonides' legal code is called *Yad haHazakah* (the Strong Hand). In the section dealing with "Murder and the Guarding of Life" he writes:

> It is a positive commandment to remove any stumbling block which constitutes a danger and to be on guard against it. The sages have prohibited many things because they endanger one's life. If one disregards any of them and says, "I am only endangering myself, what business do others have with me; or I don't care [if they are dangerous], I use them (that is, harmful things)," he can be subjected to disciplinary flogging.[1]

Maimonides reflects the Judaic ethos that sees life as not being the exclusive possession of the individual. A person must avoid harm to self and must also avoid being a source of harm to others. One should not feel that if self-inflicted harm affects oneself, it is of no concern to the community. We are all part of each other. The community has a stake in the well-being of the community. Both the community and the individual have responsibilities to the Creator. Life is too precious deliberately to expose it to dangerous and harmful effects.

DANGER TO LIFE IS STRICTER THAN A PROHIBITION

The Talmud states that a person is not permitted to wound himself.[2] The rabbis derive this law from the biblical admonition that sees the Nazarite who voluntarily deprives himself of the legitimate goods of the world as a sinner. They reason if a person who deprives himself

> ### From the Sources
>
> The classical writer Rabbi Moses Isserles (1525–1572), whose notes on the *Shulchan Aruch* are seen as binding, writes: "one should avoid all things that might lead to danger because a danger to life is stricter than a prohibition. One should be more concerned about a possible danger to life than a possible prohibition. . . . And it is prohibited to rely on a miracle or to put one's life in danger."[3]

of wine is considered in a bad light, certainly one who causes himself to suffer (by bodily harm) is culpable in God's eye.

The concept that Rabbi Isserles expounds ("a danger to life is stricter than a prohibition. . . . One should be more concerned about a possible danger to life than [about a] prohibition") is of special importance. Judaism exhorts the Jew to be careful in avoiding anything that might be prohibited according to ancient Jewish prescription. Therefore, an observant Jewish person would make sure that he does not eat anything about which there would be the slightest suspicion that anything forbidden, for example, swine's flesh, might be in the food he eats. Rabbi Isserles says that he should be even more careful about eating or taking into his body anything that might be dangerous. The application of this exhortation to the problem of cigarette smoking seems obvious.

DO NOT RELY ON MIRACLES

It is also interesting to note that Rabbi Isserles says: "In these matters it is forbidden to rely on miracles." This means that an individual should not deceive himself in thinking that, although others are harmed, he might escape the consequences. It is a divine commandment to preserve the health of your body and spirit. These exhortations apply, even when the risk appears to be minimal. This is illustrated in the following way. In ancient times, people were warned not to drink water that had been left uncovered for a period of time.

The water might have become contaminated in some way. The rabbis prohibited the drinking of "uncovered water." What if the risk is minimal? The rabbis ruled: "If a jar was uncovered, even though nine persons drank of its contents without any fatal consequences, the tenth person is still forbidden to drink from it."

Even a minimal risk should not be taken. Life is too precious; health is too important; well-being is too vital to be risked.

AVOID RISK

The attitude of Judaism toward possible risk to health can be summed up as follows:

1. Life is precious. It is given to us as a trust. We may, therefore, not do anything that would possibly impair our health, shorten our lives, or cause us harm and pain.
2. As we may not do this to ourselves, so, of course, we may not do harm to others. All human lives are precious in God's sight.
3. The responsibility to avoid danger to ourselves or others applies, even when it is not certain that harm will ensue. We are forbidden even to take the risk.
4. The harm is to be avoided, even if the bad effects are not immediately evident but will show up in the long run.

CONCLUSION

In regard to smoking, there is little difficulty in applying these principles to the question of smoking. Scientific evidence has now established beyond doubt that smoking, especially cigarette smoking, is injurious to our health. It is now evident, too, that the nonsmoker can be harmed when he or she has to suffer the smoke of those who use tobacco. The smoking habit is dirty, harmful, and antisocial. It would, therefore, follow that Jewish ethics and Jewish law would prohibit the use of cigarettes. Smoking should, at least, be discouraged in synagogues, Jewish schools, and in Jewish gathering places. The rabbinate and community leaders should discourage smoking.

This would help us live longer and healthier. In doing so, we would be fulfilling our responsibilities to God and humanity.

One aspect of this question is of special interest. According to Jewish law, the observance of the Sabbath is of paramount importance. One of the Ten Commandments exhorts us to cease from labor every seventh day. The rabbis have long and complicated discussions of what is "work." The kindling of fire and the extinction of fire is forbidden on the Sabbath. Thus from sundown Friday to sundown Saturday, Jewish law forbids smoking. I have personally known many people who were heavy smokers who did not touch tobacco the entire Sabbath day. What is remarkable is that in most of these cases, all smoke hunger ceases during the Sabbath day. It is only as the sun begins to wane and the end of the Sabbath day approaches that the yearning for tobacco returns. I myself experienced this phenomenon when I was a habitual smoker. As far as I know, scientists have not fully investigated the fact that the religious prohibition against smoking on the Sabbath seems to distract habitual smokers from their addiction. It means that determination and commitment can overcome the desire to smoke. Surely, religious people seek to do God's will. When they accept the idea that it is forbidden to smoke on the Sabbath day, they are freed from the compulsion. We fervently hope that the considerations of the danger to health by smoking might become internalized so that those who now shorten their lives by the use of cigarettes will hear God's command and will stop smoking.

Rabbi Seymour Siegel

Notes

1. *MT Hilkhot Rotzeah* 11:4–5.
2. *B. Bava Kama* 80a.
3. *Rama*, YD 116:5.

Chapter 78

Abortion: What Jewish Law Says

As abortion frequently resurfaces as a contentious issue in U.S. politics, it is worthwhile to investigate the Jewish approach to the issue. The traditional Jewish view of abortion does not fit conveniently into any of the major camps in the current American abortion debate. We neither ban abortion completely, nor do we allow indiscriminate abortion on demand.

A woman may feel that until the fetus is born, it is a part of her body, and therefore she retains the right to abort an unwanted pregnancy. Does Judaism recognize a right to "choose" abortion? In what situations does Jewish law sanction abortion? To gain a clear understanding of when abortion is permitted (or even required) and when it is forbidden requires an appreciation of certain nuances of halakhah (Jewish law), which govern the status of the fetus.[1]

The easiest way to conceptualize a fetus in halakhah is to imagine it as a full-fledged human being—but not quite.[2] In most circumstances, the fetus is treated like any other "person." Generally, one may not deliberately harm a fetus. But although it would seem obvious that Judaism holds accountable one who purposefully causes a woman to miscarry, sanctions are even placed upon one who strikes a pregnant woman causing an unintentional miscarriage.[3] That is not to say that all rabbinical authorities consider abortion to be murder. The fact that the Torah requires a monetary payment for causing a miscarriage is interpreted by some rabbis to indicate that abortion is not a capital crime[4] and by others as merely indicating that one is not executed for performing an abortion, even though it is a type of murder.[5]

There is even disagreement regarding whether the prohibition of abortion is biblical or rabbinic. Nevertheless, it is universally agreed that the fetus will become a full-fledged human being, and there must be a very compelling reason to allow for abortion.

As a general rule, abortion in Judaism is permitted only if there is a direct threat to the life of the mother by carrying the fetus to term or through the act of childbirth. In such a circumstance, the baby is considered tantamount to a *rodef* (pursuer)[6] after the mother with the intent to kill her. Nevertheless, as explained in the Mishnah,[7] if it would be possible to save the mother by maiming the fetus, such as by amputating a limb, abortion would be forbidden. Despite the classification of the fetus as a pursuer, once the baby's head or most of its body has been delivered, the baby's life is considered equal to the mother's, and we may not choose one life over another, because it is considered as though they are both pursuing each other.

It is important to point out that the reason the life of the fetus is subordinate to the mother is that the fetus is the *cause* of the mother's life-threatening condition, whether directly (for example, due to toxemia, placenta previa, or breech position) or indirectly (for example, exacerbation of underlying diabetes, kidney disease, or hypertension).[8] A fetus may not be aborted to save the life of any other person whose life is not directly threatened by the fetus, such as use of fetal organs for transplant.

Judaism recognizes psychiatric as well as physical factors in evaluating the potential threat that the fetus poses to the mother. However, the danger posed by the fetus (whether physical or emotional) must be both probable and substantial to justify abortion.[9] The degree of mental illness that must be present to justify termination of a pregnancy has been widely debated by rabbinic scholars,[10] without a clear consensus of opinion regarding the exact criteria for permitting abortion in such instances.[11] Nevertheless, all agree that were a pregnancy to cause a woman to become truly suicidal, there would be grounds for abortion.[12] However, several modern rabbinical experts ruled that since pregnancy-induced and postpartum depressions are treatable, abortion is not warranted.[13]

As a rule, Jewish law does not assign relative values to different lives. Therefore, most major *poskim* (rabbis qualified to decide matters of Jewish law) forbid abortion in cases of abnormalities or

DID YOU KNOW?

Judaism recognizes psychiatric as well as physical factors in evaluating the potential threat that the fetus poses to the mother.

deformities found in a fetus. Rabbi Moshe Feinstein, one of the greatest *poskim* of the past century, rules that even amniocentesis is forbidden if it is performed only to evaluate for birth defects for which the parents might request an abortion. Nevertheless, a test may be performed if a permitted action may result, such as performance of amniocentesis or drawing alpha-fetoprotein levels for improved peripartum or postpartum medical management.

While most *poskim* forbid abortion for "defective" fetuses, Rabbi Eliezar Yehuda Waldenberg is a notable exception. Rabbi Waldenberg allows first-trimester abortion of a fetus that would be born with a deformity that would cause it to suffer, and termination of a fetus with a lethal fetal defect such as Tay-Sachs up to the seventh month of gestation.[14] The rabbinic experts also discuss the permissibility of abortion for mothers with German measles and babies with Down syndrome confirmed prenatally.

There is a difference of opinion regarding abortion for adultery or in other cases of impregnation from a relationship with someone biblically forbidden. In cases of rape and incest, a key issue would be the emotional toll exacted from the mother in carrying the fetus to term. In cases of rape, Rabbi Shlomo Zalman Auerbach allows the woman to use methods that prevent pregnancy after intercourse.[15] The same analysis used in other cases of emotional harm might be applied here. Cases of adultery interject additional considerations into the debate, with rulings ranging from prohibition to its being a *mitzvah* to abort.[16]

I have attempted to distill the essence of the traditional Jewish approach to abortion. Nevertheless, every woman's case is unique and special, and the parameters determining the permissibility of abortion within halakhah are subtle and complex.

It is crucial to remember that when faced with an actual patient, a competent halakhic authority must be consulted in every case.

✍ *Daniel Eisenberg, M.D.*

Notes

1. Although there is debate among the rabbis as to whether abortion is a biblical or rabbinical prohibition, all agree on the fundamental concept that abortion is only permitted to protect the life of the mother or in other extraordinary situations. Jewish law does not sanction abortion on demand without a pressing reason.
2. *Igros Moshe, Choshen Mishpat* II:69B.
3. *Shulchan Aruch, Choshen Mishpat*, 423:1.
4. Rabbi Yehuda Ashkenazi, *Be'er Hetiv, Choshen Mishpat* 425:2.
5. *Igros Moshe*, op. cit.
6. Maimonides, *Mishneh Torah*, Laws of Murder 1:9; Talmud *Sanhedrin* 72B.
7. *Oholos* 7:6.
8. See Dr. Abraham Steinberg's article, "Abortion and Miscarriage," in the *Encyclopedia of Jewish Medical Ethics*, for an extensive discussion of the maternal indications for abortion.
9. *Igros Moshe*, op. cit.
10. See *Encyclopedia of Jewish Medical Ethics*, p. 10, for references.
11. See Moshe Spero's *Judaism and Psychology*, pp. 168–180.
12. Rabbi Yitzchak Zilberstein, "Emek Halacha," *Assia*, 1986, *1*, 205–209.
13. Rabbi Shlomo Zalman Auerbach and Rabbi Yehoshua Neuwirth, cited in *English Nishmat Avraham, Choshen Mishpat*, 425:11, p. 288.
14. *Tzitz Eliezer*, vol. 13:102.
15. Rabbi Shlomo Zalman Auerbach and Rabbi Yehoshua Neuwirth, cited in *English Nishmat Avraham, Choshen Mishpat*, 425:23, p. 294.
16. See the excellent chapter in *English Nishmat Avraham, Choshen Mishpat* 425, by Dr. Abraham Abraham, particularly p. 293.

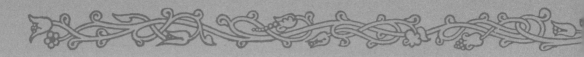

Chapter 79

Abortion: The Controversy over Jewish Religious Rights and Responsibilities

Jewish law (halakhah) presents a fairly consistent view regarding abortion in cases where a mother's life is or is not in danger. However, when the danger to a mother's health may be present but less easily defined, the issue is more complex. Here are some guiding principles in halakhic discussions of the issue:

A basic text for this stance is in the Mishnah: "If a woman has [life-threatening] difficulty in childbirth, one dismembers the embryo within her, limb by limb, because her life takes precedence over its life. However, once its head (or its "greater part") has emerged, it may not be touched, for we do not set aside one life for another" (*Ohalot* 7:6). Later commentators argue regarding the status of the child from the time the head emerges until the birth is complete (at which time it no longer poses a danger to the mother). However, most cases of therapeutic (life-saving) abortion are covered clearly and concisely by this Mishnah, which posits that existing life takes precedence over potential life.

 DID YOU KNOW?

Halakhah clearly permits, and even mandates, abortion in any case where there is danger to the mother's life, from conception at least until the head of an infant emerges in childbirth.

432

DID YOU KNOW?

The Torah draws an important distinction: causing a miscarriage of the fetus is a civil wrong resulting in monetary compensation (implying the fetus is not a person), while killing the mother is considered to be homicide.

THE STATUS OF A FETUS

In the modern debate on abortion, many religious traditions view a fetus as equivalent to an existing human life, even from conception. While Judaism sees the fetus as valuable and sacred as potential life, the sources indicate that it is not equivalent to a person.

One source for understanding this attitude comes from the Torah in Exodus 21:22–23: "If two men are fighting and wound a pregnant woman so that the pregnancy is lost, but no 'great harm' occurs, he will be fined as much as her husband assesses, and the matter will be placed before a court." Such a case is not considered murder. However, "If 'great harm' does occur, it is a case of *nefesh tahat nefesh*, 'life for life.'"

Some later commentators have interpreted Judaism's view of a fetus as representing an actual life, therefore, prohibiting abortion in all cases but those in which the mother's life is endangered by the pregnancy. For example, Maimonides understood this Mishnah to be based on the idea that the fetus is a "pursuer" of the mother's life. This would allow the fetus to be killed in an attempt to save the mother, as an act of "self-defense." By this reasoning, the status of personhood is conveyed to the fetus. However, if it is not a pursuer, that is, it does not constitute a threat to the mother's life, we may not permit its destruction. Maimonides' view, however, is unique and did not gain general acceptance among Jewish legal authorities.

Finally, there are opinions that differentiate the "potentiality" of life, depending on how far along the pregnancy is. Several sources regard a fetus as a partial person after the first forty days (before which some Talmudic sources regard it as "mere fluid" and are more permissive). However, after forty days, if a spontaneous or induced abortion occurs, a woman is required to undergo the purification process identical to that which follows giving birth, implying that some aspect of "personhood" has been attained.

However, cases in which abortion might be considered do not always fall into such clearly defined categories. What about cases where a test indicates the child may have a genetic disorder, such as Tay-Sachs? Does a family's ability to economically support an additional child have any relevancy? If a pregnancy or additional child may result in psychological harm to the mother, is this comparable to physical harm? Is abortion following rape or incest allowable?

Individuals, as well as the rabbis they consult in attempting to deal with such situations, weigh all the attitudes described, as

---

 Committee on Jewish Law and Standards Position on Abortion

Jewish tradition is sensitive to the sanctity of life, and does not permit abortion on demand. However, it sanctions abortion under some circumstances because it does not regard the fetus as an autonomous person. This is based partly on the Bible (Exodus 21:22–23), which prescribes monetary damages when a person injures a pregnant woman, causing a miscarriage. The Mishnah (*Ohalot* 7:6) explicitly indicates that one is to abort a fetus if the continuation of pregnancy might imperil the life of the mother. Later authorities have differed as to how far we might go in defining the peril to the mother in order to justify abortion. The Rabbinical Assembly Committee on Jewish Law and Standards takes the view that an abortion is justifiable if a continuation of pregnancy might cause the mother severe physical or psychological harm, or when the fetus is judged by competent medical opinion as severely defective. The fetus is a life in the process of development, and the decision to abort should never be taken lightly. Before reaching her final decision, the mother should consult with the father, other members of her family, her physician, her spiritual leader, and any other person who can help her in assessing the many grave legal and moral issues involved.

 Reproductive Choice: Hadassah Health Care Policy Statement

Hadassah, the Women's Zionist Organization of America, calls upon its nationwide membership to reaffirm this organization's mandate for freedom of choice. We support the right of women everywhere to full and complete access to reproductive health care services.

Hadassah calls upon its nationwide membership to significantly increase its advocacy on behalf of the Freedom of Choice Act, a bill which restores the protection of *Roe* v. *Wade* by prohibiting state legislatures from interfering with the fundamental right of choice.

Further, we urge our regions and chapters to educate their respective members with regard to any attempt by their own legislatures to restrict or interfere with a woman's right to choose in accordance with her religious, moral, and ethical values.

Hadassah opposes any attempts to restrict, through state administrative regulations, legislation, or court action, the right to reproductive choice and/or use of family planning programs delivering any and all services.

Hadassah urges chapters to join in coalitions with freedom of choice advocacy groups, participating as full members in pro-choice activities.

---

expressed in many additional source texts. In particular, although the sources are clear regarding abortion due to a physical threat to the mother's health, sources are divided regarding situations that cause psychological harm. Some sources tend to be lenient in such cases, especially early on in pregnancy. On the other hand, there is a strong tendency to be as restrictive as possible, lest lenience be seen as minimizing the seriousness of the act of abortion.

✐ *United Synagogues of Conservative Judaism*

Statement of the Women of Reform Judaism 30th Biennial Assembly on the Rights of Individuals and Legal Abortion (1975)

The National Federation of Temple Sisterhoods affirms our previously adopted strong support for the right of a woman to obtain a legal abortion, under conditions now outlined in the 1973 decision of the United States Supreme Court. The Court's position established that during the first two trimesters the private and personal decision of whether or not to continue to term an unwanted pregnancy should remain a matter of choice for the woman; she alone can exercise her ethical and religious judgment in this decision. Only by vigorously supporting this individual right to choose can we also ensure that every woman may act according to the religious and ethical tenets to which she adheres.

We oppose laws which would remove abortion from the category of medical assistance, as well as any discriminatory laws which would effectively prevent women from making the choice which is their right, by denying them access to proper medical care.

NFTS reaffirms our commitment to *taharat hamishpachah*—the purity of the family—and supports the dissemination of birth control information as well as other education for family planning as a contribution to responsible family life. Such education and parallel efforts to eradicate ignorance and poverty would substantially reduce the need to make the choice for abortion.

Chapter 80

Eating Disorders: Perceptions and Perspectives in Jewish Life Today

Food is the classic symbol of Jewish culture. Tradition teaches that since the destruction of the Temple, every table in every Jewish home has become an altar, that is, a center for the sacred in our lives. Even today, all of our holiday celebrations are identified through the abundance of foods we eat. We joke with other Jews about our cultural focus on food, yet for those with eating disorders in our community, food is no laughing matter. For them the table has ceased to be a sacred place. Rather than being an object of holiness, food for them has become an instrument of self-destruction.

The prevalence of anorexia, bulimia, and binge eating or compulsive overeating disorder is increasing in North America, especially among white, well-educated, middle-class young women. The Jewish community is a prime target for eating disorders. Indeed, many of our daughters and sisters and mothers, as well as a rising

From the Sources

The body is the soul's house. Shouldn't we therefore take care of our house so that it will not fall into ruin?

Philo, Jewish philosopher (20 B.C.E.–50 C.E.)

number of our sons and brothers and fathers, are afflicted with eating disorders. We must ask ourselves: Why has this issue become a dangerous phenomenon in our community?

This is a complex question, mainly because eating disorders are not about food per se but about emotions and a person's sense of self-esteem. One answer may lie in the Jewish community's emphasis on success. We are a community of achievers. We strive for academic, economic, and professional success. People with eating disorders are often unaware of how intensely they feel the pressure to measure up to a standard of excellence. They are perceived as highly competent and successful by their friends, families, classmates, and coworkers, but what they see in the mirror does not reflect this dynamic image.

What's more, many Jews believe that they do not conform to what is considered to be the classic American image of model-thin beauty—a sentiment that is often underscored by the mixed messages we receive as children: "Eat, eat, but don't get too fat!"

This strikes yet another blow to our self-esteem. Sometimes, perhaps more often than we'd like to admit, Jewish families do not want to accept the fact that a loved one is using excessive bingeing or the restriction of food to mask deep-seated pain.

Families, too, must struggle and come to terms with the factors that have contributed to their loved one's eating disorder. As a community, we have begun to chip away at the denial that compels us to say, "not my loved one" or "not in my synagogue," when we see someone engaged in self-destructive behaviors.

TO NOURISH HOPE

Litapayach Tikvah: To Nourish Hope, a publication of the Women of Reform Judaism and the Union of American Hebrew Congregations, is a first step toward guiding people with eating disorders in our community toward recovery. Because of the pressure to perform and excel *and* the cultural focus on food, for many Jews food becomes a tool we use to regulate control over our lives, suppress anger, and attend to our feelings of low self-esteem. Yet, as Rabbi Akiva teaches, "Human beings are loved because they are made in God's image."

Litapayach Tikvah: To Nourish Hope strives to help people with eating disorders discover their own holiness so that they, too, can find a center for the sacred in their lives.

WHAT ARE EATING DISORDERS?

The first step in helping someone or getting help is understanding what we mean by "eating disorders," which generally fall under three categories: anorexia nervosa, bulimia nervosa, and binge eating or compulsive overeating disorder. Although the root issues may be the same for all three, each disorder manifests itself in a unique way.

Anorexia is characterized by significant weight loss, often as a result of self-imposed starvation. People with anorexia cannot maintain their body at the minimum ideal weight for their age and height. They are intensely fearful of gaining weight, perceive themselves as fat, and deny the seriousness of their weight loss. Their intense fear of gaining weight often becomes a preoccupation with food, calories, and exercising. More people die from anorexia than from any other psychiatric disorder.

Bulimia is marked by a cycle of binge eating (consuming a large amount of food in short time periods with an accompanying sense of being out of control), followed by some form of purging— behaviors that compensate for the experience of binge eating. Purging behaviors run the gamut from vomiting to excessive use of laxatives or diuretics to obsessive exercising. Bulimia can result in a variety of medical problems from dental and esophageal disorders to kidney and gastrointestinal damage. In some cases, bulimia nervosa leads to death.

Binge eating, or compulsive overeating, is like bulimia in that this disorder entails consuming a large amount of food in short time periods with an accompanying sense of being out of control. However, in this case, the food binge *is not* followed by a purging episode. Often people with this disorder eat very quickly or until they are uncomfortably full, after which they feel intense shame. Binge eaters or compulsive overeaters often exhibit such classic symptoms of depression as lethargy, isolation, and mood swings.

WHAT ARE THE WARNING SIGNS?

The purpose of this list is to help raise awareness about eating disorders. You may notice that the list is not broken down into individual disorders. That's because it is intended to be a guide and not a diagnostic tool. It is also not exhaustive. The warning signs listed next are only some of the signals that accompany eating disorders. A person may exhibit one, some, or all of these signs.

People with eating disorders *can* recover. The first step is to heed the warning signs. If, after reading this list, you are concerned that you or a loved one has an eating disorder, the most important thing to do is to seek professional help (see the following sections).

A person with eating disorders

- Gains or loses an excessive amount of weight during a short period of time
- Exhibits significant changes in eating behavior, such as excessive dieting, eating alone behind closed doors, refusing to eat certain foods, or hurrying to the bathroom after meals
- Is preoccupied with food, weight, counting calories, and cooking for others
- Experiences an irregular menstrual cycle
- Complains about being "too fat," even if thin
- Is overly self-deprecating and unable to accept compliments
- Believes that she or he will be "better," "happier," "more attractive," "more successful" when she or he reaches the desired goal weight
- Has difficulty eating in public
- Wears baggy clothes in order to hide body
- Feels guilty about eating habits and ashamed or tormented by body
- Displays signs of depression, such as irritability or mood swings
- Gives the impression of withdrawing from relationships
- Steps on the scale more than once a day

HOW CAN YOU HELP?

A caring community goes a long way in helping a person with eating disorders. If you are concerned that someone you love is afflicted with anorexia, bulimia, or binge eating or compulsive overeating disorder, there are tangible ways in which you can be of assistance. The most important thing to remember is that you cannot cure the eating disorder by yourself. The ultimate goal is for the person with eating disorders to consult specialists in the medical and therapeutic fields.

Eating disorders are complex, and people with eating disorders are unique—a difficult combination for anyone trying to help. Here are a few hints to guide you in your discussions with your loved one. First, *do* the following:

- Express your concern in a sensitive, nonjudgmental way. It's important to choose carefully the time and place for your conversation.
- Be prepared for a denial of the problem. It's often difficult for people with eating disorders to acknowledge that they are ill.
- Encourage the family to seek professional help together. Eating disorders in an individual often signal a problem within the family system.
- Be patient and understanding. Because of the complexity of eating disorders, no single factor is to "blame."
- Be aware of your own biases regarding food, eating, and body image.

And *don't do* the following:

- Ignore the problem. If it is left unchecked, an eating disorder can endanger a person's physical and emotional health and perhaps lead to death.
- Try to force your loved one to eat or insist that she or he gain or lose weight.
- Make comments about appearance, dieting, weight, or calorie counting. Such comments can be misinterpreted and used to reinforce the eating disorder.
- Agree to keep the eating disorder a secret. In some settings, confidentiality is key, but if someone's health is threatened, it is OK to reach out to others for help.

EATING DISORDERS RESOURCES

The organizations listed here will be happy to provide you with information about eating disorders or inform you about resources in your community. Many of the Web sites have excellent links to other online resources.

American Anorexia/Bulimia Association (AABA)
165 West 46 Street, Suite 1108
New York, NY 10036
(212) 575-6200
http://members.aol.com/amanbu/index.html

Anorexia Nervosa and Related Eating Disorders, Inc. (ANRED)
*This is an excellent, anonymous online resource affiliated with
    NEDO.*
http://www.anred.com

Eating Disorder Awareness and Prevention (EDAP)
603 Stewart Street, Suite 803
Seattle, WA 98101
(206) 382-3587
http://members.aol.com/edap.inc

National Association of Anorexia Nervosa and Associated Disorders
    (ANAD)
P.O. Box 7
Highland Park, IL 60035
(847) 831-3438
http://members.aol.com/anad20/index.html

National Eating Disorders Organization (NEDO)
665 South Yale Avenue
Tulsa, OK 74136
(918) 481-4044; (800) 322-5173, ext. 5600
http://www.laureate.com/nedointro.html

Overeaters Anonymous
World Service Office
6075 Zenith Court NE
Rio Ranch, NM 87124
(505) 891-2664
http://www.overeatersanonymous.org

Renfrew Center
475 Spring Lane
Philadelphia, PA 19128
(800) RENFREW
http://www.renfrew.org

For more information, contact the UAHC Department of Jewish Family Concerns at (212) 650-4294, fax (212) 650-4239, or e-mail: deptjewfamcom@uahc.org.

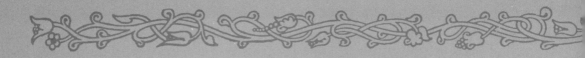

Chapter 81

Eating Disorders: The Jewish Community's Perspective

At the Jewish New Year, observant Jews the world over antici-pate days of fasting to achieve clarity of thought, personal self-awareness, and moral cleansing. As a Jew and as a psychotherapist specializing in the treatment of eating disorders in children and their families for the past twenty-eight years, I have been witness to Jewish self-starvation of another sort, for less lofty and more tragic purposes. Anorexia nervosa and bulimia nervosa represent a misuse of food to resolve emotional problems and cope with anxiety and stress; these diseases strike 5 percent of adolescents, with an addi-tional 15 percent suffering from subclinical forms of disordered eat-ing. At ever younger ages, children in increasing numbers are succumbing to disorders marked by body image concerns and pro-pelled by the underlying drive to be thin and a pathological fear of weight gain.

All too frequently, these diseases go unnoticed until they dam-age life quality, affecting the physical and emotional functioning and well-being of its victims. To those who are aware of the impact and magnitude of these problems that afflict millions of American youth and adults alike, what is particularly disturbing is the dispro-portionate number of Jews with eating disorders.

In a "shoot the messenger" analysis of the situation, it is com-monly presumed that there is something within the practice, values, and culture of Judaism that is responsible for this phenomenon. Jewish parents, by virtue of their carrying out the traditions and val-ues of their faith, are chastised. The stereotypic image of the Jewish

HEALTH FACTS

The Renfrew Center of Philadelphia reports that at one point 12 percent of their inpatient eating disorder population was Jewish, despite the fact that Jews make up only 2 percent of the general population. Dr. Ira Sacker reports that in a study of Orthodox Jewish girls in Brooklyn, one out of nineteen was found to be eating disordered—a statistic 50 percent greater than the occurrence of these disorders in the general population.

mother forcing food on her child—"*Ess, ess, mein Kind!*"—gives rise to the image of the controlling intrusiveness of a demanding and judgmental parent, giving credence to the Jewish child's acting out in response. In addition, Judaism's focus on food as the centerpiece of Jewish celebration and tradition implicates Jewish observance.

It is my belief that Judaism has gotten an unfair shake. The Renfrew Center study was conducted in a large urban metropolis, one that happens to be situated close to one of the world's largest Jewish populations; this, in my mind, renders the study's conclusions questionable. The high incidence of eating disorders in the Orthodox community probably has less to do with religiosity or the culture of Judaism than with the fact that the self-discipline, mastery, and precision required for Orthodox observance, when turned against or applied to the self, can result in harmful consequences for those individuals who are genetically predisposed.

HEALTH FACTS

Scientific research now points conclusively to evidence of the roots of these diseases being in genetics, in brain and body chemistries, and in personality structure and temperament, in addition to environmental factors.

Scientists are not entirely certain what gives rise to eating disorders. Upward mobility—a characteristic that has always defined the Jewish people—has been determined to be a causal factor among ethnic and minority groups. Contributing secular influences may include the restructuring of the American family in divorce, remarriage, and family blending; more parents entering the workforce with kids left to their own devices—to the television or their peers to determine how to live and behave, what to eat, think, and believe. Bombarded by a fickle and toxic media, people have come to deify thinness and, most significantly, have lost track of what healthy eating is. They have forgotten that regular and moderate eating that includes all the food groups at least three times a day is as much a part of healthy living as is sleeping, learning, studying, working, exercising, or praying.

If there is any correlation between Judaism and eating disorders, I believe it is not the Jewish culture, traditions, values, and laws that lie at the root of the eating disorder phenomenon, as much as it is the turning away from these verities by the Jewish people. A recent study of a group of Jewish women showed that secular Jews scored higher than Orthodox Jews on measures of body dissatisfaction and eating disorders, indicating that high levels of religious observance may, in fact, serve as a protective factor. The values and mores of our wider society expressly contradict those of Torah, which have reliably taught us what to value, how to live, and how to raise our children through the generations. On second look, we, as Jews, might just find that the solutions we seek for ourselves and our children about problems that we face today are, and have been, available to us for the past five thousand years.

Abigail Natenshon, M.A., L.C.S.W., G.C.F.P.

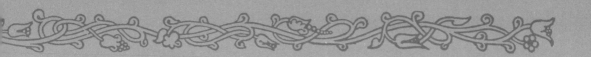

Chapter 82

Eating Disorders: Six Ways to Boost Girls' Self-Esteem

Do you know a teenage girl who has low self-esteem? Chances are that you know several. According to groups such as the Commonwealth Fund and the American Association of University Women (AAUW), girls entering junior high school feel less self-confident than they do in elementary school, and they become less self-assured with each successive year of school. In contrast, boys become more confident with each passing year.

Parents, teachers, mentors, and other concerned adults can have a significant impact on how girls see themselves. Here are six concrete things that an adult can do to help a girl:

1. *Focus on the person she is instead of her appearance.* Girls are harshly judged by other girls, as well as written off by boys, if they don't fit within the bounds of our society's narrow definition of beauty. As a result, a girl's body becomes the focus of her attention and energies. This is borne out by two startling statistics: one out of every five girls between the ages of twelve and nineteen has an eating disorder, and one-fifth of cosmetic surgery performed in the United States is on teens. To help a girl develop a healthier self-image, compliment her for her achievements, thoughts, and actions. Remind her in various ways that she is a smart, valuable person with great ideas and lots of potential.

2. *Call her attention to media deception.* One reason girls feel so negative about themselves is that they are continuously barraged by picture-perfect images of girls and women in magazines and

on television. Teens compare themselves to these images, either consciously or unconsciously, and feel dissatisfied when they inevitably don't "measure up." One way to help a girl feel better is to expose unrealistic media images for what they are: retouched, computer-manipulated photos of models—a group that makes up only 5 percent of the population. As supermodel Cindy Crawford admits, "Even I don't wake up looking like Cindy Crawford." Once a girl knows that most people look like the ones she sees in her everyday life, she will likely feel more satisfied with her own looks.

3. *Give her a journal.* Girls experience many conflicting emotions during their preteen and adolescent years, and expressing their thoughts and feelings by writing in a diary or journal is a proven way for them to boost their self-esteem. According to Mary Pipher, in *Reviving Ophelia,* "In their writing, [girls] can clarify, conceptualize, and evaluate their experiences . . . and strengthen their sense of self." You can simply give a girl a blank book—there are many decorative ones available—or present her with a more structured journal that asks her to answer open-ended questions. These can be found in the "teen issues" section of local bookstores.

4. *Encourage her to share her thoughts and opinions.* Studies show that girls are more frequently interrupted than boys. Over the course of many conversations, they also get the message that what they have to say is not necessarily as compelling or valued as what boys have to say. Compounding this subtle conditioning is the fact that boys often feel threatened by smart, outspoken girls. It's no wonder some girls "go underground" and clam up when they enter their teens. However, adults can help girls move forward on this front by conveying that their thoughts are important and that their unique viewpoints should be shared. If a girl learns to use her voice confidently on a regular basis, and people listen and respect her, she starts charting a course for higher self-esteem.

5. *Encourage her to take risks.* Individuals develop self-reliance when they're given the space to solve problems and make mistakes in the process. What happens with girls? Researchers have found that teachers are more likely to intervene and solve problems for girls who are stuck than they are for boys. In addition, girls are rewarded for being good and behaving well, as opposed to being adventurous in their thinking, as boys are. Girls need to be given time and permission to creatively complete what they start. We can

praise them for considering new problem-solving options, allow them to make mistakes, and refrain from "rescuing" them.

6. *Suggest that she get involved in a sport.* Research shows that female athletes are more self-reliant and get better grades and higher test scores, than girls who don't participate in sports. Being on a team or playing an individual sport is also a way for a girl to divert some of the energy focused on superficial concerns, such as appearance, toward healthy physical activity and personal achievement. With the right kind of support and encouragement from key adults, girls can potentially avoid many common problems (such as low motivation and underachievement) that are rooted in low self-esteem. Commenting on an accomplishment, making an observation about her skills, or giving her an opportunity to push through frustration and solve a problem on her own can start the ball rolling. In many everyday ways, we can help girls transform the ways they think about themselves so that they begin to think, feel, and act more confident.

Catherine Dee

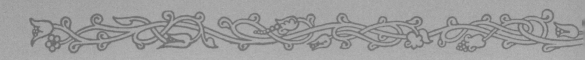

Chapter 83

Eating Disorders: A Young Woman's Story

Try my chocolate cake, it's delicious!" These simple words once struck terror in my heart. As a young woman with an eating disorder, I was terrified to eat anything, especially rich chocolate cake.

I was a skinny thirteen-year-old when my fear of gaining weight first surfaced. I had just recovered from a bout of mononucleosis and had lost more than fifteen pounds from the illness. Dimly conscious of the fact that I was extremely thin, I had only recently become more aware of concepts such as dieting, calories, and fat content.

> Gitty's mother is baking cookies for Shabbat. Gitty and I eat at least ten each when they come out of the oven. They are delicious. Gitty says something about the cookies being fattening. I ask her whether she thinks I am fat. She says no. But I worry. She tells me not to worry, just to be careful not to eat too much. I feel panicky, and make up my mind to carefully watch what I eat. I'm a shy, insecure girl, dealing with my parents' difficult divorce, my father's illness, and my brother's death in an accident a few years earlier. I'm especially vulnerable to the pressures of adolescence. I yearn to look perfect, to be one of the "popular" girls, to fit in. I don't eat any more cookies that Shabbat.

Throughout high school, I obsessed about my weight.

I worried that I was "too fat" and felt inferior and unattractive compared to my classmates at the girls' religious school in New York that I attended. I would lose weight, gain it back, panic, and lose the weight again. When I graduated from high school, I was a normal size 10 but felt desperate to lose weight.

> I attend a prestigious seminary in Europe. I don't have a good "seminary experience." I feel insecure, troubled throughout the year. I do well with the class work and function during the day, but at night I sneak into the kitchen and eat whole boxes and containers full of food. I am worried about family issues and about the pressures of adulthood. My parents' divorce worries me; how will it affect me in regards to *shidduchim*?
>
> I fall into a depression, buy huge quantities of food, and eat it all in one sitting. I gain some weight and feel frantic about losing it.

I simply didn't feel attractive or good enough.

In retrospect, I see that I simply didn't feel attractive or good enough. All I saw was imperfection and I felt an almost desperate need to "do something" about it.

> After my year of seminary, I return to New York where I have a great job and excel at my work. I go on *shidduchim*, and my fears regarding dating are, for the most part, unfounded: I am set up with really "good" boys. But something holds me back. Although I am proposed to three times, I can't make a commitment. I contract the measles at age twenty and lose twenty pounds. Anorexia, lurking within for so many years, finds its way to the surface.

After recovering from the measles, I weighed 100 pounds. Proud of my new thinness, I ate almost nothing. To stave off hunger and simulate eating, I chewed low-calorie gum and ate watermelon, cantaloupe, lettuce, and other vegetables. At night, I couldn't sleep because of the hunger pangs.

I monitored my social activities and made decisions based on the demands of my illness: What kind of food would be available at this or that place or event? Would I be tempted to eat the "wrong" foods? My friends stopped inviting me to eat out at restaurants and to Shabbat meals because they knew I wouldn't come. The eating disorder took up so much internal space that it crowded out everyone else. I could only give a small part of myself to those I was with; I was living half a life.

By the time I was twenty-six years old, I weighed eighty-nine pounds; I was skinnier, and unhappier than I had ever been before. But I was convinced that if I gained any weight at all I'd be even more unhappy.

I kept telling myself that I wouldn't let the eating disorder interfere with my ability to have children, have a life. I would stop when I was "thin enough." But even when I became anemic and felt like I was dying, I couldn't stop. It was only getting worse. As soon as I got to one "magic" number, I felt the urge to lose even more.

Ironically, as much as I had originally wanted people to notice how thin I was, it was difficult once they did. My friends and family members began to express worry, but I shrugged them off and told them that I was "handling it."

I knew I was playing with life and death, but in some horrifying way, death and fat seemed equally terrifying. But after one particularly horrendous bulimic episode that landed me in the emergency room with heart palpitations and a doctor warning me that I was going to die before long, I began seeing a therapist. My therapist—a wonderful and compassionate woman who had struggled with an eating disorder herself—recommended that I enter a hospital that specializes in eating disorders and depression. She and I both recognized that I would not stop the behaviors on my own.

My eating patterns had become firmly entrenched, and it would take a lot of work—hundreds of hours of therapy, much self-introspection, and many tears—to relearn how to eat normally.

In the hospital, if I didn't eat my entire plate of food, I was forced to sit in the nurses' station for two hours. It was a relief not to have to make decisions about what foods to eat; I no longer had to feel guilty about eating.

I avoided fashion magazines and the stick-thin models displayed in them. When around extremely thin people, I told myself that they had made a choice to be that thin and that they probably were not very happy.

Being around other anorexics in the hospital was difficult: we all wanted to be the "best anorexics." When I saw a skinnier patient,

I became jealous; I was no longer the best, I could still be skinnier. After a while, I recognized that I needed some distance from others in the throes of an eating disorder and gravitated toward people who were already in recovery and accepting of their bodies.

Through spending time in the hospital (this was to be the first of three hospitalizations) and exploring issues in therapy, I realized that when I starved, binged, and purged, I was expressing pain and self-hatred. During my hospitalizations, I met many people struggling with eating disorders. While we came from different backgrounds and had very different life stories, we shared one thing in common: a lack of self-acceptance.

Like many sufferers of eating disorders, I needed to work on feeling OK with myself, regardless of what I looked like on the outside. I tried to come to terms with my unhappy childhood. My father had been physically and emotionally abusive and left me with many scars. He had given me the message that I was not OK the way I was, that I was not making him happy, and that I was the cause of my parents' divorce. He nearly destroyed me with his anger. Being deprived of a mother further damaged me. (I lived with my father, who did not allow me to have contact with my mother while I was growing up.) I had a lot of healing to do. In time, I got to know my mother again, and today we are very close. This added a measure of happiness and well-being that helped me along in recovery. As I got healthier, I slowly learned to replace the pain of my childhood with positive people and experiences. Thinness, I slowly learned, was not the answer.

During the recovery period, I read lots of books about eating disorders and found them to be very helpful, especially those written by recovered anorexics and bulimics. I took pictures of myself at my thinnest, right before entering the hospital. This helped me let go of the eating disorder since it was a way to document, for myself and others, how deep my pain once was. Today, the pictures remind me of where I never want to go again.

When I first left the hospital, it was a challenge to continue to eat normally. I began to notice a pattern. Whenever I felt especially insecure, I would revert back to the old desperation to lose weight. I began to recognize that I equated outer appearance with inner worth and being a successful anorexic with being a successful person.

For almost ten years, my life was ruled by the eating disorder.

I am now in my early thirties, have gained back most of the weight I lost, and have allowed my favorite foods back into my life. I have been doing well for a number of years, although I struggle occasionally. The road to health has been rocky and painful. But whereas the eating disorder once took over 99 percent of my life, it now only occasionally checks in during times of stress or discomfort to remind me that it's there if I want it. I don't want it, that's for sure. I love the freedom that I have today. I am happy with my attractive body size, and it feels wonderful to fit in with the rest of the crowd once again. Instead of the old tapes in my head that said, "That was too much food. I must eat less next time!" I have replaced them with new ones: "If I eat normally I'll be able to participate more fully in life, enjoy the company of others, bear healthy children, and make a difference in the world." It took a long time before I could listen to the new messages. But I am listening to them and am finally becoming that happy person I've always wanted to be.

⨕ *Rina Stein*

A Note from the Editors

We would like to note that science and medical recommendations change frequently. As a result, we want to caution you that any questions you have should be addressed by your health care practitioner. Here are a few items that have been addressed most recently as examples.

1. Regarding dietary intake of fats, there are many different kinds of fats, some excellent for the body, others not. Theories are rapidly changing. It is important to seek the advice of a physician who is knowledgeable and up to date, and the advice must be targeted to your own personal health situation.

2. Regarding the use of hormone replacement, there are highly respected physicians who practice complementary medicine, such as Dr. Andrew Weil (Harvard Medical School, University of Arizona) and numerous others, all of whom have offered as an alternative to synthetic hormones, bio-identical hormone therapies that purportedly do not carry the same risks as the synthetic hormones. The advice of a physician who is knowledgeable in these matters should be sought if you'd like to explore this option.

3. Regarding the issue of "bad foods," there are some foods that are bad for some people, based on biochemical individuality.

This should be discussed with a health professional knowledgeable in these areas.

Robin E. Berman, M.D.
Arthur Kurzweil
Dale L. Mintz, M.P.A., C.H.E.S.

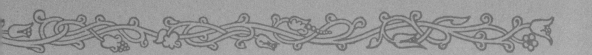

About Hadassah

Hadassah, the Women's Zionist Organization of America, Inc. (HWZOA), is an American not-for-profit voluntary organization. Founded in 1912, Hadassah retains the passion and timeless values of its founder, Henrietta Szold, Jewish scholar and activist, who was dedicated to Judaism, Zionism, and the American ideal. HWZOA's mission is to motivate and inspire its members to strengthen their partnership with Israel, ensure Jewish continuity, and realize their potential as a dynamic force in American society. In Israel, Hadassah projects benefit people throughout the country. These projects are the Hadassah Hebrew University Medical Center, Hadassah College Jerusalem, the Hadassah Career Counseling Institute, Youth Aliyah/Children at Risk, and land reclamation and water conservation projects.

NEEDS ADDRESSED, POPULATION SERVED, CURRENT PROGRAMS

In the United States, the Learning, Education, and Training Division develops peer-led family-based health education and awareness programs for women and their families, dealing with self-esteem for girls, breast cancer, testicular cancer, genetic discrimination, nutrition, heart disease, and osteoporosis, with particular attention given to prevention and wellness. Hadassah advocates on issues of concern to women and their families, such as the importance of clinical research

457

and the inclusion of women. Young Judaea offers Zionist youth activities and summer camps; summer and yearlong Israel abroad programs; and campus-based Jewish, Zionist, and pro-Israel advocacy programs and Jewish education programs.

In Israel, Hadassah provides professional career education at Hadassah College Jerusalem. Vocational testing, counseling, and job placement assistance are provided at the Hadassah Career Counseling Institute, and through Youth Aliyah/Children at Risk, children in need of special assistance are supported in day schools and residential programs for immigrants, refugees, and children of dysfunctional or at-risk families.

The Hadassah Hebrew University Medical Center (Hadassah) is recognized around the world for excellence in patient care, research, and teaching. The center is comprised of two hospitals in Jerusalem—Hadassah Hebrew University Medical Center at Ein Kerem and Hadassah Hospital at Mount Scopus. Hadassah strives to be a leader in patient care. Hadassah established Israel's first trauma unit, first bone marrow transplantation unit, first comprehensive burns unit, first biohazard unit, and the first Jewish hospice in Jerusalem. Since the *intifada* began in 2000, Hadassah's Center for Emergency Medicine has treated half of the more than four thousand victims of terrorism.

RECENT ACHIEVEMENTS

The ultramodern Charlotte Bloomberg Mother and Child Center opened at Ein Kerem in 1996. It houses many specialized medical services for mothers and children in one building. Since the center is overflowing its current premises, Hadassah is in the process of adding three floors to the building. The floors will meet the specialized needs of children with cancer (pediatric oncology), women undergoing high-risk pregnancies, and children requiring psychiatric care.

When the Emergency Room and Trauma Unit at Hadassah opened at Ein Kerem in 1979, the facilities were designed to accommodate forty-one thousand patients annually. As the number of emergency trauma referrals continued to grow over the years, due in part to the *intifada,* the overcrowded conditions made it imperative that a new facility be designed and built as soon as possible. On March 25, 2005, the Judy and Sidney Swartz Center for Emergency

Medicine (CEM) was officially dedicated. The new CEM is more than three times the size of the old center and has the capacity to treat 100,000 to 120,000 patients annually, an increase of 41 percent. It is equipped with the latest technology in the field of emergency medicine, including on-site imaging technology and safeguards against biological and chemical attacks. During crisis situations, when the hospital is receiving mass casualties, large sections of the ground-floor areas of buildings adjacent to the ER have the capacity for conversion into temporary supplemental emergency room units through the use of mobile intensive care islands, highly specialized and sophisticated stretchers that include mobile X-ray equipment, an emergency care monitor, a respiratory and metabolic monitor, a respirator, infusion pumps, a syringe pump, a feeding pump, a blood warmer, and a patient warming blanket, all built directly into the stretcher. Other innovations include the use of "digital diagnosis," whereby paramedics at the accident scene use digital cameras to relay pictures directly to a computer in the trauma unit at the CEM so that doctors may prepare for incoming casualties.

Beyond their devotion to patient care, the medical staff at Hadassah Hebrew University Medical Center are also world-renowned for their commitment to research. Fifty percent of all medical research in Israel is conducted at Hadassah. Recent achievements in research include a breakthrough discovery in cystic fibrosis treatment, the linking of a specific gene to posttraumatic stress disorder, and the identification of the protein particle responsible for mad cow disease. The Hadassah Hebrew University Medical Center is also a teaching center. The faculty of Hadassah instructs doctors, nurses, and other medical personnel in the latest U.S. protocols and clinical techniques for health care.

Since its founding in 1912, Hadassah, through Hadassah Hebrew University Medical Center, has set the standards for medical care in the state of Israel, setting Hadassah apart from other organizations in Israel and elsewhere in the Middle East. Hadassah provides equal treatment to all who come to it for assistance.

STAFF AND VOLUNTEERS

Hadassah is the largest national women's organization, the largest Jewish membership organization, and the largest Zionist organization in the United States. It is unique among organizations in that it is both volunteer-led and professionally managed, offering personally relevant opportunities for members to volunteer, grow, and make a difference. Its members' contributions of time and money are devoted to projects and initiatives directly associated with Hadassah. HWZOA has 316 paid staff in its New York headquarters and other offices throughout the country. Hadassah volunteers are culled from a membership of three hundred thousand women who reside in every congressional district.

Hadassah Hebrew University Medical Center's combined service, research, and teaching facilities employ more than five thousand people, making it the largest nongovernmental employer in Jerusalem.

RELATIONSHIPS WITH OTHER ORGANIZATIONS

Hadassah Hebrew University Medical Center is responsible for the clinical training of students in five Hadassah Hebrew University schools—Medicine, Occupational Therapy, Dentistry, Nursing, and Public Health. Hadassah has cooperative relationships with hospitals around the world for staff exchanges, fellowships, and joint research projects. The Hadassah School of Nursing has an internship with New York University (NYU) School of Nursing, for its master's degree students in clinical nursing. The Braun School of Public Health has an international master's program that prepares physicians to return to their home countries to work in public health. In this way, Hadassah is able to prepare well-trained health care personnel who serve in Israel and its neighboring countries as well as around the world.

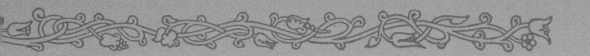

The Editors and Contributors

THE EDITORS

Robin Ely Berman, M.D., the founder, president, CEO, and medical director of the National Gaucher Foundation (NGF), is a woman, and a physician, with a purpose. A graduate of Yale University and Georgetown Medical School, she is married and the mother of six children, three of whom have Gaucher's disease. She also has one grandchild.

Berman, who lives in a suburb of Washington, D.C., worked as a family practice physician until one of her children was diagnosed with Gaucher's disease. She quit her private practice and began to work with physicians Roscoe Brady and John Barranger at the National Institutes of Health (NIH), where they were seeking a treatment for the disease. In 1984, together with her husband and her brother-in-law, Berman organized the National Gaucher Foundation, a nonprofit, tax-exempt organization.

When it came time for the new treatment to be tested on a human subject, Berman volunteered her son, then four years old and severely afflicted with the disease, to be infused with an enzyme replacement developed by Brady and Barranger. Brian Berman thus became the very first person to be treated with the experimental drug that was eventually approved in 1991 by the Food and Drug Administration and marketed by Genzyme Corporation as Ceredase.

Berman currently practices family medicine at the Center for Integrative Medicine in Rockville, Maryland.

Arthur Kurzweil (www.arthurkurzweil.com) is the publisher at *Parabola: The Search for Meaning,* a nondenominational quarterly devoted to the exploration of universal themes through the world's great spiritual traditions (www.parabola.org).

Trained as a professional librarian, for seventeen years he was editor-in-chief of the Jewish Book Club, where he was responsible for over seven hundred volumes of Jewish interest that were published by Jason Aronson Inc. Kurzweil is also past president of the Jewish Book Council, and has been a Judaica acquisitions editor and literary agent. As the Coordinator of the Talmud Circle Project, under the direction of Rabbi Adin Steinsaltz, Kurzweil's mission has been to introduce the Talmud to Jewish spiritual seekers. He has been the catalyst for many individuals as well as synagogue groups who now study Talmud regularly.

Kurzweil is an accomplished magician. A member of the Society of American Magicians (founded by Harry Houdini) as well as a member of the International Brotherhood of Magicians, Kurzweil often performs his show, "Searching for God in a Magic Shop," before Jewish audiences, blending his spiritual interests with magical effects, adding his own insights and weaving together an entertaining and informative presentation for his audiences.

Often described as America's foremost Jewish genealogist, Kurzweil's highly praised book, *From Generation to Generation: How to Trace Your Jewish Genealogy and Family History,* has become known as the definitive guidebook to the field. Kurzweil is the recipient of the Distinguished Humanitarian Award from the Melton Center of Ohio State University for his unique contributions to the field of Jewish education. He also received a Lifetime Achievement Award from the International Association of Jewish Genealogical Societies.

Kurzweil serves as Jewish Interest consultant for Jossey-Bass, an imprint of John Wiley Publishers. He lives in New Jersey and is the father of three children, Malya, Miriam, and Moshe.

Dale Leibson Mintz, MPA, CHES, has been educating women about the importance of taking care of themselves for more than twenty-five years. She and her husband, Steve, have two children, Eric, a behavioral neurobiologist who is a professor at Kent State University, and Jaclyn, a former lawyer and currently a yarn shop owner married to Adam, a physical therapist. Eric and his wife, Paige, made them grandparents in 2005 with the birth of Jordan Isaac.

Mintz graduated from Purchase College with a B.A. and Baruch College with an MPA and the designation as a certified health education specialist. She received her college degree when her children were twelve and nine. She has been active in her community, as a member of the board of directors of the Rye Art Center, Rye Historical Society, and Community Synagogue, in addition to the many years she spent starting a chapter of the American Medical Center at Denver, Tree of Life, in memory of Jack Leibson, her dad, to raise funds for cancer research.

Early in her career, Mintz worked for the American Heart Association and the National Hemophilia Foundation. For the past ten years she has been an advocate for women and their families as part of her professional activities at Hadassah. She is the founding national director of Women's Health and Advocacy. She has developed the curriculum for Healthy Women, Healthy Lives, a women's health program disseminated by Hadassah volunteers throughout the United States through symposia. She is a member of the Steering Committee of the National Colorectal Cancer Roundtable, which is a Centers for Disease Control and American Cancer Society funded organization advocating screening for colorectal cancer, a ninety-five percent preventable disease.

Through Mintz's efforts, Hadassah is a partner with the National Heart Lung and Blood Institute dedicated to educating women everywhere about nutrition, exercise, risks, and symptoms, through Hadassah's Healthy Women Healthy Lives symposiums. As the founding director of Women's Health and Advocacy, Mintz has realized her dream of reaching out to women to help them realize the importance of advocating on behalf of themselves and their families.

THE CONTRIBUTORS

Rabbi Richard F. Address, D.Min., directs the Department of Jewish Family Concerns for the Union for Reform Judaism. He teaches courses in issues related to the family at Hebrew Union College in New York.

Rabbi Bradley Shavit Artson is the dean, Ziegler School of Rabbinic Studies. He may be reached at Vice President, University of Judaism; 15600 Mulholland Drive, Los Angeles, California 90077-1599; http://www.bradartson.com

Elizabeth A. Battaglino, R.N., is the director of marketing and consumer affairs for the National Women's Health Resource Center and has worked more than thirteen years in coordinating outreach programs at the state, local, and national levels.

Shoshana Matzner Bekerman is a graduate of Bar Ilan University, Israel, and Hofstra University, New York. She is the author of the *International Directory of Child Development Research Centers*, distributed internationally by UNICEF, and of *The Jewish Child: A Halakhic Perspective* (Ktav Publications, 1984), which outlines the biblical perspective on child development and child rearing. She taught ethics and sociology at the Israeli campuses of Fairleigh-Dickinson University and Touro College and is the founder of the Global Ethics Resource Center (GERC), affiliated with Touro College USA. Among the initiatives of the GERC is a project to promote parenting education and school systems geared toward peace and ethics.

Adena K. Berkowitz, Ph.D., an independent consultant in New York, is an attorney with her doctorate in Jewish ethics. A prolific writer whose articles have appeared in a host of publications, she helped found the Hadassah National Center for Attorneys' Councils.

Rabbi Sandra Rosenthal Berliner serves as the chaplain for Federation Housing Inc. and the JCC Klein Branch Senior Adult Department under the auspices of the Joan Grossman Center for Chaplaincy and Healing of the Jewish Family and Children's Services of Greater Philadelphia. Rabbi Berliner directed Yedid Nefesh, the Jewish Hospice Program of Philadelphia, for eleven years, as well as serving Congregation Temple Menorah Kenesseth Chai in Philadelphia. She is a past president of the National Association of Jewish Chaplains.

Rabbi Berliner is a graduate of the Reconstructionist Rabbinical College, where she received her rabbinical ordination and Master of Hebrew Letters degree. She earned a master's degree in social work at Case Western Reserve University and a bachelor's degree in Near Eastern and Judaic studies and education from Brandeis University. She has written many articles for the *Philadelphia Jewish Press* and consults on aspects of Jewish healing, especially as it relates to aging, dying, and bereavement. She is the wife of Roy Berliner and the mother of Benjamin, Jonathan, and Jacob.

Diane Bloomfield is the creator of Torah Yoga and the author of *Torah Yoga: Experiencing Jewish Wisdom Through Classic Postures* (Jossey Bass, 2004). She has been studying Torah since the mid-1980s. She began her yoga studies shortly thereafter at the Kripalu Institute in Massachusetts in a wide range of styles. She is a certified Phoenix Rising Yoga Therapist.

Bloomfield lives in Jerusalem with her husband and daughter. She teaches Torah yoga classes throughout North America, Western Europe, and Israel. She is the codirector of the Yoga and Jewish Spirituality Teacher Training Program at Elat Chayyim (http://www.elatchayyim.org) and the founder of the Torah Yoga Association (http://www.torahyoga.org).

Rabbi Barry H. Block has served Temple Beth-El in San Antonio since 1992 and became the congregation's senior rabbi in 2002. He is chair of the Central Conference of American Rabbis' Resolutions Committee and treasurer of the Southwest Association of Reform Rabbis. He represents his colleagues throughout Texas and Oklahoma as rabbinic adviser of the Union of American Hebrew Congregations' Greene Family Camp for Living Judaism in Bruceville, Texas. Locally, Rabbi Block is a director of Methodist Healthcare Ministries and serves on the board of governors of the Methodist Healthcare System. He served as chair of Planned Parenthood of San Antonio and South Central Texas and serves on the boards of the American Jewish Society for Service, the Jewish Federation of San Antonio, and United Way of San Antonio and Bexar County. Rabbi Block has been a member of the Ethics Committee of the Bexar County Medical Society and the Steering Committee of Leadership San Antonio.

Rick Blum, Ph.D., is a licensed psychologist in the state of Connecticut, pursuing a full-time psychotherapy practice since opening his West Hartford office in 1986. A graduate of Brandeis University, he completed graduate degrees in comparative religion and the psychology of religion (Iowa and Syracuse). He went on to receive his Ph.D. in psychology (Saybrook) and achieved a rank in the top ten percent of doctors of psychology in the national testing program. In consulting work, he has been helpful in settings as diverse as the San Francisco Police Department and the Power Authority of the State of New York. He later developed a full, non-HMO practice. The two chapters he contributed to this book reflect his ongoing project focusing on psychological issues in Jewish continuity, under the working title *God for People with Brains: A Psychologist Puts Judaism on the Couch*. To learn more of his perspectives on psychology or to contact him, go to http://www.dr-rick.com.

Rear Admiral Susan J. Blumenthal, M.D., M.P.A, a champion and a pioneer in improving women's health, served as the country's first deputy assistant secretary for women's health and as assistant surgeon general of the United States in the U.S. Department of Health and Human Services. She is clinical professor of psychiatry at Georgetown and Tufts Schools of Medicine and distinguished visiting professor of women's studies at Brandeis University.

Leslie Bonci, M.P.H., R.D., L.D.N., is director of sports medicine nutrition at the University of Pittsburgh Medical Center.

Roscoe O. Brady, M.D., is chief of the Developmental and Metabolic Neurology Branch in the National Institute of Neurological Disorders and Stroke. He is a graduate of Harvard Medical School. He interned at the Hospital of the University of Pennsylvania and was a postdoctoral fellow in biochemistry at that medical school. He is an innovator in the identification of the causes and treatment of Gaucher's disease, Niemann-Pick disease, Fabry disease, and Tay-Sachs disease. He is currently exploring enzyme replacement, gene therapy, and other treatment strategies for Gaucher's and Fabry. He is the recipient of numerous awards and a member of the National Academy of Sciences USA and its Institute of Medicine.

Rabbi Yitzchok Breitowitz is the rabbi of the Woodside Synagogue in Silver Spring, Maryland, and a professor of law at the University of Maryland School of Law in Baltimore. He received his rabbinical ordination from Ner Israel Rabbinical College in 1976, and his J.D.

(magna cum laude) from Harvard Law School in 1979. He is a frequent lecturer on medical, legal, and family ethics and their interface with halakhah. He has written extensively on medical ethics, including articles on cloning, assisted reproduction, organ transplantation, and brain death. He is also the author of *Between Religious and Civil Law: The Plight of the Agunah* (Greenwood Press, 1993).

Deborah Bright, Ph.D., is president of Bright Enterprise, formerly in New York, headquartered now in Tucson, Arizona. Speaker and author of *On the Edge* and *In Control* (McGraw-Hill). She may be contacted at dbright@brightent.com or 520-620-3500.

Aggie Casey, R.N., M.S., is a clinical nurses specialist and director of the Cardiac Wellness Program at the Mind/Body Medical Institute in Boston, Massachusetts. She is coauthor of *Mind Your Heart: A Mind/Body Approach to Stress Management, Exercise, and Nutrition* (2004) and *The Medical School Guide to Lowering Your Blood Pressure* (forthcoming, 2006).

Lisa C. Cohn, M.M.Sc., M.Ed., R.D., is founder of Park Avenue Nutrition Spa and Consulting in New York. She may be reached at Park Avenue Nutrition, 1108 Park Avenue, NY, NY 10128. Tel: 212-831-7900, www.parkavenutrition.com and lccnutrition@aol.com.

Debra P. Cohen first learned of Gaucher when trying to understand exactly what was causing her daughter's mysterious illness. Since learning of Gaucher, she has become passionate in writing articles and speaking about Gaucher, the most common genetic disorder carried by individuals of Eastern European Jewish descent. Cohen lives in Atlanta, Georgia, with her husband and two children.

Bonnie Cramer is the Hillel adviser for Union College and has worked for the past twelve summers at Camp Ramah in New England. She is currently head of the art department at Ramah and oversees the specialty staff. She has taught in the Schenectady, New York, Midrasha and has for many years co-led the Art and Spirituality Project for the Greater New England Women's annual retreat. She is a Reiki master and is deeply committed to teaching Kabbalah to young people. She has made many presentations on Jewish spirituality, including a recent presentation at the Albany Capital District Hadassah "Mind Body Spirit" conference on the subject of Reiki and Judaism. Cramer lives in Schenectady with her husband Steve, son Dan, and daughter Shira. She may be contacted at SepSci@msn.com.

Catherine Dee is the award-winning author of five inspirational non-fiction titles for girls ages nine to fifteen, including *The Girls' Guide to Life* and *The Girls' Book of Wisdom*. For information about the books, please visit www.empowergirls.com.

Andrea M. Denicoff, R.N., M.S., C.A.N.P., is a senior program manager with twenty years of experience in cancer clinical trials at the National Cancer Institute, part of the National Institutes of Health within the U.S. Department of Health and Human Services.

Margo A. Denke, M.D., practices at Sid Peterson Memorial Hospital in Kerrville, Texas. She received her M.D. from Harvard Medical School, Boston, Massachusetts and is a member of the American Board of Internal Medicine and the American Board of Endocrinology.

Rabbi Amy Eilberg was a cofounder of the Bay Area Jewish Healing Center, where she directed the center's Jewish Hospice Care Program. She currently serves as codirector of the Morei Derekh Training Program for Jewish Spiritual Direction, a program of the Yedidya Center for Jewish Spiritual Direction, which is dedicated to introducing the practice of Jewish spiritual direction to the American Jewish community through training, public education, and professional support. She offers spiritual direction in Saint Paul, Minnesota (http://www.yedidyacenter.org; rebamy@yedidyacenter.org).

Daniel Eisenberg, M.D., is an attending radiologist at Albert Einstein Medical Center in Philadelphia and a Jewish medical ethics lecturer. He serves as the scholar in residence for the yearly Jewish Medical Ethics and Israel Experience Program in Jerusalem. He has taught a weekly medical halakhah class for fifteen years, most recently at the Philadelphia Community Kollel, and lectures widely on the Jewish approach to medical ethics. His articles can be found on his Web site (http://www.daneisenberg.com), as well as at Aish HaTorah (http://www.aish.com), Jewish Law (http://www.jlaw.com), and many other sites.

Wendy Elliman was born in London, England, and has lived in Jerusalem for over thirty years. She is a prize-winning feature writer, specializing in science and technology.

Rabbi Nancy Flam is a pioneer in the field of Jewish healing. Having cofounded the Jewish Healing Center in 1991, she then directed the Jewish Community Healing Program of Ruach Ami: Bay Area Jewish Healing Center in San Francisco. She was the founding director and is now codirector of programs of the Institute for Jewish Spirituality, a retreat-based learning program for Jewish leaders. She has served as a consultant for Synagogue 2000 and the National Center for Jewish Healing. Rabbi Flam earned her B.A. degree in religion from Dartmouth College in 1982, earned her M.A. degree in Hebrew literature from the Hebrew Union College–Jewish Institute of Religion in 1986, and was ordained in 1989. Rabbi Flam lectures widely on the topic of Judaism and healing and has written on the issue for such publications as *Reform Judaism* magazine and *Sh'ma: A Journal of Jewish Responsibility.* She has also contributed to such works as *Wrestling with the Angel: Jewish Insights on Death and Mourning* (Schocken Books, 1995), edited by Jack Riemer; *Jewish Pastoral Care* (Jewish Lights, 2nd ed., 2005), edited by Dayle A. Friedman; and *Best Contemporary Jewish Writing* (Jossey-Bass, 2001), edited by Michael Lerner. She is the series editor for *LifeLights,* a series of informational, inspirational pamphlets on challenges in the emotional and spiritual life. She lives in Northampton, Massachusetts, with her husband and two children.

Tamar Frankiel, Ph.D., is the dean of students and a professor of comparative religion at the Academy for Jewish Religion, California, in Los Angeles. She is the author of *The Voice of Sarah: Feminine Spirituality and Traditional Judaism* (HarperCollins, 1990) and *The Gift of Kabbalah: Discovering the Secrets of Heaven, Renewing Your Life on Earth* (Jewish Lights, 2001) and coauthor with Judy Greenfeld of *Minding the Temple of the Soul* (Jewish Lights, 1997) and *Entering the Temple of Dreams* (Jewish Lights, 2000). She earned her doctorate in the history of religions at the University of Chicago and is a life member of Hadassah.

Michael Freund is founder and chairman of Shavei Israel (http://www.shavei.org), a Jerusalem-based group that reaches out and assists "lost Jews" seeking to return to the Jewish people. He writes a syndicated column and feature stories for the *Jerusalem Post,* Israel's leading English-language daily, and he previously served as deputy director of communications and policy planning in the prime minister's office under Benjamin Netanyahu. A native of New York, he holds an M.B.A. in finance from Columbia University and a B.A. from the Woodrow Wilson School of Public and International Affairs at Princeton University. Freund has a special connection with Hadassah: his late grandmother, Miriam Freund-Rosenthal, served as its national president from 1956 to 1960. He can be contacted at michael@shavei.org.

Rabbi Barry Freundel has been the rabbi of Kesher Israel Congregation, Washington, D.C., since 1989. He also serves as assistant professor of rabbinics, Baltimore Hebrew University and adjunct professor of law at Georgetown University. Freundel is the author of *Contemporary Orthodox Judaism's Response to Modernity* and many articles on Judaism and contemporary issues.

Ruth Gassner is a nurse, born in Tel Aviv, and graduated from the Hadassah nursing school in Ein Karem. She worked as a head nurse at the Oncology Pediatric ward in Ein Karem until 1985 and since then at the Ina and Jack Kay Hospice on Scopus as a director.

Ya'akov Gerlitz is the founder and director of the Jewish Healing Foundation (http://www.JewishHealing.com), a resource and support center dedicated to the development and practice of authentic Jewish healing systems based on Torah and Kabbalah. He can be reached yaakovg@Jewishhealing.com.

Rabbi Moshe Goldberger is the author of more than fifteen popular books, including *Be a Friend*, *Treat Yourself Right*, *The Road to Greatness*, *Master Your Thoughts*, and *Watch Your Wealth* (all published by Feldheim). He teaches at the Yeshiva of Staten Island and gives the Daf Yomi Shiur, a daily Talmud class, in a number of places.

Joel Lurie Grishaver is a coowner of Torah Aura Productions and the Alef Design Group. He is a writer, a teacher, a cartoonist, and a storyteller. He coedits three weekly publications: *Bim Bam*, *C.Ha* (pronounced "see-kha"), and the *Torah Aura Bulletin Board*. He has written or cowritten more than sixty books, including *Shema Is for Real* (Torah Aura, 1994) and *Forty Things You Can Do to Save the Jewish People* (Alef, 1997). Grishaver has degrees from Boston University and the University of Chicago. He has pursued graduate studies at the Hebrew Union College and the University of Southern California. He is a founding board member of the Coalition for the

Advancement of Jewish Education, a consultant to the Whizin Institute for Jewish Family Life, and a faculty member for the Department of Continuing Education of the University of Judaism. More than twenty weekends a year, Grishaver teaches Jewish learners of all ages as a scholar in residence in communities all over North America and Europe. In 1998, he was awarded the Covenant Award for outstanding contributions to Jewish education. He can be contacted at grishaver@torahaura.com.

Rachel Gurevich specializes in empowering parents through her books and magazine articles. She is the author of *The FabJob Guide to Become a Doula* (FabJob.com, 2000) and *The Doula Advantage: Your Complete Guide to Having an Empowering and Positive Childbirth with the Help of a Professional Labor Assistant* (Prima, 2003). *The Doula Advantage* received endorsements from Dr. William Sears, America's pediatrician and author of more than thirty books, and Ann Douglas, author of several books, including *The Mother of All Pregnancy Books*. *The FabJob Guide* and *The Doula Advantage* have become part of many doula training programs. Gurevich's articles have appeared in nearly two dozen publications, including *Pregnancy Magazine*, *Low Carb Energy*, *ePregnancy Magazine*, and *North West Baby and Child*. She is also an award-winning poet and an experienced book and magazine editor who currently teaches for the Long Ridge Writer's Group. Visit her Web site at http://www.doyoudoula.com, or e-mail her at Rachel@doyoudoula.com.

Edith Diament Gurewitsch, M.D., is assistant professor of gynecology and obstetrics at the Johns Hopkins University School of Medicine.

Rickie M. Haas M.S., R.D., C.D.N., is a registered dietitian in private practice in Rye Brook, New York.

Andrea Y. Hart is a program associate in the United Hospital Fund's Division of Education and Program Initiatives. She is responsible for coordinating research and programmatic activities for the Families and Health Care Project and the Medicine as a Profession Forum, a collaboration of the Fund and the Open Society Institute.

Lisa Hoffman, M.A., is an exercise physiologist and the founder and president of Solo Fitness, Inc., an in-home personal training company in New York City. She is the author of *Better Than Ever: The 4-Week Workout Program for Women Over 40* and *The Healing Power of Movement: How to Benefit from Physical Activity During Your Cancer Treatment.* She can be reached at lisahoffman@solofitness.com.

Hospice Foundation of America (http://www.hospicefoundation.org) provides leadership in the development and application of hospice and its philosophy of care with the goal of enhancing the American health care system and the role of hospice within it. The foundation meets its mission by conducting programs in professional development, public education and information, research, and health policy issues. Programs for health care professionals assist those who cope personally or professionally with terminal illness, death, and the process of grief and are offered on a national or regional basis. Programs for the public assist individual consumers of health care who are coping with issues of caregiving, terminal illness, and grief.

Rabbi Richard J. Israel, z"l, was a rabbi, marathon runner, beekeeper, and mentor to college students and colleagues during his career as a Hillel director and Jewish educator. He served Hillels at UCLA and Yale University and was regional director of Hillel for metropolitan Boston and New England. After retiring, he wrote, lectured, taught, and served as a consultant to and interim director of several Jewish organizations, including the Hillels at Princeton and Brandeis Universities. He died in July 2000.

Yoel Julian Jakobovits, M.D., was born in Dublin, Ireland, in 1950. He studied at Ner Israel Rabbinical College and John Hopkins University, both in Maryland, and then returned to the British Isles, joining his father, then chief rabbi of England, and pursuing his medical studies at the University of London. Since 1982, Jakobovits has been on the staff of the Sinai Hospital in Baltimore, where he is currently an attending physician in the Division of General Medicine and the Division of Gastroenterology. He is an assistant professor of medicine at the John Hopkins University School of Medicine and maintains a busy private and teaching practice. He resides with his wife and family on the campus of the Ner Israel Rabbinical College, Baltimore, where he is the resident physician. He travels extensively to teach, lecture, and conduct Jewish seminars and medical clinics.

Jewish AIDS Trust (JAT) (http://jat-uk.org) was established as a charity in 1988 to provide the Jewish community with HIV education, counseling, and support. JAT has now extended its work to include education and raising awareness of all matters of sexual health, including HIV. Its services are extended to the entire Jewish community, and it is not allied with any particular branch. JAT's sexual health and HIV educational programs and workshops are tailored to the needs of individuals and groups in the community, including youth groups, schools, students, parents, social welfare organizations, friends, and rabbis. Confidential and professional face-to-face counseling is provided for Jewish people with HIV/AIDS as well as their partners, friends, and family members. JAT provides financial support for Jewish people with symptomatic HIV who cannot meet essential bills and provides short-term social and economic support to meet the needs of people living with or affected by HIV.

Lisa Katz has managed online sites that focus on Judaism, Jewish culture, and Israel since 1994. First she ran sites for CompuServe and Microsoft Network, and currently she manages the About Judaism site (http://judaism.about.com). In 1996, she produced the first Net chat with a major head of state, Prime Minister Benjamin Netanyahu, for MSNBC. In addition, Katz comanages two companies: WPI (http://www.webpresentit.com) is a Web design company, and Shemot (http://www.shemot.com) offers personalized Hebrew name gifts. Katz lives in Israel with her husband and four children.

Alexis Kuerbis, C.S.W., is a project director of the onsite CASAWORKS for Families research project of the National Center on Addiction and Substance Abuse at Columbia University, at the Mount Sinai Medical Center Alcohol and Other Drug Treatment Program, where she also provides individual, group, and family addiction treatment. Kuerbis teaches courses on alcoholism and on bioethical issues at St. Joseph's College of New York in Brooklyn. Formerly, she was the program associate at the United Hospital Fund's Families and Health Care Project.

Esther D. Kustanowitz is a full-time freelance writer and editor whose areas of expertise include dating and relationships, Jewish life, and pop culture. She can be reached via her website, www.estherk.com.

Carol Levine joined the United Hospital Fund in 1996 as director of its Families and Health Care Project. She continues to direct the Orphan Project: Families and Children in the HIV Epidemic, which she founded in 1991. She was director of the Citizens Commission on AIDS in New York City from 1987 to 1991. As a senior staff associate of the Hastings Center, she edited the *Hasting Center Report.* In 1993 she was awarded a MacArthur Foundation Fellowship for her work in AIDS policy and ethics.

Fran Levine is the former media relations manager for Hadassah and wrote for the Hadassah *Health Memo.*

Yaakov Levinson holds a bachelor of arts degree in biology from Hamilton College and a master of science degree in clinical nutrition from Case Western Reserve University. He was a member of the American Dietetic Association. In Israel, Levinson was for five years the director of the Nutrition Department of the Rebecca Sieff Hospital in Tzefat, during which time he also taught dietetic interns from the Hebrew University of Rechovot and lectured at the Tzefat School of Nursing and to hospital physicians on nutrition topics. He has been the nutritionist of the Surgery and Orthopedics Departments at Hadassah Hospital, Ein Karem; nutritionist for the Radiology Department of the Sharett Cancer Institute at Hadassah; the head dietitian at Hadassah Hospital, Mount Scopus; and nutrition consultant at the Neve Simcha Geriatric Hospital in Mattersdorf. Levinson has presented original research at international nutrition congresses in the Philippines and in Scotland. He is the author of *The Jewish Guide to Natural Nutrition* (Feldheim, 1995). A Torah-observant Jew, Levinson has studied at both Chasidic and Lithuanian yeshivas in Brooklyn, Tzefat, and Jerusalem.

Litapayach Tikvah (To Nourish Hope) is part of the program of the Union for Reform Judaism's Department of Jewish Family Concerns. This program department develops programs for congregations that deal with issues of how Judaism and Jewish values affect current issues facing the Jewish family. The Eating Disorders program is now part of the larger *K'dushat HaGuf* (Sanctity of the Body) program of Jewish Family Concerns, which deals with self-destructive behaviors. The department of Jewish Family Concerns is directed by Rabbi Richard F. Address, D.Min., who can be reached at raddress@urj.org.

Chaim Lotan, M.D., was born and trained in Israel. Since 2000, he has been the director of The Heart Institute of Hadassah Hospital in Jerusalem, Israel (e-mail: lotan@hadassah.org.il; Web site: http://www.hadassah.org.ill/English/Eng_SubNavBar/Departments/Medical+departments/Cardiology/).

Rabbi Goldie Milgram, D.Min., M.S.W., travels internationally as a teacher of Torah and Jewish spiritual practices. She is founder and director of ReclaimingJudaism.org and author of *Meaning and Mitzvah: Daily Practices for Reclaiming Judaism Through God, Prayer, Torah, Mitzvot, Hebrew, and Peoplehood* (Jewish Lights, 2005); *Reclaiming Judaism as a Spiritual Practice: Holy Days and Shabbat* (Jewish Lights, 2004); and *Make Your Own Bar/Bat Mitzvah: A Personal Guide to a Meaningful Rite of Passage* (Jossey-Bass, 2004). "Reb Goldie" is a 2006 Covenant Award nominee for excellence as a Jewish educator and holds the American Cancer Society's Distinguished Citizen Award for her innovation and coanchoring of NBC's *Health Watch*, America's first health-based television programming.

Rabbi Avis Dimond Miller, who holds the longest pulpit tenure of any woman in the Conservative movement, has served Adas Israel Congregation, Washington, D.C., since 1986. She is chair of the Rabbinical Assembly's Committee on Outreach and Conversion, as well as immediate past president of its Washington/Baltimore Region. A Life Member of Hadassah, she is married to Ralph Miller, the mother of five sons, and the grandmother of nine.

Abigail Natenshon, M.A., L.C.S.W., G.C.F.P., is a psychotherapist and author of *When Your Child Has an Eating Disorder: A Step-by-Step Workbook for Parents and Other Caregivers* (Jossey-Bass, 1999) and of the e-book *Doing What Works: The Professional's Guide to Treating Eating Disorders.* As founder and director of Eating Disorder Specialists of Illinois, Natenshon is also a guild-certified Feldenkrais practitioner. She can be visited on the Web at http://www.empoweredparents.com and contacted at anatenshon@empoweredparents.com.

National Center for Jewish Healing (NCJH) helps communities meet the spiritual needs of Jews living with illness and loss. Working closely with a network of Jewish healing centers and programs, both nationally and internationally, NCJH develops Jewish healing resources and leadership and offers consultation, publications, training, and referrals to community resources.

National Niemann-Pick Disease Foundation, Inc. (NNPDF), is an international voluntary nonprofit organization made up of parents, medical and educational professionals, friends, relatives, and others who are committed to finding a cure for Niemann-Pick disease (NPD). Its primary goals are to promote medical research into the cause of NPD in order to eventually find a cure, provide medical and educational information to assist in the correct diagnosis and referral of children with NPD, provide support to families of NPD patients, facilitate genetic counseling for parents who are known carriers of NPD, encourage the sharing of research information among scientists, and support legislation that positively affects patients and families with NPD. NNPDF has close ties with other Niemann-Pick foundations, allowing for efficient planning for research. Its Website is http://www.nnpdf.org.

Nishmat Women's Online Information Center is a public service of Nishmat, the Jerusalem Center for Advanced Jewish Study for Women. The school was established in 1990 and offers women the opportunity to immerse themselves in Torah study. In 1997, Nishmat established the Keren Ariel Women's Halachic Institute to train Yoatzot Halacha (Women Halachic Consultants), under the direction of Rabbi Yaacov Varhaftig, dean of the institute, and Rabbi Yehuda Herzl Henkin. These women are certified by a panel of Orthodox rabbis to be a resource for women with questions regarding *Taharat Hamishpachah* (an area of Jewish law that relates to marriage, sexuality, and women's health) who are more comfortable discussing these personal issues with another woman than with a man. Each consultant devotes two years (over one thousand hours) to intensive study with rabbinic authorities and experts in psychology, gynecology, infertility, women's health, family dynamics, and sexuality. The Yoatzot Halacha Web site is http://www.yoatzot.org; there is also a Web site for women's health professionals, http://www.jewishwomenshealth.org.

Vanessa L. Ochs is director of Jewish studies and associate professor of religious studies at the University of Virginia. Her books include *Sarah Laughed, The Jewish Dream Book, Safe and Sound,* and *Words on Fire.*

Ohr Somayach (http://www.ohr.org.il) was founded in 1972 in Jerusalem by a group of experienced Torah educators from America. Deeply concerned about the vast number of Jews who were growing up with little or no knowledge of their heritage, these dedicated teachers sought to shine a ray of hope into the darkness of ignorance—the light of Torah knowledge. They understood that the beauty and truth of Torah study, which has united and inspired Jews throughout the ages, would kindle the interest and excitement of the next generation as well. They created a school to stimulate bright young minds with the collected wisdom of three thousand years, in a format geared for students of contemporary higher education. From modest origins—an unheated, rented room, with no dining facilities—blossomed an institution for the intellectually sophisticated newcomer to Jewish thought and learning, and the age-old philosophy of the Jewish people, brought forward into today's turbulent world. That original school has grown into an international network of schools, facilities, and outreach programs on six continents, serving thousands of Jewish students of all ages. The philosophy, however, has not changed: teach Jews about their heritage by giving them direct access into its source, the Torah.

Gregory M. Pastores, M.D., G.M.P., is an associate professor of neurology and pediatrics at New York University School of Medicine and director of the Neurogenetics Laboratory, Department of Neurology, NYU SOM.

Rebecca Phillips is assistant managing editor of Beliefnet (http://www.beliefnet.com), the multifaith religion and spirituality Web site. She is a frequent contributor to JBooks.com and has written for the *Forward*, the *Jewish Telegraphic Agency*, and other publications. She lives in Brooklyn, New York.

Thea Pugatsch, Ph.D., T.P., grew up in Switzerland. In 1979 she earned her Ph.D. in molecular biology at the ETH-Zurich. She joined the Heart Institute at Hadassah in 2001 as research coordinator in basic science. (e-mail: pthea@hadassah.org.il).

Rabbinical Council of America (http://www.rabbis.org) was established in 1935 to advance the cause and the voice of Torah and the rabbinic tradition by promoting the welfare, interests, and professionalism of Orthodox rabbis around the world. Membership is held by close to one thousand rabbis in fourteen countries, including numerous rabbinic authorities. It has been led by outstanding personalities, most notably Rabbi Joseph B. Soloveitchik, who died in 1993. The council frequently partners with other Jewish organizations. It publishes Torah and intellectual journals, holds annual conventions and conferences, and issues occasional position papers and statements on current issues. The council also provides services for the Orthodox rabbinate.

Rabbi Yisrael Rutman was born and raised in New York City. He graduated from the City University of New York, where he served as an editor of the weekly student newspaper on the Lehman College campus. After some years of wandering, he took an interest in Judaism and received rabbinical ordination in Israel. Nowadays, he does his wandering in one place—Zichron Yaakov, Israel—where he teaches Jewish studies and writes for various publications.

Ellen Schulman is a career woman, Jewish communal volunteer, and advocate for organ donor awareness. Raised in Hartford, Connecticut, she graduated from Hofstra University in Hempstead, New York. Ellen's business career began as an operations manager for Bloomingdale's in Manhattan. Following her marriage to Douglas, she entered the family business in the position of sales manager for Manhattan Shade and Glass.

Ellen is part of a family that has been involved with Hadassah for many years. She is the third link of four generations of life members, three generations of Hadassah presidents, and is a third generation Founder. Ellen was instrumental in forming a Young Leaders Group in Bayside, New York, and is currently a member of the Kochivim Group in Great Neck, New York.

Ellen epitomizes today's young woman successfully balancing family, career, and Jewish communal life. She has always been actively involved in the life of her community and her synagogue, and has now added advocate for organ donation to her efforts.

Richard H. Schwartz, Ph.D., is the author of *Judaism and Vegetarianism, Judaism and Global Survival,* and *Mathematics and Global Survival.* He has over 130 articles on the Internet at http://jewishveg.com/schwartz and frequently speaks and contributes articles on environmental, health, and other current issues. He is pro-fessor emeritus of mathematics at the College of Staten Island, president of the Jewish Vegetarians of North America (JVNA), and coordinator of the Society of Ethical and Religious Vegetarians (SERV). He was inaugurated into the Hall of Fame of the North American Vegetarian Society (NAVS) at its 2005 Summerfest. He and his wife, Lisa Schwartz, have four children: Akiva, Hillel, Eitan, and Ilana.

Cantor Philip L. Sherman, *Mohel,* was trained by Rabbi Yosef Halperin (of blessed memory) in Jerusalem and was certified by the Chief Rabbinate of Israel in June 1977. Cantor Sherman is also certi-fied by the Brith Milah Board of New York. He is familiar with both Ashkenazi and Sephardic customs and traditions. Cantor Sherman has been invited to Japan, Singapore, Hong Kong, and Bermuda to perform brisses. He is located in Manhattan and Westchester and performs brisses in New York, New Jersey, and Connecticut. Cantor Sherman serves as one of the *hazzanim* at Congregation Shearith Israel, the Spanish and Portuguese Synagogue in New York City, and is a member of the Cantorial Council of America and the Screen Actor's Guild.

Rabbi Seymour Siegel, **z"l,** was a noted theologian, writer, teacher, and specialist in the field of medical and biological ethics. He headed the Department of Philosophies of Judaism at the Jewish Theological Seminary of America and held numerous other university posts. He was for a decade the chairman of the Committee on Jewish Law and Standards of the Rabbinical Assembly, the international organization of Conservative rabbis. He wrote many articles and wrote or edited many books, including *Conservative Judaism and Jewish Law* and *Medical Ethics in a Jewish Perspective.* He died in 1988.

Rina Stein is a pseudonym.

Rabbi Chaim Steinmetz has been the spiritual leader of Tifereth Beth David Jerusalem in Montreal, Canada, since September 1996. He writes a regular column for the *Canadian Jewish News.* Rabbi Steinmetz is the past president of the Montreal Board of Rabbis and past vice-president of the Quebec Region of the Canadian Jewish Congress. He serves on the executive board of the Quebec Israel Committee, the Rabbinical Council of America, and the Kollel

Torah MiTzion and also on the board of the Federation/CJA of Montreal and Hillel-Jewish Students Center of Montreal. He was the recipient of the Federation/CJA's 2001 Gertrude and Henry Plotnick Young Leadership Award. He received his ordination from Yeshiva University, where he was a fellow of the elite Gruss Kollel Elyon. He has a master's degree in Jewish philosophy from the Bernard Revel Graduate School, and a master's in education from Adelphi University. He has completed Leadership Education and Development and Meorot Rabbinic fellowships.

Elaine Sugarman, M.S., is a board-certified genetic counselor and a project manager for Genzyme Genetics' Molecular Diagnostic Laboratory. She is active in providing education and publications related to carrier screening, particularly for conditions that occur with increased frequency in the Ashkenazi Jewish population.

Rabbi Moshe David Tendler, Ph.D., is professor of medical ethics, senior professor of biology, and professor of Talmudic law at Yeshiva University, New York, New York.

Union for Reform Judaism (URJ) is the central body of Reform Judaism in North America, uniting 1.5 million Reform Jews in more than nine hundred synagogues. URJ services include camps, music and book publishing, outreach to unaffiliated and intermarried Jews, educational programs, and the Religious Action Center in Washington, D.C.

United Synagogue of Conservative Judaism represents and supports the synagogues of the Conservative movement. The organization works with lay leaders and Jewish professionals at the national, regional, and grassroots levels to teach, inspire, and motivate Conservative Jews to live lives increasingly filled with Jewish learning, ethical behavior, spirituality, and *mitzvot*.

Miryam Z. Wahrman, Ph.D., is professor of biology, director of general education, and codirector of the Center for Holocaust and Genocide Studies at William Paterson University of New Jersey. Wahrman earned her doctorate in biochemistry at Cornell University and did biomedical research at Sloan-Kettering Institute, Cornell University Medical College, Rockefeller University, and Mount Sinai School of Medicine. She is author of *Brave New Judaism: When*

Science and Scripture Collide (University Press of New England/ Brandeis University Press, 2nd ed., 2004) and is an award-winning journalist who publishes extensively on science, medical ethics, and Judaism.

Rabbi Simkha Y. Weintraub, C.S.W., is rabbinic director of the National Center for Jewish Healing (http://www.ncjh.org), a program of the Jewish Board of Family and Children's Services in New York City.

Judy Wertheimer teaches writing to children at an elementary school. She has published occasional articles in the *Pittsburgh Post-Gazette* and completed her first novel, and is working on her second. She lives in Pittsburgh with her husband and two sons.

Rabbi Gerald I. Wolpe, M.A., M.H.L., D.D., is a rabbi emeritus of Har Zion Temple, Penn Valley, Pennsylvania, where he served as senior rabbi for thirty years, until retiring in 1999. He is the director of the Jewish Theological Seminary's Louis Finkelstein Institute of Social and Religious Studies, and a senior fellow of the University of Pennsylvania's Center for Bioethics. He is also a member of the Aphasia Society of America's board of directors, and of the National Institute of Health Commission on Genetics and the Community.

Women of Reform Judaism (WRJ) (http://wrj.rj.org), an affiliate of the Union for Reform Judaism, is the collective voice and presence of women in congregational life. WRJ brings together more than seventy-five thousand Jewish women in 550 sisterhoods throughout North America, with affiliated women's groups around the world. Founded in 1913 as the National Federation of Temple Sisterhoods (NFTS), the organization was established during a historic period of advancing struggle for recognition and equality for women. Empowered by the Reform movement's precept of placing Jewish women on a plane of religious equality with men, NFTS became active in areas that continue to define its work today. The founder of NFTY (the North American Federation of Temple Youth) and a founder of the Jewish Braille Institute, WRJ is a member of the World Union for Progressive Judaism and works on behalf of the Hebrew Union College–Jewish Institute of Religion.

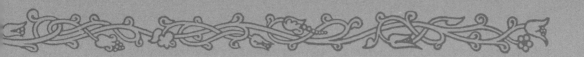

Credits

PART ONE: HEALTH IN THE JEWISH TRADITION

Chapter 1, "Hadassah's Commitment: Jewish Perspective on Health," by Edith Diament Gurewitsch.

Chapter 2, "The Jewish Way of Healing," by Nancy Flam. From www.parkridgecenter.org/Page94.html

Chapter 3, "Ten Jewish Psychological Insights," by Rick Blum. With permission from Dr. Rick Blum.

Chapter 4, "Why Are So Many Hospitals Named After Mount Sinai?" by Yisrael Rutman. From http://www.aish.com/societyWork/sciencenature/Judaisms_Mind-Body_Connection.asp

Chapter 5, "The Healing Path of Jewish Tradition Is Entering Upon an Awakening," by Tamar Frankel. From www.judaism.com/12paths/sciencemedicine.htm

PART TWO: TAKING CARE OF THE BODY

Chapter 6, "Whose Body Is It Anyway?" by Rabbi Barry H. Block. From www.beth-elsa.org/bb030703.htm

Chapter 7, "Jewish Stress Management," by Rick Blum. With permission from Dr. Rick Blum.

Chapter 8, "Nurturing the Nurturer: Be Good to Yourself," by Leslie Bonci. From *Health Memo*, Hadassah, Fall 2003.

Chapter 9, "The People of the Treadmill," by Michael Freund. From *The Jerusalem Post*, September 14, 2004.

Chapter 10, "Finally, Kosher Yoga," by Rebecca Phillips. From www.beliefnet.com/story/144/story_14473_1.html

Special Focus: Specific Health Care Issues

Chapter 11, "How to Talk to Your Doctor: An Rx for M.D. Visits," by Fran Levine. From *Health Memo*, Hadassah, Spring 2001.

Chapter 12, "Women and Heart Disease," by Chaim Lotan and Thea Pugatsch. Originally "HMO—Women and Heart Disease." From *Health Memo*, Hadassah, Spring 2002.

Chapter 13, "Take Control of Your Heart's Health," by Susan Blumenthal. Originally "Women and Heart Disease: Take Control of Your Heart's Health." From *Health Memo* Hadassah, Spring 2002.

Chapter 14, "Stress and Heart Disease," by Aggie Casey. From *Health Memo*, Hadassah, Spring 2002.

Chapter 15, "Menopause and Hormones," by Dale L. Mintz. From http://www.fda.gov/womens/menopause/mht-FS.html

PART THREE: NUTRITION

Chapter 16, "You Are What You Eat," by Yaakov Levinson. From *Jewish Guide to Natural Nutrition*, Feldheim Publishers, 1995. www.feldheim.com

Chapter 17, "Making Your Kitchen Healthy: Food, Halakhah, and Hygiene," by Rabbi Moshe Goldberger. Reprinted with permission of *Kashrus Magazine, The Periodical for the Kosher Consumer*; PO Box 204, Brooklyn, NY 11204; 718-336-8544; www.kashrusmagazine.com.

Chapter 18, "Vegetarianism and Judaism: Frequently Asked Questions," by Richard H. Schwartz. Originally "Frequently Asked Questions About Judaism and Vegetarianism." From www.jewishveg.com/schwartz/faq_vegetarianism.html

Chapter 19, "Tips on Fasting," by Rabbi Richard J. Israel. From www.joi.org/celebrate/yomkippur/fasting.shtml

Special Focus: Health Habits for Kids

Chapter 20, "Children and Exercise: A Lifelong Habit Starts Young," by Lisa Hoffman. From *Health Memo*, Hadassah, Winter 2001.

Chapter 21, "Healthy Children Today, Healthy Adults Tomorrow: A Formula for Heart Health," by Rickie M. Haas. From *Health Memo*, Hadassah, Spring 2002.

PART FOUR: JEWISH GENETIC DISEASES

Chapter 22, "Genetic Diseases Among Individuals of Ashkenazi Jewish Heritage," by Gregory Pastores. From *Health Memo*, Hadassah, Winter 2003.

Chapter 23, "Therefore Choose Life," by Rabbi Avis Miller. From *Health Memo*, Hadassah, Spring 2001.

Chapter 24, "Testing Genetic Tests for Jewish Values," by Rabbi Barry Freundel. From *It's in the Genes*, Hadassah, 2000.

Chapter 25, "Ethics and Genetic Testing," by Rabbi Moshe David Tendler. Originally "Ethical Questions—The Genome Project." From *Health Memo*, Hadassah, Winter 2003.

Chapter 26, "Hadassah Policy Statement on Genetic Testing"

Special Focus: Specific Genetic Conditions

Chapter 27, "Gaucher's Disease, Type 1," by Lisa Katz. From http://judaism.about.com/od/health/p/gaucher.htm. © 2005, by Lisa Katz (http://judaism.about.com). Used with permission of About, Inc., which can be found on the Web at www.about.com. All rights reserved.

Chapter 28, "Living with Gaucher's Disease: A Guide for Patients, Parents, Relatives, and Friends," by Robin Berman and Roscoe O. Brady. From http://gaucher.mgh.harvard.edu/living.html. © Copyright 1991 Genzyme Corporation.

Chapter 29, "Hadassah Saved My Daughter," by Debra Cohen. From *Health Memo*, Hadassah, Winter 2003.

Chapter 30, "Niemann-Pick Disease, Type A," by Lisa Katz. From http://judaism.about.com/od/health/p/niemannpick.htm. © 2005, by Lisa Katz (http://judaism.about.com). Used with permission of About, Inc., which can be found on the Web at www.about.com. All rights reserved.

PART FIVE: RAISING OUR CHILDREN

into Mensches," by Joel Lurie Grishaver, ©Torah Aura Productions. Call Making Connections for a copy of the complete article or for information about the book, *40 Things You Can Do to Save the Jewish People*, by Joel Grishaver. From http://www. chsweb.org/mc/raising.html

Special Focus: Infertility

Chapter 41, "Infertility and the Jewish Couple," by Judy Wertheimer. From www.jewishaz.com/jewishnews/ 980529/infert.shtml

Chapter 42, "Assisted Reproduction in Judaism," by Miryam Z. Wahrman. From www.jewishvirtuallibrary.org/jsource/ Judaism/ivf.html

PART SIX: CAREGIVING

Chapter 43, "The Physician's Daily Prayer," by Rabbi Simkha Y. Weintraub. From www.ncjh.org/downloads/PrayerPhysician.doc. Permission to reprint. Rabbi Y. Weintraub, LCSW, Rabbinic Director, National Center for Jewish Healing, a program of the Jewish Board of Family and Children's Services, 850 Seventh Avenue, Suite 1201, New York, NY 10019. 212-399-2320. Visit us at www.ncjh.org.

Chapter 44, "The Many Worlds of Family Caregivers," by Carol Levine. Reprinted with permission from *Always on Call: When Illness Turns Families into Caregivers*, edited by Carol Levine, 214 pages (New York: United Hospital Fund, 2000). To order a copy of the book, please call 888-291-4161; for more information about the United Hospital Fund's Families and Health Care Project, visit www.uhfnyc.org.

Chapter 45, "Honoring the Elderly," by Rabbi Sandra R. Berliner. From http://www.chsweb.org/mc/tikun_olam02.html#. Reprinted with permission from Jewish Outreach Partnerships Publication: *Making Connections Home Study Guide*. For more information, erivel@jopp.org or www.jopp.org.

Special Focus: Hospice Care

PART SEVEN: VISITING THE SICK

Chapter 53, "*Bikkur Cholim:* Visiting the Sick," by Rabbi Bradley Shavit Artson. From *It's a Mitzvah! Jewish Living Step-by-Step*, Behrman House, 1995, pp. 62–73. Reprinted with permission Behrman House, Inc. www.behrmanhouse.com

Chapter 54, "What to Say When Visiting the Ill," by Nancy Flam. Originally "Visiting Those Who Are Ill . . . What Do I Say?" From www.ncjh.org/downloads/BikurWhatDoISay.doc

Chapter 55, "Jewish Folk Traditions That You Can Use," by Vanessa L. Ochs. Originally "Rituals." From "Jewish Healing, Ritual and Psalms," *Take My Hand*, Hadassah, 2000, pp. 59–61.

PART EIGHT: PRAYER AND MEDITATION IN PRACTICE

Chapter 56, "Eight Possible Ways in Which Prayer May 'Work,'" by Amy Eilberg. From www.ncjh.org/downloads/PrayerEightWays.doc. Originally prepared for the National Center for Jewish Healing.

Chapter 57, "Healing at Bedtime: The Traditional *Kriat Sh'ma*," by Rabbi Simkha Y. Weintraub. From *The Outstretched Arm*, National Center for Jewish Healing, Winter 1992–93. Permission to reprint. Rabbi Y. Weintraub, LCSW, Rabbinic Director, National Center for Jewish Healing, a program of the Jewish Board of Family and Children's Services, 850 Seventh Avenue, Suite 1201, New York, NY 10019. 212-399-2320. Visit us at www.ncjh.org.

Chapter 58, "The Lubavitcher Rebbe on Health and Healing," by Ya'akov Gerlitz. Originally "The Lubavitcher Rebbe's Healing Philosophy." From http://www.jewishhealing.com/rebbehealing.html

Chapter 59, "Meditation," by Rabbi Goldie Milgram. Originally "Introduction to Jewish Meditation." From www.ReclaimingJudaism.org

Chapter 60, "What Is Reiki, and Is It 'Jewish'?" by Bonnie Cramer. Used with permission by Bonnie Cramer.

PART NINE: KEEPING HEALTHY
IN A CHANGING WORLD

Chapter 61, "The Challenges of Maintaining a Healthy Lifestyle in Today's Society," by Elizabeth Battaglino. From *Questions to Ask About Women's Health Screenings*, National Women's Health Report, December 2001.

Chapter 62, "Alternative Versus Complementary: What's the Difference?" by Esther D. Kustanowitz. From *Health Memo*, Hadassah, Fall 2003.

Special Focus: Medical Research

Chapter 63, "Clinical Trials: The Way We Make Progress Against Cancer," by Andrea M. Denicoff. *Health Memo*, Hadassah, Fall 2001.

Chapter 64, "Judaism and Stem Cell Research," by Yoel Julian Jakobovits. From http://www.torah.org/features/secondlook/ stemcell.html. Reprinted with permission from Jewish Action, the magazine of the Orthodox Union. www.ou.org/publications/ ja, ja@ou.org.

Chapter 65, "Stem Cell Research in Jewish Law," by Daniel Eisenberg. From www.jlaw.com/Articles/stemcellres.html#4. For more information, www.daneisenberg.com or eisenber@pol.net.

PART TEN: ORGAN DONATION

Chapter 66, "Judaism and Organ Donation" from "A Sampling of Views of the World's Religions on Organ Donation and Transplantation" in *Program Guide IX*, UAHC Committee on Bio-Ethics, Spring 1997, pages 56–67. Reprinted by permission of the UAHC Department of Jewish Family Concerns.

Chapter 67, "The Gift of Life," by Ellen Schulman. From *Health Memo*, Hadassah, Spring 2001.

Chapter 68, "The Myth of Organ Donation," from *Pikuah Nefesh— To Save a Life*, Hadassah, 2000.

Chapter 69, "Tradition, Transcendence, and Transplantation," by Rabbi Barry Freundel. From *Pikuah Nefesh—To Save a Life*, Hadassah, 2000.

Chapter 70, "Jews and Organ Donations: All Take and No Give?" by Adena K. Berkowitz. From *Moment*, August 1995/Av 5755, pp. 32–25.

Chapter 71, "When Is Death?" by Adena K. Berkowitz. From *Moment*, August 1995/Av 5755, pp. 58–59.

Chapter 72, "Coordinating *Mitzvah* and Miracle," by Wendy Elliman. *Hadassah Magazine*, November 1999.

PART ELEVEN: JEWISH VIEWS ON AIDS, SMOKING, ABORTION, AND EATING DISORDERS

Chapter 73, "AIDS: The Basics from the Jewish AIDS Trust," by the Jewish AIDS Trust. From "The Basics" at http://www.jat-uk.org/index1024x768.php?page=basics and "Jewish Values" at http://www.jat-uk.org/index1024x768.php?page=jewishvalues.

Chapter 74, "AIDS: A Jewish Perspective," by Yitzchok Breitowitz. From www.jlaw.com/Articles/aids.html

Chapter 75, "Smoking: Is It Kosher?" by Rabbi Chaim Steinmetz. From www.jlaw.com/Commentary/smoking.html

Chapter 76, "Smoking: The Rabbinical Council of America Roundtable's Proposal," by Jeffrey R. Woolf, Rabbi Reuven Bulka, Rabbi Saul J. Berman, Rabbi Daniel Landes. Originally "R.C.A Roundtable: Proposal on Smoking." From http://ash.org/rabbitext.html

Chapter 77, "Smoking: A Jewish Perspective," by Rabbi Seymour Siegel. From http://www.koach.org/Smoking.doc. Permission of the Rabbinical Assembly. www.rabbinicalassembly.org

Chapter 78, "Abortion: What Jewish Law Says," by Daniel Eisenberg. Originally "Abortion in Jewish Law." From http://www.aish.com/societyWork/sciencenature/Abortion_in_Jewish_Law.asp. For more information, www.daneisenberg.com or eisenber@pol.net.

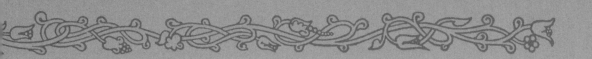

Index